a LANGE medical boo

W9-BLP-226

CURRENT

ESSENTIALS

of MEDICINE

Third Edition

Edited by

Lawrence M. Tierney, Jr., MD
Professor of Medicine
University of California, San Francisco
Associate Chief of Medical Services
Veterans Affairs Medical Center
San Francisco, California

Sanjay Saint, MD, MPH
Research Investigator and Hospitalist
Ann Arbor Veterans Affairs Medical Center
Associate Professor of Internal Medicine
University of Michigan Medical School
Director, VA/UM Patient Safety Enhancement Program
Ann Arbor, Michigan

Mary A. Whooley, MD
Associate Professor of Medicine
University of California, San Francisco
Section of General Internal Medicine
Veterans Affairs Medical Center
San Francisco, California

Lange Medical Books/McGraw-Hill
Medical Publishing Division

New York   Chicago   San Francisco   Lisbon   London   Madrid   Mexico City
Milan   New Delhi   San Juan   Seoul   Singapore   Sydney   Toronto

Current Essentials of Medicine, Third Edition

4 5 6 7 8 9 0   DOC/DOC   0 9 8 7

ISSN: 97-70188
ISBN: 0-07-143832-7

NOTICE

Medicine is an ever-changing science. As new research and clinical experience broaden our knowledge, changes in treatment and drug therapy are required. The authors and the publisher of this work have checked with sources believed to be reliable in their efforts to provide information that is complete and generally in accord with the standards accepted at the time of publication. However, in view of the possibility of human error or changes in medical sciences, neither the editors nor the publisher nor any other party who has been involved in the preparation or publication of this work warrants that the information contained herein is in every respect accurate or complete, and they disclaim all responsibility for any errors or omissions or for the results obtained from use of the information contained in this work. Readers are encouraged to confirm the information contained herein with other sources. For example and in particular, readers are advised to check the product information sheet included in the package of each drug they plan to administer to be certain that the information contained in this work is accurate and that changes have not been made in the recommended dose or in the contraindications for administration. This recommendation is of particular importance in connection with new or infrequently used drugs.

This book was set in Times Roman by International Typesetting and Composition.
The editors were Janet Foltin, Robert Pancotti, and Mary E. Bele.
The production supervisor was Catherine H. Saggese.
The cover designer was Mary McKeon.
The indexer was Pat Perrier.
RR Donnelley was printer and binder.

This book is printed on acid-free paper.

To Katherine Tierney: a sister whose absolute commitment to her parents at the ends of their lives provides a model for anyone fortunate enough to know her.

Lawrence M. Tierney, Jr.

In memory of Dr. Jacob P. Deerhake (1973–2004): a fabulous physician, a gifted teacher, a role model to the very end, who has already committed each clinical pearl to memory while watching over us in Heaven.

Sanjay Saint

In memory of my mother, Mary Aquinas Whooley (1940–2003).

Mary A. Whooley

Contents

Contributors

Harold R. Collard, MD
Clinical Instructor, Pulmonary Sciences and Critical Care Medicine,
  University of Colorado Health Sciences Center
collardh@njc.org
Pulmonary Diseases; References

Jeffrey Critchfield, MD
Vice Chief of Medicine, Clinical Services, San Francisco General
  Hospital; Assistant Clinical Professor of Medicine, University
  of California, San Francisco
jeff@itsa.ucsf.edu
Rheumatologic & Autoimmune Disorders

Neal A. Fischbach, MD
Adjunct Assistant Professor, University of California, San Francisco;
  Attending Physician, University of California, San Francisco
  Medical Center
fischba@itsa.ucsf.edu
Hematologic Diseases; Oncologic Diseases

Jennifer C. Hirsch, MD
Cardiothoracic Surgery Fellow, University of Michigan Medical
  Center, Ann Arbor
jhirsch@med.umich.edu
Common Surgical Disorders

Rebecca Ann Jackson, MD
Assistant Clinical Professor, University of California, San Francisco;
  Medical Director, Women's Health Center, San Francisco General
  Hospital
jacksonr@obgyn.ucsf.edu
Gynecologic, Obstetric, & Breast Disorders

Jacob Johnson, MD
Assistant Clinical Professor, University of California, San Francisco
jacobj@itsa.ucsf.edu
Common Disorders of the Ear, Nose, & Throat

Catherine Bree Johnston, MD, MPH
Associate Professor of Clinical Medicine, Division of Geriatrics,
    Department of Medicine, San Francisco Veterans Affairs Medical
    Center & University of California, San Francisco
bree526@itsa.ucsf.edu
Geriatric Disorders

Stephanie L. Jun, MD
Resident, University of California, San Francisco
stephaniejun@yahoo.com
Gastrointestinal Diseases; Hepatobiliary Disorders

Daniel R. Kaul, MD
Assistant Professor, University of Michigan Medical School,
    Ann Arbor
kauld@med.umich.edu
Infectious Diseases

Kewchang Lee, MD
Associate Clinical Professor of Psychiatry, University of California,
    San Francisco; Director of Psychiatry Consultation, San Francisco
    Veterans Affairs Medical Center
kewlee@itsa.ucsf.edu
Psychiatric Disorders

Joan C. Lo, MD
Assistant Professor of Medicine, University of California,
    San Francisco
jlo@itsa.ucsf.edu
Endocrine Disorders

Michael P. Lukela, MD
Associate Director, Medicine–Pediatrics Program,
    University of Michigan; Clinical Instructor, University
    of Michigan, Ann Arbor
mlukela@umich.edu
Common Pediatric Disorders

Timothy M. Miller, MD, PhD
Clinical Instructor, Research Fellow, University of California,
    San Diego
timiller@ucsd.edu
Neurologic Diseases

Brahmajee K. Nallamothu, MD, MPH
Assistant Professor, Division of Cardiology, University of Michigan
    Medical Center, Ann Arbor
bnallamo@umich.edu
Cardiovascular Diseases

Vikas I. Parekh, MD
Clinical Instructor of Medicine, University of Michigan Medical
    School, Ann Arbor
viparekh@umich.edu
Fluid, Acid-Base, & Electrolyte Disorders

Uptal D. Patel, MD
Assistant Professor of Internal Medicine and Pediatrics, Divisions of
    Nephrology and Pediatric Nephrology, Duke University, Durham
patelu@umich.edu
Genitourinary & Renal Disorders

Stephanie T. Phan, MD
Clinical Instructor/Faculty, Wilmer Eye Institute, Johns Hopkins
    Bayview Medical Center, Baltimore
steph_phan@yahoo.com
Common Disorders of the Eye

James M. Pribble, MD
Lecturer, Department of Emergency Medicine, University
    of Michigan, Ann Arbor
jpribb@umich.edu
Poisoning

Jack Resneck, Jr., MD
Assistant Professor of Dermatology & Health Policy, University
    of California, San Francisco
resneckj@derm.ucsf.edu
Dermatologic Disorders

Michael Rizen, MD, PhD
Cornea Fellow, Department of Ophthalmology, University
    of California, Davis
mrizen@yahoo.com
Common Disorders of the Eye

Sanjay Saint, MD, MPH
Research Investigator and Hospitalist, Ann Arbor Veterans Affairs
    Medical Center; Associate Professor of Internal Medicine,
    University of Michigan Medical School; Director, VA/UM
    Patient Safety Enhancement Program, Ann Arbor
saint@umich.edu
Selected Genetic Disorders

Lawrence M. Tierney, Jr., MD
Professor of Medicine, University of California, San Francisco;
    Associate Chief of Medical Services, Veterans Affairs Medical
    Center, San Francisco
vaspa@itsa.ucsf.edu
Pearls

Louise C. Walter, MD
Assistant Professor of Medicine, University of California,
    San Francisco; Staff Physician, Veterans Affairs Medical Center,
    San Francisco
louisew@itsa.ucsf.edu
Geriatric Disorders

Mary A. Whooley, MD
Associate Professor of Medicine, University of California,
    San Francisco; Section of General Internal Medicine, Veterans
    Affairs Medical Center, San Francisco
Mary.Whooley@med.va.gov

Preface

The third edition of *Current Essentials of Medicine* (formerly titled *Essentials of Diagnosis & Treatment*) continues a popular feature introduced in the second edition: a Clinical Pearl for each diagnosis. The Pearl is a timeless part of clinical medicine, and it has been our experience that learners at every level, and in many countries where we have taught, remember the Pearls as a crucial adjunct to more detailed information about disorders of every type. At its best, the Pearl is succinct, witty, and indeed colloquial at times. Similarly, it is stated with a certitude suggesting 100% accuracy. Everyone knows that nothing in medicine is so, yet Pearls such as "If you diagnose multiple sclerosis over the age of fifty, diagnose something else" are easily committed to memory. Thus, the Pearls should be accepted as they are offered, and in fact, many have been changed since the second edition. We continue to urge readers to provide Pearls of their own, which may prove to be more useful than our current ones.

The third edition, like the previous edition, uses a single page to discuss each disease, thereby providing the reader with a concise yet usable bolus of information about most of the common diseases seen in clinical practice. In addition, we provide a current reference for each disease for those readers seeking more detailed information. We have expanded the number of diseases from the previous edition and have updated the clinical manifestations, diagnostic tests, and treatment considerations throughout with the help of our contributing subject-matter experts.

We hope that you enjoy this edition as much as, if not more than, the previous ones.

Lawrence M. Tierney, Jr., MD
San Francisco, California

Sanjay Saint, MD, MPH
Ann Arbor, Michigan

Mary A. Whooley, MD
San Francisco, California

Cardiovascular Diseases

Acute Myocardial Infarction

- **Essentials of Diagnosis**
  - Prolonged (> 30 minutes) chest pain, associated with shortness of breath, nausea, left arm or neck pain, and diaphoresis; can be painless in diabetics
  - S_4 common; S_3, mitral insufficiency on occasion
  - Cardiogenic shock, ventricular arrhythmias may complicate
  - Non–Q wave infarct may mean ongoing jeopardized myocardium

- **Differential Diagnosis**
  - Stable or unstable angina; aortic dissection; pulmonary emboli
  - Tietze's syndrome (costochondritis)
  - Cervical or thoracic radiculopathy, including pre-eruptive zoster
  - Esophageal spasm or reflux; cholecystitis
  - Pericarditis
  - Pneumococcal pneumonia; pneumothorax

- **Treatment**
  - Monitoring, aspirin, and analgesia for all; heparin for most
  - Reperfusion by thrombolysis early or angioplasty in selected patients with either ST segment elevation or new left bundle-branch block on ECG
  - Glycoprotein IIb/IIIa inhibitors considered in non–Q wave infarcts
  - Nitroglycerin for recurrent ischemic pain; also useful for relieving pulmonary congestion and reducing blood pressure
  - ACE inhibitors, angiotensin II receptor blockers, and aldosterone blockers improve ventricular remodeling after infarcts

- **Pearl**

Proceed rapidly in consideration of thrombolysis in ST-segment elevation infarct; time is muscle.

Reference

Fox KA: Management of acute coronary syndromes: an update. Heart 2004; 90:698. [PMID: 15145891]

1

Acute Pericarditis

- **Essentials of Diagnosis**
  - Inflammation of the pericardium due to viral infection, drugs, recent myocardial infarction, autoimmune syndromes, renal failure, cardiac surgery, trauma, or neoplasm
  - Common symptoms include pleuritic chest pain radiating to the shoulder (trapezius ridge) and dyspnea; pain improves with sitting up and expiration
  - Examination may reveal fever, tachycardia, and an intermittent friction rub; cardiac tamponade may occur in any patient
  - Electrocardiography usually shows PR depression, diffuse ST-segment elevation followed by T-wave inversions
  - Echocardiography may reveal pericardial effusion

- **Differential Diagnosis**
  - Acute myocardial infarction
  - Aortic dissection
  - Pulmonary embolism
  - Pneumothorax
  - Pneumonia
  - Cholecystitis and pancreatitis

- **Treatment**
  - Aspirin or nonsteroidal anti-inflammatory agents such as ibuprofen or indomethacin to relieve symptoms; rarely, steroids for recurrent cases
  - Hospitalization for patients with symptoms suggestive of significant effusions or cardiac tamponade

- **Pearl**

Uremic pericarditis commonly exhibits normal ST segments; concomitant epicardial injury causes the elevation and is not present in renal failure.

Reference

Troughton RW, Asher CR, Klein AL: Pericarditis. Lancet 2004;363:717. [PMID: 15001332]

Acute Rheumatic Fever

■ Essentials of Diagnosis
- A systemic immune process complicating group A beta-hemolytic streptococcal pharyngitis
- Usually affects children between the ages of 5 and 15; rare after 25
- Occurs 1–5 weeks after throat infection
- Diagnosis based on Jones' criteria (two major or one major and two minor) and confirmation of recent streptococcal infection
- Major criteria: Erythema marginatum, migratory polyarthritis, subcutaneous nodules, carditis, and Sydenham's chorea; the latter is the most specific, least sensitive
- Minor criteria: Fever, arthralgias, elevated erythrocyte sedimentation rate, elevated C-reactive protein, PR prolongation on ECG, and history of pharyngitis

■ Differential Diagnosis
- Juvenile or adult rheumatoid arthritis
- Endocarditis
- Osteomyelitis
- Systemic lupus erythematosus
- Lyme disease
- Disseminated gonococcal infection

■ Treatment
- Bed rest until vital signs and ECG become normal
- Salicylates and nonsteroidal anti-inflammatory drugs reduce fever and joint complaints but do not affect the natural course of the disease; rarely, corticosteroids may be used
- If streptococcal infection is still present, penicillin is indicated
- Prevention of recurrent streptococcal pharyngitis in patients < 25 years old (a monthly injection of benzathine penicillin is most commonly used)

■ Pearl

Inappropriate tachycardia in a febrile child with a recent sore throat suggests this diagnosis.

Reference

Rullan E, Sigal LH: Rheumatic fever. Curr Rheumatol Rep 2001;3:445.

1

Angina Pectoris

- **Essentials of Diagnosis**
    - Generally caused by atherosclerotic coronary artery disease; cigarette smoking, diabetes, hypertension, hypercholesterolemia, and family history are established risk factors
    - Pressure-like episodic precordial chest discomfort, precipitated by exertion or stress, relieved by rest or nitrates
    - S_4, S_3, mitral murmur, paradoxically split S_2 may occur transiently with pain
    - Electrocardiography usually normal between episodes (or may show evidence of old infarction); electrocardiography with pain may show evidence of ischemia, classically ST depression
    - Diagnosis from history and stress tests; confirmed by coronary arteriography

- **Differential Diagnosis**
    - Other coronary syndromes (myocardial infarction, unstable angina, vasospasm)
    - Tietze's syndrome (costochondritis)
    - Intercostal neuropathy, especially caused by herpes zoster
    - Cervical or thoracic radiculopathy, including pre-eruptive zoster
    - Esophageal spasm or reflux disease
    - Cholecystitis
    - Pneumothorax
    - Pulmonary embolism
    - Pneumococcal pneumonia

- **Treatment**
    - Address reversible risk factors
    - Sublingual nitroglycerin for individual episodes
    - Ongoing treatment includes aspirin, long-acting nitrates, beta-blockers, and calcium channel blockers
    - Angioplasty with or without stenting considered in patients with anatomically suitable stenoses who remain symptomatic on medical therapy
    - Bypass grafting for patients with refractory angina on medical therapy, three-vessel disease (or two-vessel disease with proximal left anterior descending artery disease), and decreased left ventricular function, or left main coronary artery disease

- **Pearl**

An unchanged ECG does not exclude angina; up to 20% of patients with ischemic episodes do not show electrocardiographic changes with pain.

Reference

DeJongste MJ, Tio RA, Foreman RD. Chronic therapeutically refractory angina pectoris. Heart 2004;90:225. [PMID: 14729809]

Aortic Coarctation

- ■ Essentials of Diagnosis
  - • Elevated blood pressure in the aortic arch and its branches with reduced blood pressure distal to the left subclavian artery
  - • Lower extremity claudication or leg weakness with exertion in young adults is characteristic
  - • Systolic blood pressure is higher in the arms than in the legs, but diastolic pressure is similar compared with radial
  - • Femoral pulses delayed and decreased, with pulsatile collaterals in the intercostal areas; a harsh, late systolic murmur may be heard in the back; an aortic ejection murmur suggests concomitant bicuspid aortic valve
  - • Electrocardiography with left ventricular hypertrophy; chest x-ray may show rib notching inferiorly due to collaterals
  - • Transesophageal echo with doppler or MRI is diagnostic; angiography confirms gradient across the coarctation

- ■ Differential Diagnosis
  - • Essential hypertension
  - • Renal artery stenosis
  - • Renal parenchymal disease
  - • Pheochromocytoma
  - • Mineralocorticoid excess
  - • Oral contraceptive use
  - • Cushing's syndrome

- ■ Treatment
  - • Surgery is the mainstay of therapy; balloon angioplasty in selected patients
  - • All patients require endocarditis prophylaxis even after correction
  - • Twenty-five percent of patients remain hypertensive after surgery

- ■ Pearl

Listen to the back in a hypertensive young patient with an aortic out-flow murmur; this may be the diagnosis.

Reference

Hornung TS, Benson LN, McLaughlin PR: Interventions for aortic coarctation. Cardiol Rev 2002;10:139. [PMID: 12047792]

1

Aortic Dissection

- **Essentials of Diagnosis**
  - Most patients between age 50 and 70; risks include hypertension, Marfan's syndrome, bicuspid aortic valve, coarctation of the aorta, and pregnancy
  - Type A involves the ascending aorta or arch; type B does not
  - Sudden onset of chest pain with interscapular radiation in at-risk patient
  - Unequal blood pressures in upper extremities, new diastolic murmur of aortic insufficiency occasionally seen in type A
  - Chest x-ray nearly always abnormal; ECG unimpressive unless right coronary artery compromised
  - CT, transesophageal echocardiography, MRI, or aortography usually diagnostic

- **Differential Diagnosis**
  - Acute myocardial infarction
  - Angina pectoris
  - Acute pericarditis
  - Pneumothorax
  - Pulmonary embolism
  - Boerhaave's syndrome

- **Treatment**
  - Nitroprusside and beta-blockers to lower systolic blood pressure to approximately 100 mm Hg, pulse to 60/min
  - Emergent surgery for type A dissection; medical therapy for type B is reasonable, with surgery or percutaneous intra-aortic stenting reserved for high-risk patients

- **Pearl**

Severe hypertension in a patient appearing to be in shock is aortic dissection until proved otherwise.

Reference

Nienaber CA, Eagle KA: Aortic dissection: new frontiers in diagnosis and management. Circulation 2003;108:628. [PMID: 12900496]

Aortic Regurgitation

- **Essentials of Diagnosis**
  - Causes include congenital bicuspid valve, endocarditis, rheumatic heart disease, Marfan's syndrome, aortic dissection, ankylosing spondylitis, reactive arthritis, and syphilis
  - Acute aortic regurgitation: Abrupt onset of pulmonary edema
  - Chronic aortic regurgitation: Asymptomatic until middle age, when symptoms of left heart failure develop insidiously
  - Soft, high-pitched, decrescendo holodiastolic murmur in chronic aortic regurgitation; occasionally, an accompanying apical low-pitched diastolic rumble (Austin Flint murmur) in nonrheumatic patients; in acute aortic regurgitation, the diastolic murmur can be short (or not even heard) and harsh
  - Acute aortic regurgitation: Reduced S_1 and an S_3, along with signs of pulmonary edema
  - Chronic aortic regurgitation: Reduced S_1, wide pulse pressure, water-hammer pulse, subungual capillary pulsations (Quincke's sign), rapid rise and fall of pulse (Corrigan's pulse), and a diastolic murmur over a partially compressed femoral artery (Duroziez's sign)
  - ECG shows left ventricular hypertrophy, and x-ray shows left ventricular dilation
  - Echo doppler confirms diagnosis, estimates severity

- **Differential Diagnosis**
  - Pulmonary hypertension with Graham Steell murmur
  - Mitral, or rarely tricuspid stenosis
  - Left ventricular failure due to other cause
  - Dock's murmur of left anterior descending artery stenosis

- **Treatment**
  - Vasodilators (eg, nifedipine and ACE inhibitors) delay the progression to valve replacement
  - In chronic aortic regurgitation, surgery reserved for patients with symptoms, or mild left ventricular dysfunction or ventricular cavity enlargement (> 55 mm) on echocardiography
  - Acute regurgitation caused by aortic dissection or endocarditis consistently requires surgical replacement of the valve

- **Pearl**

The Key-Hodgkin murmur of aortic regurgitation is harsh and raspy, caused by leaflet eventration typical of luetic aortopathy.

Reference

Borer JS, Bonow RO: Contemporary approach to aortic and mitral regurgitation. Circulation 2003;108:2432. [PMID: 14623790]

1

Aortic Stenosis

■ Essentials of Diagnosis

- Causes include congenital bicuspid valve and progressive calcification with aging of a normal three-leaflet valve; rheumatic fever rarely, if ever, causes isolated aortic stenosis
- Dyspnea, angina, and syncope singly or in any combination; sudden death in less than 1% of asymptomatic patients
- Weak and delayed carotid pulses; a soft, absent, or paradoxically split S_2; a harsh diamond-shaped systolic ejection murmur to the right of the sternum, often radiating to the neck, but on occasion heard apically (Gallivardin's phenomenon)
- Left ventricular hypertrophy by ECG and chest x-ray may show calcification in the aortic valve
- Echo confirms diagnosis and estimates valve area and gradient; cardiac catheterization confirms severity, documents concomitant coronary atherosclerotic disease, present in 50%

■ Differential Diagnosis

- Mitral regurgitation
- Hypertrophic obstructive or dilated cardiomyopathy
- Atrial or ventricular septal defect
- Syncope due to other causes
- Ischemic heart disease without valvular abnormality

■ Treatment

- Surgery is indicated for all symptomatic patients, ideally before heart failure develops
- Asymptomatic patients with declining left ventricular function considered for surgery if echo doppler demonstrates an aortic valve gradient > 80 mm Hg or severely reduced valve areas (≤ 0.7 cm^2)
- Percutaneous balloon valvuloplasty for temporary (6 months) relief of symptoms in poor surgical candidates

■ Pearl

The later the peak of the systolic ejection murmur, the more severe the stenosis.

Reference

Stouffer GA, Lenihan DJ, Lerakis S, et al: Timing of aortic valve surgery in chronic aortic stenosis and regurgitation. Am J Med Sci 2004;327:348. [PMID: 15201649]

Atrial Fibrillation

- ■ Essentials of Diagnosis
  - The most common chronic arrhythmia
  - Causes include mitral valve disease, hypertensive and ischemic heart disease, dilated cardiomyopathy, alcohol use, hyperthyroidism, pericarditis, cardiac surgery; many idiopathic ("lone" atrial fibrillation)
  - Complications include precipitation of cardiac failure, arterial embolization
  - Palpitations, shortness of breath, chest pain; however, commonly asymptomatic
  - Irregularly irregular heartbeat, variable intensity S_1, occasional S_3; S_4 absent in all
  - Electrocardiography shows ventricular rate of 80–170/min in untreated patients; if associated with an accessory pathway (ie, Wolff-Parkinson-White), the ventricular rate can be > 200/min with wide QRS and antegrade conduction through the pathway

- ■ Differential Diagnosis
  - Multifocal atrial tachycardia
  - Atrial flutter or tachycardia with variable block
  - Sinus arrhythmia
  - Normal sinus rhythm with multiple premature contractions

- ■ Treatment
  - Control ventricular response with AV-nodal blockers such as digoxin, beta-blocker, calcium channel blocker—choice depending upon contractile state of left ventricle
  - Cardioversion with countershock in unstable patients with acute atrial fibrillation; elective countershock or antiarrhythmic agents (eg, ibutilide, procainamide, amiodarone, sotalol) in stable patients once a left atrial thrombus has been ruled out or effectively treated
  - Chronic warfarin or aspirin in all patients not cardioverted
  - With elective cardioversion, anticoagulation for 4 weeks prior to and 4 weeks after the procedure unless transesophageal echocardiography excludes a left atrial thrombus
  - Radiofrequency ablation of pulmonary vein sources of atrial fibrillation increasingly used in appropriate patients

- ■ Pearl

Consider accessory pathway in atrial fibrillation when rates exceed 200/min, and remember that AV-nodal blockers favor antegrade conduction without rate control.

Reference

McNamara RL, Tamariz LJ, Segal JB, Bass EB: Management of atrial fibrillation: review of the evidence for the role of pharmacologic therapy, electrical cardioversion, and echocardiography. Ann Intern Med 2003;139:1018. [PMID: 14678922]

1

Atrial Flutter

- **Essentials of Diagnosis**
  - Common in COPD; also seen in dilated cardiomyopathy, especially in alcoholics
  - Atrial rate between 250 and 350 beats/min with every second, third, or fourth impulse conducted by the ventricle; 2:1 most common
  - Patients may be asymptomatic, complain of palpitations, or have evidence of congestive heart failure
  - Flutter (*a*) waves visible in the neck in occasional patients
  - Electrocardiography shows "sawtooth" P waves in V_1 and the inferior leads; ventricular response usually regular; less commonly, irregular due to variable atrioventricular block

- **Differential Diagnosis**
  With regular ventricular rate:
  - Automatic atrial tachycardia
  - Atrioventricular nodal reentry tachycardia
  - Atrioventricular reentry tachycardia with accessory pathway
  - Sinus tachycardia
  With irregular ventricular rate:
  - Atrial fibrillation
  - Multifocal atrial tachycardia

- **Treatment**
  - Often spontaneously converts to atrial fibrillation
  - Electrical cardioversion is reliable and safe
  - Conversion may also be achieved by drugs (eg, ibutilide)
  - Risk of embolization is lower than for atrial fibrillation, but anticoagulation still recommended
  - Radiofrequency ablation is highly successful (> 90%) in patients with chronic atrial flutter

- **Pearl**

A regular heart rate of 140–150 in a patient with COPD is flutter until proven otherwise.

Reference

Cosio FG: Atrial flutter update. Card Electrophysiol Rev 2002;6:356. [PMID: 12438813]

Atrial Myxoma

1

- ■ Essentials of Diagnosis
  - • Most common cardiac tumor, usually originating in the interatrial septum, with 80% growing into the left atrium; 5–10% bilateral
  - • Symptoms fall into one of three categories: (1) systemic—fever, malaise, weight loss; (2) obstructive—positional dyspnea and syncope; and (3) embolic—acute vascular or neurologic deficit
  - • Diastolic "tumor plop" or mitral stenosislike murmur; signs of congestive heart failure and systemic embolization in many
  - • Episodic pulmonary edema, classically when patient assumes an upright position
  - • Leukocytosis, anemia, accelerated erythrocyte sedimentation rate
  - • MRI or echocardiogram demonstrates tumor

- ■ Differential Diagnosis
  - • Subacute infective endocarditis
  - • Lymphoma
  - • Autoimmune disease
  - • Mitral stenosis
  - • Cor triatriatum
  - • Parachute mitral valve
  - • Other causes of congestive heart failure

- ■ Treatment
  - • Surgery usually curative (recurrence rate is approximately 5%)

- ■ Pearl

An apical diastolic murmur that varies dramatically in intensity with positional changes should raise concern; few similar conditions are curable.

Reference

Percell RL Jr, Henning RJ, Siddique Patel M: Atrial myxoma: case report and a review of the literature. Heart Dis 2003;5:224. [PMID: 12783636]

1

Atrial Septal Defect

- ■ Essentials of Diagnosis
  - Patients with small defects are usually asymptomatic and have a normal life span
  - Large shunts symptomatic by age 40, including exertional dyspnea, fatigue, and palpitations
  - Paradoxical embolism may occur (ie, upper or lower extremity venous thrombus embolizing to brain or extremity rather than lung) with transient shunt reversal
  - Right ventricular lift, widened and fixed splitting of S_2, and systolic flow murmur in the pulmonary area
  - Electrocardiography may show right ventricular hypertrophy and right axis deviation (in ostium secundum defects), left anterior hemiblock (in ostium primum defects); complete or incomplete right bundle-branch block in 95%
  - Atrial fibrillation commonly complicates
  - Echo doppler with agitated saline contrast injection is diagnostic; radionuclide angiogram or cardiac catheterization estimates ratio of pulmonary flow to systemic flow (PF:SF)

- ■ Differential Diagnosis
  - Left ventricular failure
  - Left-sided valvular disease
  - Primary pulmonary hypertension
  - Chronic pulmonary embolism
  - Sleep apnea
  - Chronic obstructive pulmonary disease
  - Eisenmenger's syndrome
  - Pulmonary stenosis

- ■ Treatment
  - Small defects do not require surgical correction
  - Surgery or percutaneous closure devices indicated for patients with PF:SF > 1.7 or smaller shunts if there is right ventricular failure
  - Surgery contraindicated in patients with pulmonary hypertension and right-to-left shunting

- ■ Pearl

Endocarditis seldom occurs given low interatrial gradient; endocarditis prophylaxis is thus unnecessary.

Reference

Brickner ME, Hillis LD, Lange RA: Congenital heart disease in adults. First of two parts. N Engl J Med 2000;342:256. [PMID: 10648769]

Atrioventricular Block

■ Essentials of Diagnosis

- First-degree block: Delayed conduction at the level of the atrioventricular node; PR interval > 0.20 s
- Second-degree block: Mobitz I—progressive prolongation of the PR interval and decreasing R—R interval prior to a blocked sinus impulse; Mobitz II—fixed PR intervals before a beat is dropped
- Third-degree block: Complete block at or below the node; P waves and QRS complexes occur independently of one another, both at fixed rates
- Clinical manifestations of third-degree block include chest pain, syncope, and shortness of breath; cannon *a* waves in neck veins; first heart sound varies in intensity

■ Differential Diagnosis

Causes of first-degree and Mobitz I atrioventricular block:
- Increased vagal tone
- Drugs that prolong atrioventricular conduction
- All causes of second- and third-degree block

Causes of Mobitz II and third-degree atrioventricular block:
- Chronic degenerative conduction system disease (Lev's and Lenégre's syndromes)
- Acute myocardial infarction: Inferior myocardial infarction causes complete block at the node, anterior myocardial infarction below it
- Acute myocarditis (eg, Lyme disease, viral myocarditis, rheumatic fever)
- Digitalis toxicity
- Congenital

■ Treatment

- In symptomatic patients with Mobitz I, permanent pacing
- For those with Mobitz II or infranodal third-degree atrioventricular block, permanent pacing unless a reversible cause (eg, drug toxicity, inferior myocardial infarction, Lyme disease) is present

■ Pearl

A "circus of atrial sounds" may be created by atrial contractions at different rates than ventricular, eg, in complete heart block.

Reference

Da Costa D, Brady WJ, Edhouse J: Bradycardias and atrioventricular conduction block. BMJ 2002;324:535. [PMID: 11872557]

Cardiac Tamponade

■ Essentials of Diagnosis

- Life-threatening disorder occurring when pericardial fluid accumulates under pressure; effusions rapidly increasing in size may cause an elevated intrapericardial pressure (> 15 mm Hg), leading to impaired cardiac filling and decreased cardiac output
- Common causes include metastatic malignancy, uremia, viral or idiopathic pericarditis, and cardiac trauma; however, any cause of pericarditis can cause tamponade
- Clinical manifestations include dyspnea, cough, tachycardia, hypotension, pulsus paradoxus, jugular venous distention, and distant heart sounds
- Electrocardiography usually shows low QRS voltage and occasionally electrical alternans; chest x-ray shows an enlarged cardiac silhouette with a "water-bottle" configuration if a large (> 250 mL) effusion is present—which it need not be if effusion develops rapidly
- Echocardiography delineates effusion and its hemodynamic significance, eg, atrial collapse; cardiac catheterization confirms the diagnosis if equalization of diastolic pressures in all four chambers occurs with loss of the normal y descent

■ Differential Diagnosis

- Tension pneumothorax
- Right ventricular infarction
- Severe left ventricular failure
- Constrictive pericarditis
- Restrictive cardiomyopathy
- Pneumonia with septic shock

■ Treatment

- Immediate pericardiocentesis
- Volume expansion until pericardiocentesis is performed
- Definitive treatment for reaccumulation may require surgical anterior and posterior pericardiectomy or percutaneous balloon pericardiotomy

■ Pearl

Pulsus paradoxus is diagnostically useful only in regular sinus rhythm.

Reference

Spodick DH: Acute cardiac tamponade. N Engl J Med 2003;349:684. [PMID: 12917306]

Congestive Heart Failure

1

- **Essentials of Diagnosis**
    - Two pathophysiologic categories: Systolic dysfunction and diastolic dysfunction
    - Systolic: The ability to pump blood is compromised; ejection fraction is decreased; causes include coronary artery disease, dilated cardiomyopathy, myocarditis, "burned-out" hypertensive heart disease, and regurgitant valvular heart disease
    - Diastolic: Heart unable to relax and allow adequate diastolic filling; normal ejection fraction; causes include ischemia, hypertension with left ventricular hypertrophy, aortic stenosis, hypertrophic cardiomyopathy, restrictive cardiomyopathy, and small-vessel disease (especially diabetes)
    - Evidence of both common in the typical heart failure patient, but up to 20% of patients will have isolated diastolic dysfunction
    - Symptoms and signs can result from left-sided failure, right-sided failure, or both
    - Left ventricular failure: Exertional dyspnea, orthopnea, paroxysmal nocturnal dyspnea, pulsus alternans, rales, gallop rhythm; pulmonary venous congestion on chest x-ray
    - Right ventricular failure: Fatigue, malaise, elevated venous pressure, hepatomegaly, abdominojugular reflux, and dependent edema
    - Diagnosis confirmed by echo, pulmonary capillary wedge measurement, or elevated levels of brain natiuretic peptide (BNP)

- **Differential Diagnosis**
    - Constrictive pericarditis
    - Nephrosis or cirrhosis
    - Hypothyroidism or hyperthyroidism
    - Noncardiogenic causes of pulmonary edema
    - Beriberi

- **Treatment**
    - Systolic dysfunction: Vasodilators (ACE inhibitors, angiotensin II receptor blockers, or combination of hydralazine and isosorbide dinitrate), beta-blockers, aldosterone blockers (eg, spironolactone), and low-sodium diet; for symptoms, use diuretics and digoxin; anticoagulation advocated by many in high-risk patients, even with sinus rhythm
    - Diastolic dysfunction: A negative inotrope (beta-blocker or calcium channel blocker), low-sodium diet, and diuretics for symptoms

- **Pearl**

Do not be misled by a normal ejection fraction if all else points to congestive heart failure; it is typical of isolated diastolic dysfunction.

Reference

Guyatt GH, Devereaux PJ: A review of heart failure treatment. Mt Sinai J Med 2004;71:47. [PMID: 14770250]

Constrictive Pericarditis

- **Essentials of Diagnosis**
  - A thickened fibrotic pericardium impairing cardiac filling and decreasing cardiac output
  - May follow tuberculosis, cardiac surgery, radiation therapy, or viral, uremic, or neoplastic pericarditis
  - Gradual onset of dyspnea, fatigue, weakness, pedal edema, and abdominal swelling; right-sided heart failure symptoms often predominate, with ascites sometimes disproportionate to pedal edema
  - Physical examination reveals tachycardia, elevated jugular venous distention with rapid y descent, Kussmaul's sign, hepatosplenomegaly, ascites, "pericardial knock" following S_2, and peripheral edema
  - Pericardial calcification on chest film in less than half; electrocardiography may show low QRS voltage; liver function tests abnormal from passive congestion
  - Echocardiography can demonstrate a thick pericardium and normal left ventricular function; CT or MRI is more sensitive in revealing pericardial pathology; cardiac catheterization demonstrates dip-and-plateau pattern to left and right ventricular diastolic pressure tracings with a prominent y descent (in contrast to restrictive cardiomyopathy)

- **Differential Diagnosis**
  - Cardiac tamponade
  - Right ventricular infarction
  - Restrictive cardiomyopathy
  - Cirrhosis with ascites (most common misdiagnosis)

- **Treatment**
  - Acute treatment usually includes gentle diuresis
  - Definitive therapy is surgical stripping of the pericardium; effective in up to half of patients
  - Evaluation for tuberculosis

- **Pearl**

Constriction should be entertained in patients with new-onset ascites; it is the most treatable cause.

Reference

Troughton RW, Asher CR, Klein AL: Pericarditis. Lancet 2004;363:717. [PMID: 15001332]

Cor Pulmonale

■ Essentials of Diagnosis

- Heart failure resulting from pulmonary disease
- Most commonly due to COPD; other causes include pulmonary fibrosis, pneumoconioses, recurrent pulmonary emboli, primary pulmonary hypertension, sleep apnea, and kyphoscoliosis
- Clinical manifestations are due to both the underlying pulmonary disease and the right ventricular failure
- Chest x-ray reveals an enlarged right ventricle and pulmonary artery; electrocardiography may show right axis deviation, right ventricular hypertrophy, and tall, peaked P waves (P pulmonale) in the face of low QRS voltage
- Pulmonary function tests usually confirm the presence of underlying lung disease, and echocardiography will show right ventricular dilation but normal left ventricular function and elevated right ventricular systolic pressures

■ Differential Diagnosis

Other causes of right ventricular failure:
- Left ventricular failure (due to any cause)
- Pulmonary stenosis
- Left-to-right shunt causing Eisenmenger's syndrome

■ Treatment

- Treatment is primarily directed at the pulmonary process causing the right heart failure (eg, oxygen if hypoxia is present)
- In frank right ventricular failure, include salt restriction, diuretics, and oxygen
- For primary pulmonary hypertension, cautious use of vasodilators (calcium channel blockers) or continuous-infusion prostacyclin may benefit some patients

■ Pearl

Oxygen is the furosemide of the right ventricle.

Reference

Weitzenblum E: Chronic cor pulmonale. Heart 2003;89:225. [PMID: 12527688]

1

Deep Venous Thrombosis

- ■ Essentials of Diagnosis
  - Dull pain or tight feeling in the calf or thigh
  - Up to half of patients are asymptomatic in the early stages
  - Increased risk: Congestive heart failure, recent major surgery, neoplasia, oral contraceptive use by smokers, prolonged inactivity, varicose veins, hypercoagulable states (eg, protein C, protein S, other anticoagulant deficiencies, nephrotic syndrome)
  - Physical signs unreliable
  - Doppler ultrasound and impedance plethysmography are initial tests of choice (less sensitive in asymptomatic patients); venography is definitive but difficult to perform
  - Pulmonary thromboembolism, especially with proximal, above-the-knee deep vein thrombosis is a life-threatening complication

- ■ Differential Diagnosis
  - Calf strain or contusion
  - Cellulitis
  - Ruptured Baker cyst
  - Lymphatic obstruction
  - Congestive heart failure, especially right-sided

- ■ Treatment
  - Anticoagulation with intravenous heparin (goal PTT twice normal) for 5 days followed by oral warfarin for 3–6 months; thrombolytics in acute phlebitis may prevent valvular damage and post-phlebitic syndrome
  - Subcutaneous low-molecular-weight heparin may be substituted for intravenous heparin
  - NSAIDs for associated pain and swelling
  - For idiopathic and recurrent cases, hypercoagulable conditions should be considered, although factor V Leiden should be sought on a first episode without risk factors in patients of European ethnicity
  - Postphlebitic syndrome (chronic venous insufficiency) is common following an episode of deep venous thrombosis and should be treated with graduated compression stockings, local skin care, and in many, chronic warfarin administration

- ■ Pearl

The left lower extremity is 1 cm greater in circumference than the right at any point of measurement in 90% of the population.

Reference

Bates SM, Ginsberg JS: Clinical practice. Treatment of deep-vein thrombosis. N Engl J Med 2004;351:268. [PMID: 15254285]

Dilated Cardiomyopathy

■ Essentials of Diagnosis

- A cause of systolic dysfunction, this represents a group of disorders that lead to congestive heart failure
- Symptoms and signs of congestive heart failure: Exertional dyspnea, cough, fatigue, paroxysmal nocturnal dyspnea, cardiac enlargement, rales, gallop rhythm, elevated venous pressure, hepatomegaly, and dependent edema
- Electrocardiography may show nonspecific repolarization abnormalities and atrial or ventricular ectopy, but is not diagnostic
- Echocardiography reveals depressed contractile function and cardiomegaly
- Cardiac catheterization useful to exclude ischemia as a cause

■ Differential Diagnosis

Causes of dilated cardiomyopathy:
- Alcoholism
- Postviral myocarditis
- Sarcoidosis
- Postpartum
- Doxorubicin toxicity
- Endocrinopathies (hyperthyroidism, acromegaly, pheochromocytoma)
- Hemochromatosis
- Idiopathic

■ Treatment

- Treat the underlying disorder when identifiable
- Abstention from alcohol
- Routine management of systolic dysfunction, including with vasodilators (ACE inhibitors, angiotensin II receptor blockers or a combination of hydralazine and isosorbide dinitrate), beta-blockers, spironolactone, and low-sodium diet; digoxin and diuretics for symptoms
- Many empirically employ chronic warfarin
- Cardiac transplant for end-stage patients

■ Pearl

Causes of death: one-third pump failure, one-third arrhythmia, and one-third stroke, of which the latter is most preventable.

Reference

Elliott P: Cardiomyopathy. Diagnosis and management of dilated cardiomyopathy. Heart 2000;84:106. [PMID: 10862601]

Hypertension

■ Essentials of Diagnosis
- In most patients (95% of cases), no cause can be found
- Chronic elevation in blood pressure (> 140/90 mm Hg) occurs in 15% of white adults and 30% of black adults in the United States; onset is usually between ages 20 and 55
- The pathogenesis is multifactorial: Environmental, dietary, genetic, and neurohormonal factors all contribute
- Most patients are asymptomatic; some, however, complain of headache, epistaxis, or blurred vision if hypertension is severe
- Most diagnostic study abnormalities are referable to "target organ" damage: heart, kidney, brain, retina, and peripheral arteries

■ Differential Diagnosis
Secondary causes of hypertension:
- Coarctation of the aorta
- Renal insufficiency
- Renal artery stenosis
- Pheochromocytoma
- Cushing's syndrome
- Primary hyperaldosteronism
- Chronic use of oral contraceptive pills or alcohol

■ Treatment
- Decrease blood pressure with a single agent (if possible) while minimizing side effects
- Many recommend diuretics or beta-blockers as initial therapy, but considerable latitude is allowed for individual patients
- Other agents useful either alone or in combination include ACE inhibitors, angiotensin II receptor blockers, and calcium channel blockers; α_1-blockers are considered second-line agents
- If hypertension is unresponsive to medical treatment, evaluate for secondary causes

■ Pearl
A disease without a pearl—30 million Americans have it, and no clinical feature is characteristic, either symptomatically or on examination.

Reference

Chobanian AV, Bakris GL, Black HR, et al: The Seventh Report of the Joint National Committee on Prevention, Detection, Evaluation, and Treatment of High Blood Pressure: the JNC 7 report. JAMA 2003;289:2560. Epub 2003 May 14. [PMID: 12748199]

Hypertrophic Obstructive Cardiomyopathy (HOCM)   **1**

- **Essentials of Diagnosis**
  - Asymmetric myocardial hypertrophy causing dynamic obstruction to left ventricular outflow below the aortic valve
  - Sporadic or dominantly inherited
  - Obstruction is worsened by increasing left ventricular contractility or decreasing filling
  - Symptoms are dyspnea, chest pain, and syncope; a subgroup of younger patients is at high risk for sudden cardiac death (1% per year), especially with exercise
  - Sustained, bifid (rarely trifid) apical impulse, S_4
  - Electrocardiography shows exaggerated septal Q waves suggestive of myocardial infarction; supraventricular and ventricular arrhythmias may also be seen
  - Echocardiography with hypertrophy, evidence of dynamic obstruction from abnormal systolic motion of the anterior mitral valve leaflet
  - Limited role for genetic testing

- **Differential Diagnosis**
  - Hypertensive heart disease
  - Restrictive cardiomyopathy (eg, amyloidosis)
  - Aortic stenosis
  - Ischemic heart disease
  - Athlete's heart

- **Treatment**
  - Beta-blockers are the initial drug of choice in symptomatic patients, especially those with evidence of dynamic obstruction
  - Calcium channel blockers may also be useful
  - Otherwise, surgical myectomy, percutaneous transcoronary septal reduction with alcohol, or dual-chamber pacing are considered; an automatic implantable cardiac defibrillator and amiodarone in patients at high risk for sudden death are often employed, but are of debatable value
  - Natural history is unpredictable; sports requiring high cardiac output should be discouraged
  - All first-degree relatives should be evaluated with echocardiography
  - Prophylaxis for infective endocarditis is required

- **Pearl**

Hypertrophic cardiomyopathy is the pathologic feature most frequently associated with sudden death in athletes.

Reference

Nishimura RA, Holmes DR Jr: Clinical practice. Hypertrophic obstructive cardiomyopathy. N Engl J Med 2004;350:1320. [PMID: 15044643]

1

Mitral Regurgitation

- Essentials of Diagnosis
  - Causes include rheumatic heart disease, infectious endocarditis, mitral valve prolapse, ischemic papillary muscle dysfunction, torn chordae tendineae
  - Acute: Immediate onset of symptoms of pulmonary edema
  - Chronic: Asymptomatic for years, then exertional dyspnea and fatigue
  - S_1 usually reduced; a blowing, high-pitched apical pansystolic murmur increased by finger squeeze is characteristic; S_3 common in chronic cases; murmur is not pansystolic and less audible in acute
  - Left atrial abnormality and often left ventricular hypertrophy on ECG; atrial fibrillation typical with chronicity
  - Echo doppler confirms diagnosis, estimates severity

- Differential Diagnosis
  - Aortic stenosis or sclerosis
  - Tricuspid regurgitation
  - Hypertrophic obstructive cardiomyopathy
  - Atrial septal defect
  - Ventricular septal defect

- Treatment
  - Acute mitral regurgitation due to endocarditis or torn chordae may require immediate surgical repair
  - Prophylaxis for infective endocarditis in chronic mitral regurgitation; surgical repair for severe symptoms, for left ventricular dysfunction (eg, ejection fraction < 55%), or for enlargement by echo
  - Mild to moderate symptoms can be treated with diuretics, sodium restriction, and afterload reduction (eg, ACE inhibitors); digoxin, beta-blockers, and calcium channel blockers control ventricular response with atrial fibrillation, and warfarin anticoagulation should be given

- Pearl

An overlooked physical sign in mitral regurgitation is a rapid up-and-down carotid pulse: this is quite useful in distinguishing it from aortic stenosis.

Reference

Borer JS, Bonow RO: Contemporary approach to aortic and mitral regurgitation. Circulation 2003;108:2432. [PMID: 14623790]

Mitral Stenosis

■ **Essentials of Diagnosis**

- Always caused by rheumatic heart disease, but 30% of patients have no history of rheumatic fever
- Dyspnea, orthopnea, paroxysmal nocturnal dyspnea, even hemoptysis—often precipitated by volume overload (pregnancy, salt load) or tachycardia
- Right ventricular lift in many; opening snap occasionally palpable
- Crisp S_1, increased P_2, opening snap; these sounds often easier to appreciate than the characteristic low-pitched apical diastolic murmur
- Electrocardiography shows left atrial abnormality, and commonly, atrial fibrillation; echo confirms diagnosis, quantifies severity

■ **Differential Diagnosis**

- Left ventricular failure due to any cause
- Mitral valve prolapse (if systolic murmur present)
- Pulmonary hypertension due to other cause
- Left atrial myxoma
- Cor triatriatum (in patients under 30)
- Tricuspid stenosis

■ **Treatment**

- Heart failure symptoms may be treated with diuretics and sodium restriction
- With atrial fibrillation, ventricular rate controlled with beta-blockers, calcium channel blockers such as verapamil or digoxin; long-term anticoagulation instituted with warfarin
- Balloon valvuloplasty or surgical valve replacement in symptomatic patients with mitral orifice of less than 1.2 cm^2; valvuloplasty preferred in noncalcified and pliable valves
- Prophylaxis for beta-hemolytic streptococcal infections until age 25 and for infective endocarditis for lifetime

■ **Pearl**

The left ventricle is not affected in pure mitral stenosis.

Reference

Berger M: Natural history of mitral stenosis and echocardiographic criteria and pitfalls in selecting patients for balloon valvuloplasty. Adv Cardiol 2004;41:87. [PMID: 15285221]

1

Multifocal Atrial Tachycardia

- **Essentials of Diagnosis**
  - Classically seen in patients with severe COPD; electrolyte abnormalities (especially hypomagnesemia or hypokalemia) occasionally responsible
  - Symptoms those of the underlying disorder, but some may complain of palpitations
  - Irregularly irregular heart rate
  - Electrocardiography shows at least three different P-wave morphologies with varying P–R intervals
  - Ventricular rate usually between 100 and 140 beats/min; if less than 100, rhythm is wandering atrial pacemaker

- **Differential Diagnosis**
  - Normal sinus rhythm with multiple premature atrial contractions
  - Atrial fibrillation
  - Atrial flutter with variable block
  - Reentry tachycardia with variable block

- **Treatment**
  - Treatment of the underlying disorder is most important
  - Verapamil particularly useful for rate control; digitalis ineffective
  - Intravenous magnesium and potassium administered slowly may convert some patients to sinus rhythm even if serum levels are within normal range; be sure renal function is normal
  - Medications causing atrial irritability, such as theophylline, should be avoided
  - Atrioventricular nodal ablation with permanent pacing is used in rare cases that are refractory to pharmacologic therapy

- **Pearl**

An irregularly irregular rhythm in COPD is multifocal atrial tachycardia far more commonly than atrial fibrillation.

Reference

Blomstrom-Lundqvist C, Scheinman MM, Aliot EM, et al: ACC/AHA/ESC guidelines for the management of patients with supraventricular arrhythmias—executive summary. A report of the American college of cardiology/American heart association task force on practice guidelines and the European society of cardiology committee for practice guidelines (writing committee to develop guidelines for the management of patients with supraventricular arrhythmias) developed in collaboration with NASPE-Heart Rhythm Society. J Am Coll Cardiol 2003;42:1493. [PMID: 14563598]

Myocarditis

■ Essentials of Diagnosis

- Focal or diffuse inflammation of the myocardium due to various infections, toxins, drugs, or immunologic reactions; viral infection, particularly with coxsackieviruses, is the most common cause
- Other infectious causes include Rocky mountain spotted fever, Q fever, Chagas' disease, Lyme disease, AIDS, trichinosis, and toxoplasmosis
- Symptoms include fever, fatigue, palpitations, chest pain, or symptoms of congestive heart failure, often following an upper respiratory tract infection
- Electrocardiography may reveal ST—T wave changes, conduction blocks
- Echocardiography shows diffusely depressed left ventricular function and enlargement
- Routine myocardial biopsy usually not recommended since inflammatory changes are often focal and nonspecific

■ Differential Diagnosis

- Acute myocardial ischemia or infarction due to coronary artery disease
- Pneumonia
- Congestive heart failure due to other causes

■ Treatment

- Bed rest
- Specific antimicrobial treatment if an infectious agent can be identified
- Immunosuppressive therapy is controversial
- Appropriate treatment of systolic dysfunction: Vasodilators (ACE inhibitors, angiotensin II receptor blockers or combination of hydralazine and isosorbide dinitrate), beta-blockers, spironolactone, digoxin, low-sodium diet, and diuretics
- Cardiac transplant for severe cases

■ Pearl

"Rule of thirds" for patients with viral myocarditis: one-third return to normal, one-third have stable left ventricular dysfunction, and one-third have a rapidly deteriorating course.

Reference

Feldman AM, McNamara D: Myocarditis. N Engl J Med 2000;343:1388. [PMID: 11070105]

1

Paroxysmal Supraventricular Tachycardia (PSVT)

- **Essentials of Diagnosis**
  - A group of arrhythmias including supraventricular or atrioventricular reentrant tachycardias (over 90% of cases), automatic atrial tachycardia, and junctional tachycardia
  - Attacks usually begin and end abruptly, last seconds to hours
  - Patients often asymptomatic with transient episodes but complain of palpitations, mild shortness of breath, or chest pain with more prolonged bouts
  - Electrocardiography between attacks normal unless the patient has Wolff-Parkinson-White syndrome or a very short PR interval
  - Unless aberrant conduction occurs, the QRS complexes are regular and narrow; the location of the P wave helps determine the origin of the PSVT
  - Electrophysiologic study establishes the exact diagnosis

- **Differential Diagnosis**

  No P:
  - Atrioventricular nodal reentry tachycardia

  Short RP:
  - Atrioventricular reentrant tachycardia
  - Intra-atrial reentry tachycardia

  Long RP:
  - Atrial tachycardia
  - Some atrioventricular nodal reentry tachycardia
  - Permanent junctional reciprocating tachycardia

- **Treatment**
  - Many attacks resolve spontaneously; if not, first try vagal maneuvers such as carotid sinus massage or adenosine to transiently block the AV node and break the reentrant circuit
  - Prevention of frequent attacks can be achieved by digoxin, calcium channel blockers, beta-blockers, or antiarrhythmics such as procainamide or sotalol
  - Electrophysiologic study and ablation of the abnormal reentrant circuit or focus, when available, is the treatment of choice (> 90% success rate)

- **Pearl**

  In Q-wave infarct computer readouts with short PR intervals, look carefully for a delta wave; this may be your diagnosis.

Reference

Blomstrom-Lundqvist C, Scheinman MM, Aliot EM, et al: ACC/AHA/ESC guidelines for the management of patients with supraventricular arrhythmias—executive summary. A report of the American college of cardiology/American heart association task force on practice guidelines and the European society of cardiology committee for practice guidelines (writing committee to develop guidelines for the management of patients with supraventricular arrhythmias) developed in collaboration with NASPE-Heart Rhythm Society. J Am Coll Cardiol 2003;42:1493. [PMID: 14563598]

Patent Ductus Arteriosus

- ■ Essentials of Diagnosis
  - • Caused by failure of closure of embryonic ductus arteriosus with continuous blood flow from aorta to pulmonary artery (ie, left-to-right shunt)
  - • Symptoms are those of left ventricular failure or pulmonary hypertension; many cases are complaint-free
  - • Widened pulse pressure, a loud S_2, and a continuous, "machinery" murmur loudest over the pulmonary area but heard posteriorly
  - • Echo doppler helpful, but contrast or MR aortography is the study of choice

- ■ Differential Diagnosis
  In patients presenting with left heart failure:
  - • Mitral regurgitation
  - • Aortic stenosis
  - • Ventricular septal defect
  If pulmonary hypertension dominates the picture:
  - • Primary pulmonary hypertension
  - • Chronic pulmonary embolism
  - • Eisenmenger's syndrome

- ■ Treatment
  - • Pharmacologic closure in premature infants, using indomethacin or aspirin
  - • Surgical or percutaneous closure in patients with large shunts or symptoms; efficacy in the presence of moderate pulmonary hypertension is debated
  - • Prophylaxis for infective endocarditis

- ■ Pearl
  Patients usually remain asymptomatic as adults if problems have not developed by age 10 years.

Reference

Brickner ME, Hillis LD, Lange RA: Congenital heart disease in adults. First of two parts. N Engl J Med 2000;342:256. [PMID: 10648769]

1

Prinzmetal's Angina

- **Essentials of Diagnosis**
  - Caused by intermittent focal spasm of an otherwise normal coronary artery
  - Associated with migraine, Raynaud's phenomenon
  - The chest pain resembles typical angina, but often is more severe and occurs at rest
  - Affects women under 50, occurs in the early morning, and typically involves the right coronary artery
  - Electrocardiography shows ST elevation, but enzyme studies are normal
  - Diagnosis can be confirmed by ergonovine challenge during cardiac catheterization

- **Differential Diagnosis**
  - Typical angina pectoris; myocardial infarction; unstable angina
  - Tietze's syndrome (costochondritis)
  - Cervical or thoracic radiculopathy, including pre-eruptive zoster
  - Esophageal spasm or reflux disease
  - Cholecystitis
  - Pericarditis
  - Pneumothorax
  - Pulmonary embolism
  - Pneumococcal pneumonia

- **Treatment**
  - Nitrates and calcium channel blockers effective acutely and are the mainstay of chronic therapy
  - Stenting in affected coronary artery (usually right) in some, but prognosis excellent given absence of atherosclerosis

- **Pearl**

Cocaine leads to myocardial ischemia or infarction from vasospasm: be sure to remember differences in history.

Reference

Wang K, Asinger RW, Marriott HJ: ST-segment elevation in conditions other than acute myocardial infarction. N Engl J Med 2003;349:2128. [PMID: 14645641]

Pulmonary Stenosis

- **Essentials of Diagnosis**
  - A congenital disorder causing symptoms only when transpulmonary valve gradient is > 50 mm Hg
  - May be associated with Noonan's syndrome
  - Exertional dyspnea and chest pain due to right ventricular ischemia; sudden death occurs in severe cases
  - Jugular venous distention, parasternal lift, systolic click and ejection murmur, delayed and soft pulmonary component of S_2
  - Right ventricular hypertrophy on ECG; poststenotic dilation of the main and left pulmonary arteries on chest x-ray
  - Echo doppler is diagnostic

- **Differential Diagnosis**
  - Left ventricular failure due to any cause
  - Left-sided valvular disease
  - Primary pulmonary hypertension
  - Chronic pulmonary embolism
  - Sleep apnea
  - Chronic obstructive pulmonary disease
  - Eisenmenger's syndrome

- **Treatment**
  - All patients require endocarditis prophylaxis
  - Symptomatic patients with gradients > 50 mm Hg: Percutaneous balloon or surgical valvuloplasty
  - Asymptomatic patients with gradients > 75 mm Hg or right ventricular hypertrophy: Treatment is controversial
  - Prognosis for those with mild disease is good

- **Pearl**

Flushing with the murmur as described raises the issue of carcinoid syndrome, especially with concomitant tricuspid valve disease.

Reference

Almeda FQ, Kavinsky CJ, Pophal SG, Klein LW: Pulmonic valvular stenosis in adults: diagnosis and treatment. Catheter Cardiovasc Interv 2003;60:546. [PMID: 14624440]

Restrictive Cardiomyopathy

- ■ Essentials of Diagnosis
  - • Characterized by impaired diastolic filling with preserved left ventricular function
  - • Causes include amyloidosis, sarcoidosis, hemochromatosis, scleroderma, carcinoid syndrome, endomyocardial fibrosis, and postradiation or postsurgical fibrosis
  - • Clinical manifestations are those of the underlying disorder; congestive heart failure with right-sided symptoms and signs usually predominates
  - • Electrocardiography may show low voltage and nonspecific ST—T wave abnormalities particularly in amyloidosis; supraventricular and ventricular arrhythmias may also be seen
  - • Echo doppler shows increased wall thickness with preserved contractile function and mitral and tricuspid inflow velocity patterns consistent with impaired diastolic filling

- ■ Differential Diagnosis
  - • Constrictive pericarditis
  - • Hypertensive heart disease
  - • Hypertrophic obstructive cardiomyopathy
  - • Aortic stenosis
  - • Ischemic heart disease

- ■ Treatment
  - • Sodium restriction and diuretic therapy for patients with evidence of fluid overload; diuresis must be cautious, as volume depletion may worsen this disorder
  - • Digitalis is not indicated unless systolic function becomes impaired or atrial fibrillation occurs
  - • Treatment of underlying disease causing the restriction if possible

- ■ Pearl

Hemochromatosis is characterized by diagnostic T2-weighted images of the heart and other involved organs; one-third of patients have dense right upper quadrants on plain chest films due to hepatic iron deposition.

Reference

Franz WM, Muller OJ, Katus HA: Cardiomyopathies: from genetics to the prospect of treatment. Lancet 2001;358:1627. [PMID: 11716909]

Sudden Cardiac Death

- **Essentials of Diagnosis**
  - Death in a well patient within 1 hour of symptom onset
  - Can be due to cardiac or noncardiac disease
  - Most common cause (over 80% of cases) is ventricular fibrillation or tachycardia in the setting of coronary artery disease
  - Ventricular fibrillation is almost always the terminal rhythm

- **Differential Diagnosis**

  Noncardiac causes of sudden death:
  - Pulmonary embolism
  - Asthma
  - Aortic dissection
  - Ruptured aortic aneurysm
  - Intracranial hemorrhage
  - Tension pneumothorax
  - Anaphylaxis

- **Treatment**
  - If sudden cardiac death occurs in the setting of acute myocardial infarction, long-term management is no different from that of other patients with myocardial infarction
  - Aggressive approach obligatory if coronary artery disease is suspected; see below
  - Electrolyte abnormalities, digitalis toxicity, or pacemaker malfunction can be the precipitant and is treated accordingly
  - Without obvious cause, echocardiography and cardiac catheterization is indicated; if normal, electrophysiologic studies thereafter
  - An automatic implantable cardiac defibrillator should be used in all patients surviving an episode of sudden cardiac death secondary to ventricular fibrillation or tachycardia without a transient or reversible cause; empiric amiodarone is often added

- **Pearl**

  In sudden cardiac death in adults, if myocardial infarction is ruled out, the prognosis is paradoxically worse than if ruled in; it suggests that active ischemia or significant structural heart disease is present.

Reference

Antezano ES, Hong M: Sudden cardiac death. J Intensive Care Med 2003;18:313. [PMID: 14984660]

1

Tricuspid Regurgitation

- **Essentials of Diagnosis**
  - Causes include infective endocarditis, right ventricular heart failure of any cause, carcinoid syndrome, systemic lupus erythematosus, and Ebstein's anomaly
  - Most cases secondary to dilation of the right ventricle from left-sided heart disease
  - Edema, abdominal discomfort, anorexia; otherwise, symptoms of associated disease
  - Prominent (v) waves in jugular venous pulse; pulsatile liver, abdominojugular reflux
  - Characteristic high-pitched blowing holosystolic murmur along the left sternal border increasing with inspiration
  - Echo doppler is diagnostic

- **Differential Diagnosis**
  - Mitral regurgitation
  - Aortic stenosis
  - Pulmonary stenosis
  - Atrial septal defect
  - Ventricular septal defect

- **Treatment**
  - Diuretics and dietary sodium restriction in patients with evidence of fluid overload
  - If symptoms are severe and tricuspid regurgitation is primary, valve repair, valvuloplasty, or removal is preferable to valve replacement

- **Pearl**

Ninety percent of right heart failure is caused by left heart failure.

Reference

Raman SV, Sparks EA, Boudoulas H, Wooley CF: Tricuspid valve disease: tricuspid valve complex perspective. Curr Probl Cardiol 2002;27:103. [PMID: 11979238]

Tricuspid Stenosis

- ■ Essentials of Diagnosis
  - Usually rheumatic in origin; rarely, seen in carcinoid heart disease
  - Almost always associated with mitral stenosis when rheumatic
  - Evidence of right-sided failure: Hepatomegaly, ascites, peripheral edema, jugular venous distention with prominent (*a*) wave
  - A diastolic rumbling murmur along the left sternal border, increasing with inspiration
  - Echo doppler is diagnostic

- ■ Differential Diagnosis
  - Atypical aortic regurgitation
  - Mitral stenosis
  - Pulmonary hypertension due to any cause with right heart failure
  - Constrictive pericarditis
  - Liver cirrhosis
  - Right atrial myxoma

- ■ Treatment
  - Valve replacement in severe cases
  - Balloon valvuloplasty may prove to be useful in many patients

- ■ Pearl

Three percent of cases of left-sided rheumatic heart disease are associated with tricuspid stenosis.

Reference

Raman SV, Sparks EA, Boudoulas H, Wooley CF: Tricuspid valve disease: tricuspid valve complex perspective. Curr Probl Cardiol 2002;27:103. [PMID: 11979238]

1

Unstable Angina

■ Essentials of Diagnosis
  • Spectrum of illness between chronic stable angina and acute myocardial infarction
  • Characterized by accelerating angina, pain at rest, or pain less responsive to medications
  • Usually due to atherosclerotic plaque rupture, spasm, hemorrhage, or thrombosis
  • Chest pain resembles typical angina but is more severe and lasts longer (up to 30 minutes)
  • ECG may show dynamic ST depression or T-wave changes during pain, but normalizes when symptoms abate; a normal ECG, however, does not exclude the diagnosis

■ Differential Diagnosis
  • Typical angina pectoris
  • Myocardial infarction
  • Coronary vasospasm
  • Aortic dissection
  • Tietze's syndrome (costochondritis)
  • Cervical or thoracic radiculopathy, including pre-eruptive zoster
  • Esophageal spasm or reflux disease
  • Cholecystitis
  • Pericarditis
  • Pneumothorax
  • Pulmonary embolism
  • Pneumococcal pneumonia

■ Treatment
  • Hospitalization with bed rest, telemetry, and exclusion of myocardial infarction
  • Low-dose aspirin (81–325 mg) immediately on admission and every day thereafter; intravenous heparin of benefit in some
  • Beta-blockers to keep heart rate and blood pressure in the low-normal range
  • In high-risk patients, glycoprotein IIb/IIIa inhibitors effective, especially if percutaneous intervention likely
  • Nitroglycerin, either in paste or intravenously
  • Cardiac catheterization and consideration of revascularization in appropriate candidates

■ Pearl
Aortic dissection should be considered in any chest pain syndrome before aggressive anticoagulation is instituted.

Reference

Fox KA: Management of acute coronary syndromes: an update. Heart 2004;90:698. [PMID: 15145891]

Ventricular Septal Defect   **1**

- ■ Essentials of Diagnosis
  - Many congenital ventricular septal defects close spontaneously during childhood
  - Symptoms depend on the size of the defect and the magnitude of the left-to-right shunt
  - Small defects in adults are usually asymptomatic except for complicating endocarditis, but may be associated with a loud murmur (maladie de Roger)
  - Large defects usually associated with softer murmurs, but commonly lead to Eisenmenger's syndrome
  - Echo doppler diagnostic; radionuclide angiogram or cardiac catheterization quantifies the ratio of pulmonary flow to systemic flow (PF:SF)

- ■ Differential Diagnosis
  - Mitral regurgitation
  - Aortic stenosis
  - Cardiomyopathy due to various causes

- ■ Treatment
  - Small shunts in asymptomatic patients may not require surgery
  - Mild dyspnea treatable with diuretics and preload reduction
  - PF:SF shunts over 2 are repaired to prevent irreversible pulmonary vascular disease
  - Surgery if patient has developed shunt reversal (Eisenmenger's syndrome) without fixed pulmonary hypertension
  - Prophylaxis for infective endocarditis

- ■ Pearl

Small defects have a higher risk of endocarditis than large ones; endothelial injury is favored by a small, localized jet.

Reference

Brickner ME, Hillis LD, Lange RA: Congenital heart disease in adults. First of two parts. N Engl J Med 2000;342:256. [PMID: 10648769]

1

Ventricular Tachycardia

- **Essentials of Diagnosis**
  - Three or more consecutive premature ventricular beats; nonsustained (lasting < 30 seconds) or sustained
  - Mechanisms are reentry or automatic focus; may occur spontaneously or with myocardial infarction
  - Other causes include acute or chronic ischemia, cardiomyopathy, and drugs (eg, antiarrhythmics)
  - Most patients symptomatic; syncope, palpitations, shortness of breath, and chest pain are common
  - S_1 of variable intensity; S_3 present
  - Electrocardiography shows a regular, wide-complex tachycardia (usually between 140 and 220 beats/min); between attacks, the ECG often reveals evidence of prior myocardial infarction

- **Differential Diagnosis**
  - Any cause of supraventricular tachycardia with aberrant conduction (but a history of myocardial infarction or low ejection fraction indicates ventricular tachycardia until proved otherwise)
  - Atrial flutter with aberrant conduction

- **Treatment**
  - Depends upon whether the patient is stable or unstable
  - If stable: intravenous lidocaine, procainamide, or amiodarone can be used initially
  - If unstable (hypotension, congestive heart failure, or angina): immediate synchronized cardioversion
  - For sustained ventricular tachycardia, automatic implantable cardiac defibrillator placement should be strongly considered
  - Treatment of recurrent asymptomatic, nonsustained ventricular tachycardia is controversial; in a patient with ischemic heart disease and a low left ventricular ejection fraction (< 35%), an implantable cardiac defibrillator may be the wisest approach

- **Pearl**

All wide-complex tachycardia should be treated as ventricular tachycardia until proven otherwise.

Reference

Talwar KK, Naik N: Etiology and management of sustained ventricular tachycardia. Am J Cardiovasc Drugs 2001;1:179. [PMID: 14728033]

Pulmonary Diseases

Acute Bacterial Pneumonia

- **Essentials of Diagnosis**
  - Fever, chills, cough with purulent sputum production; early pleuritic pain suggests pneumococcal etiology
  - Tachycardia, tachypnea; bronchial breath sounds with percussive dullness and egophony over involved lung; findings may be more pronounced after hydration
  - Leukocytosis; WBC < 5000 or > 25,000 worrisome
  - Patchy or lobar infiltrate by chest x-ray
  - Diagnosis from Gram's stain properly interpreted or culture of sputum, blood, or pleural fluid
  - Principal causes include *Streptococcus pneumoniae, Haemophilus influenzae,* gram-negative rods, *Staphylococcus*

- **Differential Diagnosis**
  - Lung abscess; atypical or viral pneumonia
  - Pulmonary embolism
  - Congestive heart failure; ARDS
  - Interstitial lung disease (acute interstitial pneumonia, diffuse alveolar hemorrhage)

- **Treatment**
  - Empiric antibiotics for common organisms after obtaining cultures
  - Hospitalize selected patients (severe hypoxemia, more than one lobe involved, poor host resistance factors, presence of coexisting illness, leukopenia or marked leukocytosis, hypotension)
  - Pneumococcal vaccine to prevent or lessen severity of pneumococcal infections

- **Pearl**

When diplococci thrive within neutrophils on Gram's stain, think staphylococci, not pneumococci.

Reference

Mandell LA, Bartlett JG, Dowell SF, et al; Infectious Diseases Society of America: Update of practice guidelines for the management of community-acquired pneumonia in immunocompetent adults. Clin Infect Dis 2003; 37:1405. [PMID: 14614663]

Acute Pulmonary Venous Thromboembolism

2

- ■ Essentials of Diagnosis
  - Seen in immobilized patients, congestive heart failure, malignancies, hypercoagulable states, and after pelvic trauma or surgery
  - Abrupt onset of dyspnea and anxiety, with or without pleuritic chest pain, cough with hemoptysis; syncope rare, but suggestive of extensive disease
  - Tachycardia, tachypnea most common; loud P_2 with right-sided S_3 characteristic but unusual; findings of peripheral venous thrombosis often absent
  - Acute respiratory alkalosis and hypoxemia
  - Characteristic segmental mismatch in ventilation and perfusion on ventilation-perfusion scan
  - Lower extremity ultrasound demonstrates deep venous thrombosis in half
  - CT scan establishes diagnosis in many, but negative predictive value not yet established
  - Quantitative D-dimer has excellent negative predictive value
  - In occasional cases, pulmonary angiography is required to confirm the diagnosis

- ■ Differential Diagnosis
  - Pneumonia
  - Myocardial infarction
  - Atelectasis
  - Any cause of acute respiratory distress (eg, pneumothorax, aspiration, pulmonary edema, or asthma) or pleural effusion
  - Early sepsis
  - Dressler's syndrome

- ■ Treatment
  - Anticoagulation: Acutely with heparin (preferably low-molecular-weight heparin in appropriate patients), instituting warfarin concurrently and continuing for a minimum of 6 months
  - Thrombolytic therapy initially in selected patients with hemodynamic compromise; effect on mortality not proven
  - Intravenous filter placement in inferior vena cava for selected patients not candidates for or unresponsive to anticoagulation; short-term value only given collateral development

- ■ Pearl

Ten percent of pulmonary emboli originate from upper extremity veins.

Reference

Goldhaber SZ: Pulmonary embolism. Lancet 2004;363:1295. [PMID: 15094276]

Acute Respiratory Distress Syndrome (ARDS)

2

- ■ Essentials of Diagnosis
  - • Rapid onset of dyspnea and respiratory distress, commonly in setting of trauma, shock, or sepsis
  - • Tachypnea, fever; crackles or rhonchi by auscultation
  - • Arterial hypoxemia refractory to supplemental oxygen; hypercapnia and respiratory acidosis in impending respiratory failure
  - • Diffuse alveolar and interstitial infiltrates by radiography, often sparing costophrenic angles
  - • Normal pulmonary capillary wedge pressure
  - • Acute lung injury defined by a Pao_2:Fio_2 ratio < 300; ARDS is defined by Pao_2:Fio_2 ratio < 200

- ■ Differential Diagnosis
  - • Cardiogenic pulmonary edema
  - • Primary pneumonia due to any cause
  - • Diffuse alveolar hemorrhage
  - • Acute interstitial pneumonia (ie, Hamman-Rich syndrome)
  - • Cryptogenic organizing pneumonia (idiopathic bronchiolitis obliterans with organizing pneumonia (BOOP)

- ■ Treatment
  - • Mechanical ventilation with supplemental oxygen; positive end-expiratory pressure often required
  - • Low-tidal-volume ventilation, using 6 mL/kg predicted body weight, may reduce mortality
  - • Supportive therapy including adequate nutrition, vigilance for other organ dysfunction, and prevention of nosocomial complications (eg, catheter-related infection, ventilator-associated pneumonia, venous thromboembolism, stress gastritis)
  - • Mortality rate is 40–60%

- ■ Pearl

Acute interstitial pneumonia is ARDS that is not preceded by trauma, shock, or sepsis.

Reference

Kallet RH: Evidence-based management of acute lung injury and acute respiratory distress syndrome. Respir Care 2004;49:793. [PMID: 15222911]

Acute Tracheobronchitis

2

- **Essentials of Diagnosis**
  - Poorly defined but common condition characterized by inflammation of the trachea and bronchi
  - Due to infectious agents (bacteria or viruses) or irritants (eg, dust and smoke)
  - Cough is most common symptom; purulent sputum production and malaise common; hemoptysis occasionally
  - Variable rhonchi and wheezing; fever often absent but may be prominent in cases caused by *Haemophilus influenzae*
  - Chest x-ray normal
  - Increased incidence in smokers

- **Differential Diagnosis**
  - Asthma
  - Pneumonia
  - Foreign body aspiration
  - Inhalation pneumonitis
  - Viral croup

- **Treatment**
  - Symptomatic therapy with inhaled bronchodilators, cough suppressants
  - Antibiotics not recommended in most; they shorten the disease course by less than 1 day
  - Patients encouraged to stop smoking

- **Pearl**

Haemophilus influenzae *and* Pseudomonas *have a tropism for large airways and are characteristic if retrieved absent underlying lung disease.*

Reference

Martinez FJ: Acute bronchitis: state of the art diagnosis and therapy. Compr Ther 2004;30:55. [PMID: 15162593]

Allergic Bronchopulmonary Mycosis (Formerly Allergic Bronchopulmonary Aspergillosis)

■ Essentials of Diagnosis

- Caused by allergy to antigens of *Aspergillus* species or other fungi colonizing the tracheobronchial tree
- Recurrent dyspnea, unmasked by corticosteroid withdrawal, with history of asthma; cough productive of brownish plugs of sputum
- Physical examination as in asthma
- Peripheral eosinophilia, elevated serum IgE level, precipitating antibody to *Aspergillus* antigen present; positive skin hypersensitivity to *Aspergillus* antigen
- Infiltrate (often fleeting) and central bronchiectasis by chest radiography

■ Differential Diagnosis

- Asthma
- Bronchiectasis
- Invasive aspergillosis
- Churg-Strauss syndrome
- Löffler's syndrome
- Chronic obstructive pulmonary disease

■ Treatment

- Oral corticosteroids often required for several months
- Inhaled bronchodilators as for attacks of asthma
- Treatment with itraconazole (for 16 weeks) improves disease control
- Complications include hemoptysis, severe bronchiectasis, and pulmonary fibrosis

■ Pearl

One of the three ways Aspergillus *causes disease—all different pathophysiologically.*

Reference

Khan AN, Jones C, Macdonald S: Bronchopulmonary aspergillosis: a review. Curr Probl Diagn Radiol 2003;32:156. [PMID: 12838261]

Asbestosis

2

■ Essentials of Diagnosis

- History of exposure to dust containing asbestos particles (eg, from work in mining, insulation, construction, shipbuilding)
- Progressive dyspnea, rarely pleuritic chest pain
- Dry inspiratory crackles common; clubbing and cyanosis occasionally seen
- Interstitial fibrosis is characteristic (lower lung greater than upper); pleural thickening and diaphragmatic calcification common but nonspecific; however, the three together with exposure history establish the diagnosis
- Exudative pleural effusion develops before parenchymal disease
- High-resolution CT scan often confirmatory
- Pulmonary function testing shows a restrictive defect; diminished D$_{LCO}$ often the earliest abnormality

■ Differential Diagnosis

- Other inhalation pneumoconioses (eg, silicosis)
- Fungal disease
- Sarcoidosis
- Idiopathic pulmonary fibrosis
- Mesothelioma

■ Treatment

- Supportive care; chronic oxygen supplementation for sustained hypoxemia
- Legal counseling regarding compensation for occupational exposure using above diagnostic criteria

■ Pearl

Remember that the highest exposures on ships come from sweeping the floor, not working on the structure of the vessel.

Reference

Cugell DW, Kamp DW: Asbestos and the pleura: a review. Chest 2004;125:1103. [PMID: 15006974]

Asthma

- **Essentials of Diagnosis**
  - Episodic wheezing and cough; chronic dyspnea or chest tightness; can present as nighttime cough
  - Some attacks triggered by cold air or exercise
  - Prolonged expiratory time, wheezing; if severe, pulsus paradoxus and cyanosis
  - Peripheral eosinophilia common; mucus casts, eosinophils, and Charcot-Leyden crystals in sputum
  - Obstructive pattern by spirometry supports diagnosis, though may be normal between attacks
  - With methacholine challenge, absence of bronchial hyperreactivity makes diagnosis unlikely

- **Differential Diagnosis**
  - Congestive heart failure
  - Chronic obstructive pulmonary disease
  - Vocal cord dysfunction
  - Pulmonary embolism
  - Foreign body aspiration
  - Pulmonary infection (eg, strongyloidiasis, aspergillosis)
  - Churg-Strauss syndrome
  - Sinusitis with postnasal drip

- **Treatment**
  - Avoidance of known precipitants, inhaled corticosteroids in persistent asthma, inhaled bronchodilators for symptoms
  - In patients not well controlled on inhaled corticosteroids, long-acting inhaled β-agonist (eg, salmeterol)
  - Treatment of exacerbations: Oxygen, inhaled bronchodilators (β_2-agonists or anticholinergics), systemic corticosteroids
  - Leukotriene modifiers (eg, montelukast) may provide an option for long-term therapy in mild to moderate disease
  - For difficult-to-control asthma, consider exacerbating factors such as gastroesophageal reflux disease and chronic sinusitis

- **Pearl**

All that wheezes is not asthma; remember conditions like vocal cord dysfunction in patients with "steroid-resistant" asthma.

Reference

Sin DD, Man J, Sharpe H, et al: Pharmacological management to reduce exacerbations in adults with asthma: a systematic review and meta-analysis. JAMA 2004;292:367. [PMID: 15265853]

Atypical Pneumonia

2

■ Essentials of Diagnosis
- Cough with scant sputum, fever, malaise, headache; gastrointestinal symptoms variable
- Physical examination of lungs may be unimpressive
- Mild leukocytosis; cold agglutinins sometimes positive but not diagnostic
- Patchy, nonlobar infiltrate by chest x-ray often surprisingly extensive
- Pathogens include *Legionella, Mycoplasma,* chlamydia, viruses
- Typical and atypical pneumonia not always distinguishable clinically or radiographically

■ Differential Diagnosis
- Bacterial pneumonia
- *Pneumocystis carinii* pneumonia
- Pulmonary embolism
- Congestive heart failure
- Diffuse alveolar hemorrhage
- Interstitial lung disease (hypersensitivity pneumonitis, cryptogenic organizing pneumonitis)

■ Treatment
- Empiric antibiotic treatment with doxycycline, erythromycin, or other macrolide (eg, azithromycin), fluoroquinolone (eg, levofloxacin)
- Hospitalize as for bacterial pneumonia

■ Pearl

Bullous myringitis is encountered in 5% of patients with Mycoplasma pneumonia: it's as diagnostically specific as serology and takes seconds rather than days to verify.

Reference

Thibodeau KP, Viera AJ: Atypical pathogens and challenges in community-acquired pneumonia. Am Fam Physician 2004;69:1699. [PMID: 15086042]

Bronchiectasis

- **Essentials of Diagnosis**
  - A congenital, or increasingly uncommonly an acquired, disorder affecting the large bronchi causing permanent abnormal dilation and destruction of bronchial walls; may be a consequence of untreated pneumonia
  - Chronic cough with copious purulent sputum, hemoptysis; weight loss, recurrent pneumonias
  - Coarse, moist crackles; clubbing
  - Hypoxemia; obstructive pattern by spirometry
  - Chest x-rays variable, may show tram-tracking, and multiple cystic lesions at bases in advanced cases
  - High-resolution CT scan necessary for diagnosis in many cases
  - Often associated with underlying systemic disorder (eg, cystic fibrosis, hypogammaglobulinemia, IgA deficiency, common variable immunodeficiency, primary ciliary dyskinesia) and chronic pulmonary infection (eg, tuberculosis, other mycobacterioses, lung abscess)
  - Complications include massive hemoptysis, cor pulmonale, amyloidosis, and secondary visceral abscesses (eg, brain abscess)

- **Differential Diagnosis**
  - Chronic obstructive pulmonary disease
  - Tuberculosis
  - Hypogammaglobulinemia
  - Ciliary dysmotility
  - Lung abscess
  - Pneumonia due to any cause

- **Treatment**
  - Antibiotics selected by sputum culture and sensitivities
  - Chest physiotherapy
  - Inhaled bronchodilators
  - Surgical resection in selected patients with unresponsive localized disease or massive hemoptysis

- **Pearl**

The only cause in medicine of three-layered sputum.

Reference

Morrissey BM, Evans SJ: Severe bronchiectasis. Clin Rev Allergy Immunol 2003;25:233. [PMID: 14716069]

Chronic Cough

2

- **Essentials of Diagnosis**
  - One of the most common reasons for seeking medical attention
  - Defined as a cough persisting for at least 4 weeks
  - Nasal and oral examination for signs of postnasal drip (eg, cobblestone appearance or erythema of mucosa), chest auscultation for wheezing
  - Chest x-ray to exclude specific parenchymal lung diseases
  - Consider spirometry before and after bronchodilator, methacholine challenge, sinus CT scan, and 24-hour esophageal pH monitoring
  - Bronchoscopy in selected cases

- **Differential Diagnosis**
  - Bronchitis
  - Respiratory bronchiolitis (smoking-related)
  - Angiotensin-converting enzyme inhibitor
  - Postnasal drip
  - Sinusitis
  - Asthma
  - Gastroesophageal reflux
  - Postinfectious cough
  - Bronchiectasis
  - Chronic obstructive pulmonary disease
  - Congestive heart failure
  - Interstitial lung disease
  - Sarcoidosis
  - Bronchogenic carcinoma
  - Psychogenic cough

- **Treatment**
  - Smoking cessation
  - Treat underlying condition if present
  - Trial of inhaled β-agonist (eg, albuterol)
  - For postnasal drip: Antihistamines (H_1-antagonists or may add nasal ipratropium bromide)
  - For suspected gastroesophageal reflux disease, proton pump inhibitors (eg, omeprazole)

- **Pearl**

In a hypertensive with chronic cough, check the medication list first; if ACE inhibitors or receptor blockers are on it, time and money will be saved by stopping them.

Reference

Holmes RL, Fadden CT: Evaluation of the patient with chronic cough. Am Fam Physician 2004;69:2159. [PMID: 15152964]

Chronic Eosinophilic Pneumonia

- Essentials of Diagnosis
  - Fever, dry cough, wheezing, dyspnea, and weight loss—all variable from transient to severe and progressive
  - Wheezing, dry crackles occasionally appreciated by auscultation
  - Peripheral blood eosinophilia present in most, but not all, cases
  - Peripheral pulmonary infiltrates on radiographs in many cases (the "radiologic negative" of pulmonary edema); > 25% eosinophils by bronchoalveolar lavage; lung biopsy shows abundant eosinophils

- Differential Diagnosis
  - Infectious pneumonia
  - Asthma
  - Idiopathic pulmonary fibrosis
  - Cryptogenic organizing pneumonitis
  - Allergic bronchopulmonary mycosis
  - Churg-Strauss syndrome
  - Other eosinophilic pulmonary syndromes (eg, drug- or parasite-related, acute eosinophillic pneumonia)

- Treatment
  - Moderate-dose corticosteroid therapy often results in dramatic improvement; but recurrence is common
  - Most patients require corticosteroids for a year, others indefinitely

- Pearl

Pause to consider strongyloidiasis before giving steroids to a patient with pulmonary disease and eosinophilia.

Reference

Khoo KL, Lim TK: Pulmonary hypereosinophilia. Ann Acad Med Singapore 2004;33:521. [PMID: 15329768]

Chronic Obstructive Pulmonary Disease (COPD)

2

- **Essentials of Diagnosis**
  - Primarily consisting of emphysema and chronic bronchitis; most patients have components of both
  - Dyspnea or chronic productive cough or both are characteristic; COPD is nearly always a disease of heavy smokers
  - Tachypnea, barrel chest, distant breath sounds, wheezes or rhonchi, cyanosis; clubbing unusual and suggests associated malignancy
  - Hypoxemia and hypercapnia more pronounced with chronic bronchitis than with emphysema
  - Hyperexpansion with decreased markings by chest radiography; variable findings of bullae, thin cardiac shadow
  - Airflow obstruction by spirometry; normal diffusing capacity (D_{LCO}) in bronchitis, reduced in emphysema
  - Ventilation and perfusion well matched in remaining lung in emphysema, not in chronic bronchitis

- **Differential Diagnosis**
  - Asthma
  - Bronchiectasis
  - α_1-Antitrypsin deficiency
  - Interstitial lung disease (eg, sarcoidosis, hypersensitivity pneumonitis, eosinophilic granuloma)
  - Congestive heart failure
  - Recurrent pulmonary emboli

- **Treatment**
  - Stopping smoking is most important intervention
  - Inhaled anticholinergic agent, eg, ipratropium bromide, for symptomatic improvement should be tried
  - Pneumococcal vaccination; yearly influenza vaccination
  - Supplemental oxygen for hypoxemic patients ($Pa_{O_2} < 55$ mm Hg) reduces mortality
  - For exacerbations, treat for asthma and identify underlying precipitant; if patient has low baseline peak flow rates, antibiotics may be beneficial
  - Lung reduction surgery in selected patients with emphysema

- **Pearl**

The blue bloater pushes the pink puffer's wheelchair; the bronchitis patient has better exercise tolerance.

Reference

Wouters EF: Management of severe COPD. Lancet 2004;364:883. [PMID: 15351196]

Cryptogenic Organizing Pneumonia (Idiopathic Bronchiolitis Obliterans with Organizing Pneumonia [BOOP])

2

- Essentials of Diagnosis
  - Cryptogenic organizing pneumonia (COP) and idiopathic BOOP are synonymous
  - COP may follow infections (eg, *Mycoplasma,* viral infection), may be due to toxic fume inhalation or associated with connective tissue disease or organ transplantation
  - Affects patients of all ages (mean is 50 years), no gender predilection, smoking not a precipitant
  - Presentation often similar to community-acquired pneumonia; up to half have abrupt onset of flulike symptoms such as fever, malaise, nonproductive cough, fatigue, and dyspnea
  - Weight loss (often more than 10 pounds) commonly observed
  - Dry crackles by auscultation; wheezing and clubbing are both unusual
  - Restrictive abnormalities with pulmonary function studies; hypoxemia typical
  - Chest radiograph shows patchy alveolar infiltrates bilaterally
  - Open or thoracoscopic lung biopsy necessary for precise diagnosis

- Differential Diagnosis
  - Pneumonia due to bacteria, fungi, or tuberculosis
  - Diffuse alveolar hemorrhage
  - Acute interstitial pneumonia
  - ARDS
  - AIDS-related lung infections (eg, *Pneumocystis carinii*)
  - Congestive heart failure
  - Hypersensitivity pneumonitis
  - Chronic eosinophilic pneumonia
  - Pulmonary toxicity due to drugs or autoimmune disorder

- Treatment
  - Corticosteroids effective in two-thirds of cases; cytotoxic agents (eg, cyclophosphamide) in steroid failures
  - Relapse common after short (< 6 months) steroid courses

- Pearl

COP is a leading diagnosis when "community-acquired pneumonia" persists despite antibiotics.

Reference

Ryu JH, Myers JL, Swensen SJ: Bronchiolar disorders. Am J Respir Crit Care Med 2003;168):1277. [PMID: 14644923]

Cystic Fibrosis

2

■ **Essentials of Diagnosis**
- A generalized autosomal recessive disorder of the exocrine glands more common than was once believed
- Cough, dyspnea, recurrent pulmonary infections often due to *Pseudomonas;* symptoms of malabsorption, infertility
- Distant breath sounds, rhonchi, clubbing, nasal polyps
- Hypoxemia; obstructive or mixed pattern by spirometry; decreased diffusion capacity
- Chest radiograph reveals bronchiectasis, upper lobe volume loss, and cystic disease
- Sweat chloride > 60 mEq/L is characteristic but false-negative results can occur
- Testing for genetic mutations can confirm diagnosis when sweat test is negative

■ **Differential Diagnosis**
- Asthma
- Bronchiectasis (primary ciliary dysmotility)
- Congenital emphysema (α_1-antiprotease deficiency)

■ **Chronic Granulomatous Disease**
- Pancreatic insufficiency
- Other causes of malabsorption

■ **Treatment**
- Comprehensive multidisciplinary therapy required, including genetic and occupational counseling
- Inhaled bronchodilators and chest physiotherapy
- Antibiotics for recurrent airway infections guided by cultures and sensitivities given high rate of resistant *Pseudomonas aeruginosa* and *Staphylococcus aureus*
- Pneumococcal vaccination; yearly influenza vaccinations
- Recombinant human deoxyribonuclease given by aerosol has modest benefit
- Chest physiotherapy with a variety of devices may be beneficial
- Lung transplantation is the definitive treatment in selected patients

■ **Pearl**

Consider cystic fibrosis in young adults with recurrent pulmonary infections; formes frustes are more common than once thought.

Reference

Yankaskas JR, Marshall BC, Sufian B, et al: Cystic fibrosis adult care: consensus conference report. Chest 2004;125(1 Suppl):1S. [PMID: 14734689]

Foreign Body Aspiration

- ■ Essentials of Diagnosis

  - Sudden onset of cough, wheeze, and dyspnea; children may be witnessed at onset of symptoms
  - Localized wheezing, hyperresonance, stridor, and diminished breath sounds
  - Localized air trapping or atelectasis on end-expiratory chest radiograph
  - Diagnostic fiberoptic bronchoscopy usually identifies and localizes the foreign body

- ■ Differential Diagnosis

  - Mucus plugging due to asthma or chronic bronchitis
  - Bronchiolitis
  - Endobronchial tumor
  - Pyogenic upper airway process (eg, Ludwig's angina, soft tissue abscess, epiglottitis)
  - Laryngospasm associated with anaphylaxis
  - Bronchial compression from mass lesion
  - Substernal goiter
  - Tracheal cystadenoma

- ■ Treatment

  - Bronchoscopic or surgical removal of foreign body, often by rigid bronchoscopy
  - Emergency attention to airway—may require endotracheal intubation

- ■ Pearl

An adult complaining of croup has a substernal goiter until proved otherwise.

Reference

Lima JA, Fischer GB: Foreign body aspiration in children. Paediatr Respir Rev 2002;3:303. [PMID: 12457600]

2

Hypersensitivity Pneumonitis (Extrinsic Allergic Alveolitis)

■ Essentials of Diagnosis

- Work and environmental history suggesting link between activities and symptoms
- Caused by exposure to microbial agents (eg, thermophilic *Actinomyces* in farmer's lung, bagassosis, sequoiosis), animal proteins (eg, bird fancier's lung), with resultant IgG complement deposition, and chemical sensitizers (eg, isocyanates, trimellitic anhydride)
- Acute form: 4–12 hours after exposure, cough, dyspnea, fever, chills, myalgias; tachypnea, tachycardia, inspiratory crackles; leukocytosis with lymphopenia and neutrophilia; eosinophilia unusual
- Subacute or chronic form: Exertional dyspnea, cough, fatigue, anorexia, weight loss; basilar crackles
- IgG precipitating antibodies against above antigens indicates exposure but does not make diagnosis
- Skin testing not useful
- Pulmonary function tests reveal either airflow limitation or a restrictive pattern and decreased D$_{LCO}$
- High-resolution thoracic CT scan reveals fine diffuse ground-glass abnormality with centrilobular nodules
- Bronchoalveolar lavage reveals marked lymphocytosis
- Transbronchial or thoracoscopic lung biopsy can confirm diagnosis in unclear cases

■ Differential Diagnosis

- Idiopathic pulmonary fibrosis
- Sarcoidosis
- Asthma
- Atypical pneumonia
- Collagen vascular disease, eg, systemic lupus erythematosus

■ Treatment

- Identification and removal of exposure
- Consider systemic corticosteroids in subacute or chronic forms

■ Pearl

Bagassosis and sequoiosis are two examples; a history of exposure to sugar cane or fallen lumber, respectively, makes the diagnosis.

Reference

Yi ES: Hypersensitivity pneumonitis. Crit Rev Clin Lab Sci 2002;39:581. [PMID: 12484500]

Idiopathic Pulmonary Fibrosis

■ **Essentials of Diagnosis**

- Insidious onset of exertional dyspnea and dry cough in patients, usually in their sixth or seventh decades
- Definition requires the histopathologic pattern of usual interstitial pneumonia
- Inspiratory crackles by auscultation; clubbing
- Hypoxemia, especially exertional
- Predominantly lower lobe, bilateral reticular abnormality by chest x-ray, which may progress to honeycombing pattern
- Restrictive pattern with decreased total lung capacity and diffusing capacity (D_{LCO})
- High-resolution thoracic CT scan may confidently establish diagnosis in many
- Biopsy via visually-assisted thoracoscopic surgery (VATS) is the best method for definitive diagnosis, demonstrating usual interstitial pneumonia

■ **Differential Diagnosis**

- Nonspecific interstitial pneumonia
- Cryptogenic organizing pneumonia (COP)
- Interstitial lung disease due to collagen vascular disease
- Drug-induced fibrosis (eg, bleomycin, nitrofurantoin)
- Sarcoidosis
- Pneumoconiosis
- Asbestosis
- Hypersensitivity pneumonitis

■ **Treatment**

- Supportive therapy, including supplemental oxygen
- Combined high-dose corticosteroids and cytotoxic therapy largely ineffective
- Antifibrotic therapies (eg, interferon gamma 1b) of unclear benefit
- Early referral to lung transplantation center is critical for good candidates

■ **Pearl**

Progression from desquamative interstitial pneumonia to usual interstitial pneumonia does not occur; the former is a distinct smoking-related interstitial lung disease.

Reference

Khalil N, O'Connor R: Idiopathic pulmonary fibrosis: current understanding of the pathogenesis and the status of treatment. CMAJ 2004;171:153. [PMID: 15262886]

Lung Abscess

2

■ Essentials of Diagnosis

- Cough producing foul-smelling sputum; hemoptysis; fever, weight loss, malaise
- Patients with periodontal disease, alcoholism, impaired deglutition (eg, neurologic or esophageal disorder or altered consciousness) predisposed
- Usual cause is mixed aerobic/anaerobic infection
- Bronchial breath sounds with dullness and egophony over involved lung; succussion splash and amphoric breathing indicate air-fluid level
- Leukocytosis; hypoxemia
- Chest x-ray density, often with central lucency or air-fluid level

■ Differential Diagnosis

- Tuberculosis
- Bronchogenic carcinoma
- Pulmonary mycoses
- Bronchiectasis
- Cavitary bacterial pneumonia
- Pulmonary vasculitis (eg, Wegener's granulomatosis)

■ Treatment

- Clindamycin or high-dose penicillin (treatment for 6 or more weeks)
- Surgery in selected cases (particularly large abscess; massive or persistent hemoptysis)
- Supplemental oxygen as needed
- Bronchoscopic exclusion of carcinoma or foreign body aspiration in patients with atypical features, especially edentulous patients

■ Pearl

A lung abscess in an edentulous patient is lung cancer until proved otherwise.

Reference

Mansharamani NG, Koziel H: Chronic lung sepsis: lung abscess, bronchiectasis, and empyema. Curr Opin Pulm Med 2003;9:181. [PMID: 12682562]

Pleural Effusion

- **Essentials of Diagnosis**

  - Many asymptomatic; pleuritic chest pain, dyspnea in some
  - Decreased breath sounds and percussive dullness; bronchial breathing above effusion
  - Layering on decubitus chest x-rays; ultrasonography or chest CT scan occasionally required for confirmation
  - Exudative effusion commonly due to malignancy, infection, autoimmune disease, pulmonary embolism, asbestosis
  - Transudative effusion caused by congestive heart failure, cirrhosis with ascites, nephrotic syndrome, hypothyroidism
  - Exudative effusions have at least one of the following: pleural fluid protein: serum protein ratio > 0.5; pleural fluid LDH: serum LDH ratio > 0.6; or pleural fluid LDH > two-thirds the upper limit of normal serum LDH
  - Markedly reduced glucose in empyema, rheumatoid effusion

- **Differential Diagnosis**
  - Atelectasis
  - Lobar consolidation
  - Chronic pleural thickening
  - Elevated hemidiaphragm

- **Treatment**
  - Diagnostic thoracentesis for evaluating cause, with pleural fluid glucose, protein, red and white cells counts, LDH, and relevant cultures
  - Therapy guided by suspected cause
  - Pleural biopsy indicated in selected cases for diagnostic purposes (eg, tuberculosis, carcinoma)
  - Bleomycin, tetracycline, and talc are the most effective sclerosing agents for malignant pleural effusion

- **Pearl**

Amesotheliocytosis in an exudative pleural effusion implies tuberculosis until proved otherwise.

Reference

Cohen M, Sahn SA: Resolution of pleural effusions. Chest 2001;119:1547. [PMID: 11348966]

Primary Pulmonary Hypertension

2

- ■ Essentials of Diagnosis
  - • A rare disorder seen primarily in young and middle-aged women
  - • Defined as pulmonary hypertension and elevated peripheral vascular resistance in the absence of parenchymal lung or heart disease
  - • Progressive dyspnea, malaise, chest pain, exertional syncope
  - • Tachycardia, right ventricular lift, increased P_2, systolic ejection click, right-sided S_3; evidence of right-sided heart failure (peripheral edema, hepatomegaly, ascites) common
  - • Right ventricular strain or hypertrophy by electrocardiography
  - • Large central pulmonary arteries by chest x-ray, with oligemia distally
  - • Characteristic plexogenic arteriopathy on pathologic examination

- ■ Differential Diagnosis
  - • Mitral stenosis
  - • Sleep apnea
  - • Chronic pulmonary embolism
  - • Autoimmune pulmonary disease
  - • Phen-fen drug-induced pulmonary hypertension
  - • Ischemic heart disease
  - • HIV-associated pulmonary hypertension
  - • Cirrhosis of the liver
  - • Pulmonary veno-occlusive disease

- ■ Treatment
  - • A minority of patients respond well to calcium channel blockers
  - • Continuous intravenous prostacyclin infusion and oral bosentan blocking of endothelin receptors on vascular endothelium may improve symptoms and survival in more severe cases
  - • Empiric anticoagulation may confer survival benefit
  - • Bilateral lung or heart-lung transplantation important options; all eligible patients should be referred to a transplant center for evaluation

- ■ Pearl

"Primary pulmonary hypertension" with a left atrial abnormality on ECG is mitral stenosis until shown otherwise.

Reference

Runo JR, Loyd JE: Primary pulmonary hypertension. Lancet 2003;361:1533. [PMID: 12737878]

Pulmonary Alveolar Proteinosis

- ■ Essentials of Diagnosis
  - May be idiopathic (congenital or acquired) or secondary (eg, postinfection, immunocompromised host, hematologic malignancy)
  - Congenital cases due to mutations in surfactant B and C or GM-CSF receptor
  - Typical patient between 30 and 50 years of age; men outnumber women by 2 to 1
  - Progressive dyspnea on exertion, low-grade fever, weight loss, fatigue, nonproductive cough; rare expectoration of gelatinous sputum; asymptomatic patients not unusual
  - Physical examination often normal; rales present in about 50%; clubbing unusual
  - Hypoxemia; bilateral alveolar infiltrates suggestive of pulmonary edema on chest radiography
  - Characteristic intra-alveolar phospholipid accumulation without fibrosis at video-assisted thoracoscopic surgery (VATS)
  - Superinfection with *Nocardia* typical

- ■ Differential Diagnosis
  - Congestive heart failure
  - Noncardiogenic pulmonary edema
  - Interstitial lung disease
  - Diffuse alveolar hemorrhage
  - Cryptogenic organizing pneumonitis
  - ARDS

- ■ Treatment
  - Up to 25% remit spontaneously
  - Periodic whole lung lavage via double-lumen endotracheal tube reduces exertional dyspnea in those with limiting symptoms
  - Treat underlying cause in secondary forms
  - GM-CSF therapy appears beneficial in selected patients

- ■ Pearl

If the lab reports faintly acid-fast organisms on a sputum screen in a patient with new-onset "pulmonary edema," this is the diagnosis.

Reference

Trapnell BC, Whitsett JA, Nakata K: Pulmonary alveolar proteinosis. N Engl J Med 2003;349:2527. [PMID: 14695413]

Pulmonary Histiocytosis X

2

■ Essentials of Diagnosis
- Uncommon interstitial lung disorder primarily affecting smokers between 20 and 40
- The pathologic cell (Langerhans' cell) is a differentiated cell within the monocyte-macrophage line
- Mid- to upper-zone lung involvement is common (as opposed to characteristic lower-zone involvement of idiopathic pulmonary fibrosis)
- Patients may present asymptomatically on chest radiography or after spontaneous pneumothorax
- Symptoms are nonspecific and may include dry cough, dyspnea, fatigue, pleuritic chest pain, weight loss, fever
- Physical exam usually normal, however, clubbing and crackles occasionally occur; labs usually normal; specifically no eosinophilia
- Complications include recurrent spontaneous pneumothorax, hemoptysis, bone pain (due to bone cysts), diabetes insipidus, malignancy
- Reticulonodular infiltrates, stellate nodules, upper zone cysts, absence of pleural effusion, normal lung volume on chest film
- High-resolution CT especially helpful; pulmonary function tests usually reveal decreased diffusion capacity; some have restrictive or obstructive findings
- Definitive diagnosis requires tissue via bronchoscopy or video-assisted thoracoscopic surgery; bronchoalveolar lavage may be suggestive if 5% or more Langerhans' cells are found
- Some patients remit, others progress to chronic lung disease

■ Differential Diagnosis
- Cystic fibrosis
- Pulmonary lymphangioleiomyomatosis
- Sarcoidosis
- Drug-induced or idiopathic pulmonary fibrosis
- Hypersensitivity pneumonitis
- Tuberous sclerosis

■ Treatment
- Smoking cessation is most important intervention
- Corticosteroids and cytotoxic agents of limited value
- Lung transplantation for advanced disease

■ Pearl

In a young smoker with bilateral recurrent pneumothoraces, this is the diagnosis unless proved otherwise.

Reference

Vassallo R, Ryu JH, Colby TV, et al: Pulmonary Langerhans'-cell histiocytosis. N Engl J Med 2000;342:1969. [PMID: 10877650]

Pulmonary Tuberculosis

- Essentials of Diagnosis
  - Lassitude, weight loss, fever, cough, night sweats, hemoptysis; some asymptomatic
  - Cachexia in many; posttussive apical rales occasionally present
  - Apical or subapical infiltrates with cavities classic in reactivation tuberculosis; pleural effusion in primary tuberculosis, likewise mid-lung infiltration, but any radiographic abnormality possible
  - Positive skin test to intradermal purified protein derivative (PPD) in most
  - *Mycobacterium tuberculosis* by culture of sputum, gastric washing, or pleural biopsy; pleural fluid culture usually sterile
  - Increasingly encountered antibiotic-resistant strains
  - Granuloma on pleural biopsy in patients with effusions; mesothelial cells usually absent from fluid
  - Miliary tuberculosis (widespread hematogenous spread of organism) has diverse clinical presentations including failure to thrive, fever of unknown origin, multiorgan system failure, ARDS; nearly all have overt pulmonary involvement with numerous small nodules

- Differential Diagnosis
  - Bronchogenic carcinoma
  - Bacterial pneumonia or lung abscess
  - Fungal infection
  - Sarcoidosis
  - Pneumoconiosis
  - Pleural effusion of asbestosis
  - Other mycobacterial infections

- Treatment
  - Combination antituberculous therapy for 6–9 months; all regimens include isoniazid, but rifampin, ethambutol, pyrazinamide, and streptomycin all have activity
  - All cases of suspected *M tuberculosis* infection should be reported to local health departments
  - Hospitalization considered for those incapable of self-care or likely to expose susceptible individuals

- Pearl

Five percent of tuberculosis is diagnosed at autopsy.

Reference

Frieden TR, Sterling TR, Munsiff SS, et al: Tuberculosis. Lancet 2003;362:887. [PMID: 13678977]

Sarcoidosis

2

- **Essentials of Diagnosis**
  - A disease of unknown cause with an increased incidence in North American blacks, Northern European whites, and Japanese
  - Malaise, fever, dyspnea of insidious onset; symptoms referable to eyes, skin, nervous system, liver, joints, or heart encountered; often presents asymptomatically
  - Iritis, erythema nodosum or granulomatous skin lesions, parotid enlargement, lymphadenopathy, hepatosplenomegaly
  - Hypercalcemia (5%) less common than hypercalciuria (20%)
  - Pulmonary function testing may show evidence of obstruction, but restriction with decreased D_{LCO} is more common
  - Symmetric hilar and right paratracheal adenopathy, interstitial infiltrates, or both seen on chest x-ray
  - Tissue reveals noncaseating granuloma; transbronchial biopsy sensitive, even without parenchymal disease on chest film
  - Increased angiotensin-converting enzyme levels are neither sensitive nor specific; cutaneous anergy in 70%
  - ECG may show heart block of varying degrees

- **Differential Diagnosis**
  - Tuberculosis
  - Lymphoma, including lymphocytic interstitial pneumonitis
  - Histoplasmosis or coccidioidomycosis
  - Idiopathic pulmonary fibrosis
  - Pneumoconiosis
  - Berylliosis

- **Treatment**
  - Systemic corticosteroid therapy for symptomatic pulmonary disease, cardiac involvement, iritis unresponsive to local therapy, hypercalcemia, central nervous system involvement, arthritis, nodular skin lesions
  - Asymptomatic patients with normal pulmonary function may not require corticosteroids—they should receive close clinical follow-up

- **Pearl**

The only disease in medicine in which steroids reverse anergy.

Reference

Wu JJ, Schiff KR: Sarcoidosis. Am Fam Physician 2004;70:312. [PMID: 15291090]

Severe Acute Respiratory Syndrome (SARS)

- ■ Essentials of Diagnosis
  - A rapidly progressive, often life-threatening, viral pneumonia first identified in 2003
  - Caused by a novel coronavirus (SARS-CoV), spread primarily via contact with mucous membranes or respiratory droplets; incubation period 4–14 days
  - Fever, cough, and malaise, progressing to respiratory failure in 20% to 30%
  - Exam like those of atypical pneumonias
  - Lymphocytopenia, thrombocytopenia, and elevation of serum ALT and LDH levels are common
  - Chest radiography reveals ground-glass abnormality in majority of cases
  - Lung biopsy reveals diffuse alveolar damage characteristic of acute lung injury/ARDS
  - Mortality in those over 65 years old greater than 50%; survival better in younger patients

- ■ Differential Diagnosis
  - Other causes of acute lung injury/ARDS (eg, sepsis, trauma, pancreatitis, transfusion reaction)
  - Atypical bacterial pneumonia (eg, *Mycoplasma, Legionella*)
  - Influenza and other viral infections
  - Hamman-Rich syndrome (acute interstitial pneumonia)
  - Congestive heart failure
  - Diffuse alveolar hemorrhage

- ■ Treatment
  - No controlled studies of therapy exist
  - Coronavirus (SARS-CoV) may be sensitive in vitro to interferon alfa, beta, and glycyrrhizin (licorice root extract)
  - Ribavirin therapy and combination therapy with interferon alfa and corticosteroids of debatable value

- ■ Pearl

Despite international anxiety due to initial rapid spread, mortality is 5%, the same as for community-acquired pneumonia.

Reference

Peiris JS, Yuen KY, Osterhaus AD, Stohr K: The severe acute respiratory syndrome. N Engl J Med 2003;349:2431. [PMID: 14681510]

Silicosis

2

- ■ Essentials of Diagnosis
  - A chronic fibrotic lung disease caused by inhalation of dusts containing silicon dioxide in foundry work, sandblasting, and hard rock mining
  - Progressive dyspnea, often over months to years
  - Dry inspiratory crackles by auscultation
  - Characteristic changes on chest radiograph with bilateral, predominantly upper lobe fibrosis often severe, nodules, and hilar lymphadenopathy with "eggshell" calcification
  - Pulmonary function studies yield mixed obstructive and restrictive pattern

- ■ Differential Diagnosis
  - Other pneumoconioses (eg, asbestosis)
  - Tuberculosis (often complicates silicosis)
  - Sarcoidosis
  - Histoplasmosis
  - Coccidioidomycosis

- ■ Treatment
  - Supportive care; chronic oxygen if sustained hypoxemia present
  - Chemoprophylaxis with isoniazid necessary for all silicotic patients with positive tuberculin reactivity

- ■ Pearl

One of the few causes of broncholithiasis; to make the diagnosis, ask the patient with suspected silicosis if the cough produces granular sputum.

Reference

Scarisbrick D: Silicosis and coal workers' pneumoconiosis. Practitioner 2002; 246:114, 117. [PMID: 11852619]

Sleep Apnea

- ■ Essentials of Diagnosis
  - • Excessive daytime somnolence or fatigue, morning headache, weight gain, erectile dysfunction; bed partner may report restless sleep, loud snoring, and witnessed apneic episodes
  - • Obesity, systemic hypertension common; signs of pulmonary hypertension or cor pulmonale may develop over time in a few patients
  - • Erythrocytosis common
  - • Diagnosis confirmed by formal polysomnography
  - • Most cases are of mixed central or obstructive cause; pure central sleep apnea is rare

- ■ Differential Diagnosis
  - • Alcohol or sedative abuse
  - • Narcolepsy
  - • Depression
  - • Seizure disorder
  - • Chronic obstructive pulmonary disease
  - • Hypothyroidism

- ■ Treatment
  - • Weight loss and avoidance of hypnotic medications mandatory
  - • Nocturnal nasal continuous positive airway pressure (CPAP) and supplemental oxygen frequently abolish obstructive apnea
  - • Protriptyline effective in minority of patients
  - • Surgical approaches (uvulopalatopharyngoplasty, nasal septoplasty, tracheostomy) reserved for selected cases

- ■ Pearl

When a plethoric clinic patient nods off during the history, it's sleep apnea until proved otherwise; if the historian does, it's a post-call resident.

Reference

Guilleminault C, Abad VC: Obstructive sleep apnea syndromes. Med Clin North Am 2004;88:611, viii. [PMID: 15087207]

Solitary Pulmonary Nodule

2

- **Essentials of Diagnosis**
  - A round or oval circumscribed lesion less than 3 cm in diameter amid normal lung tissue
  - Twenty-five percent of cases of bronchogenic carcinoma present as such; the 5-year survival rate so detected is 50%
  - Factors favoring benign lesion: Age under 35, asymptomatic, size less than 2 cm, diffuse calcification, and smooth margins
  - Factors suggesting malignancy: Age over 45, symptoms, smoking history, size greater than 2 cm, lack of calcification, indistinct margins (spiculation)
  - Skin tests, serologies, cytology rarely helpful
  - Comparison with earlier radiographs essential; follow-up with serial plain films or CT scans helpful; the latter may reveal benign-appearing calcifications
  - Positron emission tomography (PET) scans help distinguish malignancy from benign causes, but may be positive in inflammatory lesions

- **Differential Diagnosis**
  - Benign causes: Granuloma (eg, tuberculosis or fungal infection), arteriovenous malformation, pseudotumor, lipoma, hamartoma
  - Malignant causes: Primary metastatic malignancy

- **Treatment**
  - Fine-needle aspiration (FNA) biopsy, surgical resection, or radiographic follow-up over 2 years; negative FNA does not exclude malignancy due to a high percentage of false-negatives unless a specific benign diagnosis is made
  - Thoracic CT scan (with thin cuts through nodule) to look for benign-appearing calcifications and evaluate mediastinum for lymphadenopathy
  - With high-risk clinical or radiographic features, surgical resection (eg, using thoracoscopy) recommended
  - In low-risk or intermediate-risk cases, close radiographic follow-up may be justified

- **Pearl**

In calcified pulmonary nodules, the first digit of the patient's social security number (which identifies the patient's region of birth) suggests a specific infectious cause.

Reference

Ost D, Fein AM, Feinsilver SH: Clinical practice. The solitary pulmonary nodule. N Engl J Med 2003;348:2535. [PMID: 12815140]

Spontaneous Pneumothorax

- ■ Essentials of Diagnosis
    - Primary spontaneous pneumothorax occurs in the absence of clinical pulmonary disease; secondary pneumothorax complicates a preexisting disease (eg, asthma, COPD)
    - Primary spontaneous pneumothorax generally occurs in tall, thin boys and young men who smoke
    - Abrupt onset of ipsilateral chest pain (sometimes referred to shoulder or arm) and dyspnea
    - Decreased breath sounds over involved hemithorax, which may be bronchial but distant in 100% pneumothorax; hyperresonance, tachycardia, hypotension, and mediastinal shift toward contralateral side if tension is present
    - Chest x-ray diagnostic with retraction of lung from parietal pleura, often best seen by end-expiratory film

- ■ Differential Diagnosis
    - Myocardial infarction
    - Pulmonary emboli
    - Pleural effusion
    - Pericarditis

- ■ Treatment
    - Assessment for cause, eg, *P carinii* pneumonia, lung cancer, COPD
    - Immediate decompression by needle thoracostomy if tension suspected
    - Spontaneous pneumothoraces of less than 15% followed by serial radiographs and observation in the hospital; if greater than 15%, treated by aspiration of air through small catheter or by tube thoracostomy
    - Secondary pneumothoraces (eg, due to COPD, cystic fibrosis) usually require chest tube
    - Risk of recurrence is high (up to 50%) in primary spontaneous pneumothorax
    - Therapy for recurrent pneumothorax includes surgical pleurodesis or stapling of the ruptured blebs

- ■ Pearl

Pneumothorax during menstruation (catamenial pneumothorax) makes endometriosis the leading diagnosis.

Reference

Cunnington J: Spontaneous pneumothorax. Clin Evid 2002;8:1575. [PMID: 12603955]

3

Gastrointestinal Diseases

Achalasia

- **Essentials of Diagnosis**
  - Progressive dysphagia for both liquids and solids, odynophagia, and regurgitation of undigested food
  - Barium swallow demonstrates a dilated upper esophagus with a narrowed cardioesophageal junction ("bird's beak" esophagus); chest x-ray may reveal a retrocardiac air-fluid level
  - Lack of primary peristalsis by manometry or cineradiography and incomplete lower esophageal sphincter relaxation with swallowing

- **Differential Diagnosis**
  - Diffuse esophageal spasm
  - Aperistalsis
  - Benign lower esophageal stricture
  - Esophageal or mediastinal tumors (increased risk of esophageal carcinoma with achalasia)
  - Scleroderma of esophagus

- **Treatment**
  - Nifedipine, 10–20 mg sublingually or nitrates 30 minutes before meals
  - Botulinum toxin injection endoscopically in patients who are not good surgical candidates
  - Pneumatic esophageal dilation
  - Surgical extramucosal myotomy (esophagocardiomyotomy) in refractory cases
  - Consider yearly esophagoscopy to evaluate for carcinoma

- **Pearl**

In patients with retrocardiac air-fluid levels on chest x-ray, consider this diagnosis—it's not always a lung abscess.

Reference

Da Silveira EB, Rogers AI: Achalasia: a review of therapeutic options and outcomes. Compr Ther 2002;28:15. [PMID: 11894439]

Acute Colonic Pseudo-Obstruction (Ogilvie's Syndrome)

■ Essentials of Diagnosis

- Often seen in elderly hospitalized patients
- Associated with a history of trauma, fractures, cardiac disease, infection, or the use of opioids, antidepressants, and anticholinergics
- Often detected as a distended, tympanitic abdomen with abdominal x-ray revealing gross colonic dilation (usually right sided, with cecum > 10 cm), scant air-fluid levels, a gradual transition to collapsed bowel, and air and stool present in the rectum
- May mimic true obstruction, and obstruction should be evaluated with radiologic studies using diatrizoate (Hypaque) enema
- Fevers, marked abdominal tenderness, leukocytosis, and acidosis may be present in advanced cases with impending perforation

■ Differential Diagnosis

- Mechanical obstruction
- Toxic megacolon
- Chronic intestinal pseudo-obstruction

■ Treatment

- Cessation of oral intake, nasogastric and rectal suctioning, intravenous fluids
- Correction of electrolyte abnormalities (Ca^{2+}, Mg^{2+}, K^+)
- Discontinue offending medications and treat underlying infections
- Frequent enemas (tap water) and patient repositioning may be of benefit
- Neostigmine (2 mg intravenously), in patients failing conservative therapy, can be very effective for decompression. Main side effect bradycardia.
- Colonoscopic decompression for patients failing neostigmine or in whom neostigmine therapy is contraindicated
- Surgical consultation (for tube cecostomy) for patients with peritoneal signs or impending perforation

■ Pearl

Many patients with this disorder have surprisingly unimpressive examinations; sequential abdominal films in high-risk ICU patients are prudent regardless of symptoms.

Reference

Eaker EY: Update on acute colonic pseudo-obstruction. Curr Gastroenterol Rep. 2001;3:433. [PMID: 11560803]

3

Acute Pancreatitis

- ■ Essentials of Diagnosis
  - Background of alcohol binge or gallstones
  - Abrupt onset of epigastric pain, often with radiation to the back; nausea, vomiting, low-grade fever, and dehydration
  - Abdominal tenderness, distention
  - Leukocytosis, elevated serum and urine amylase; serum lipase, hypocalcemia and hemoconcentration in severe cases; hypertriglyceridemia (> 1000 mg/dL) may be causative, likewise hypercalcemia
  - Radiographic "sentinel loop" may be seen on plain films of the abdomen, signifying localized ileus
  - CT for patients highly symptomatic, not improving, or for suspected abscesses

- ■ Differential Diagnosis
  - Acute cholecystitis or cholangitis
  - Penetrating or perforating duodenal ulcer
  - Mesenteric infarction
  - Gastritis
  - Nephrolithiasis
  - Abdominal aortic aneurysm
  - Small bowel obstruction

- ■ Treatment
  - Nasogastric suction for nausea or ileus, prompt intravenous fluid and electrolyte replacement, analgesics, and antiemetics
  - Early enteral feeding orally or by jejunal nasogastric tube if patient able; parenteral nutrition if unable to tolerate
  - Antibiotics (eg, imipenem) for documented infection or evidence of necrotizing pancreatitis on CT; discontinue drugs capable of causing the disease, eg, thiazides, corticosteroids
  - Aggressive surgical debridement for sterile pancreatic necrosis without clinical improvement with conservative measures or for infected pancreatic necrosis
  - Early endoscopic retrograde cholangiopancreatography with sphincterotomy for pancreatitis with associated jaundice and cholangitis resulting from choledocholithiasis

- ■ Pearl

In "idiopathic" pancreatitis, obtain more history from someone other than the patient; in many, alcohol is in the picture.

Reference

Swaroop VS, Chari ST, Clain JE: Severe acute pancreatitis. JAMA 2004; 291:2865. [PMID: 15199038]

Anal Fissure (Fissura-in-Ano, Anal Ulcer)

- Essentials of Diagnosis
  - Linear tear of the anal epithelium usually from local trauma, usually posterior midline
  - Rectal pain with defecation; bleeding and constipation
  - Acute anal tenderness to digital examination
  - Ulceration and stenosis of anal canal, hypertrophic anal papilla, external skin tag on anoscopy

- Differential Diagnosis
  - Rectal syphilis, tuberculosis, herpes, chlamydial infections
  - Crohn's disease
  - Other anorectal disease: Abscess, fistula, hemorrhoids
  - Acute monocytic leukemia
  - Malignant epithelioma leukemia

- Treatment
  - High-fiber diet, psyllium, bran, stool softeners, sitz baths, hydrocortisone suppositories
  - Topical nitrate therapy or botulinum toxin injection, topical calcium channel blockers
  - Lateral internal sphincterotomy if no improvement with medical therapy

- Pearl

Unexplained anal fissures call for prompt white count with differential.

Reference

Lindsey I, Jones OM, Cunningham C, Mortensen NJ: Chronic anal fissure. Br J Surg 2004;91:270. [PMID: 14991625]

Barrett's Esophagus

- ■ Essentials of Diagnosis

  - Barrett's esophagus is asymptomatic but many patients present with symptoms of GERD: Dysphagia, heartburn, regurgitation in supine position
  - Upper endoscopy with biopsy reveals columnar epithelium replacing squamous epithelium
  - May be complicated by esophageal stricture, or in area of columnar epithelium, ulceration
  - Esophageal adenocarcinoma may develop in up to 10% of patients

- ■ Differential Diagnosis

  - GERD
  - Achalasia
  - Esophageal or mediastinal tumor
  - Esophageal web
  - Benign stricture
  - Left atrial enlargement or pericardial effusion

- ■ Treatment

  - Acid suppression (pH > 4) with proton pump inhibitors
  - Surgical fundoplication in selected patients
  - Endoscopic laser or photodynamic therapy in selected patients with dysplasia who are not surgical candidates
  - Surveillance esophagoscopy with biopsy at 1- to 3-year intervals, depending on presence and degree of dysplasia

- ■ Pearl

When brisk upper gastrointestinal bleeding occurs in a patient with Barrett's esophagus, consider cardioesophageal fistula–it is rare but potentially fatal.

Reference

Shalauta MD, Saad R: Barrett's esophagus. Am Fam Physician 2004;69:2113. [PMID: 15152957]

Benign Stricture of Esophagus

- ■ Essentials of Diagnosis
  - • Dysphagia for solids more than liquids; odynophagia
  - • Smooth narrowing of lumen radiographically; esophagoscopy and biopsy or cytology mandatory to exclude malignancy
  - • Onset months to years following esophageal insult, including gastroesophageal reflux, indwelling nasogastric tube, corrosive ingestion, infectious esophagitis, or endoscopic injury

- ■ Differential Diagnosis
  - • Achalasia or other esophageal motility disorders
  - • Esophageal or mediastinal tumor
  - • Esophageal web
  - • Schatzki's ring
  - • Left atrial enlargement
  - • Pericardial effusion

- ■ Treatment
  - • Repeat bougienage or endoscopic balloon dilation is definitive therapy for most patients; high-dose proton pump inhibitors may increase the interval between dilations
  - • Surgical therapy required rarely

- ■ Pearl

When reflux is the cause, be wary of adenocarcinoma developing within columnar metaplasia induced by the acid (see Barrett's Esophagus).

Reference

Spechler SJ: Esophageal complications of gastroesophageal reflux disease: presentation, diagnosis, management, and outcomes. Clin Cornerstone 2003;5:41; discussion 49. [PMID: 15101494]

Celiac Sprue

- ■ Essentials of Diagnosis
  - • Caused by an immune reaction to gluten in diet
  - • Main manifestations are of malabsorption: Bulky, pale, frothy, greasy stools (steatorrhea); abdominal distention, flatulence, weight loss, and evidence of fat-soluble vitamin deficiencies
  - • Hypochromic or megaloblastic anemia; abnormal D-xylose absorption; increased fecal fat on quantitative studies
  - • IgA endomysial antibody, tissue transglutaminase antibody and antigliadin antibodies are positive in disease; and if negative, can help exclude the diagnosis
  - • Deficiency pattern on small bowel radiographic studies; villous atrophy on small bowel biopsy

- ■ Differential Diagnosis
  - • Crohn's disease
  - • Lactose intolerance
  - • Functional blind loop (especially jejunal diverticulosis)
  - • Intestinal tuberculosis (may be associated with celiac sprue)
  - • Intestinal lymphoma (may also complicate celiac sprue)
  - • Whipple's disease
  - • Pancreatic insufficiency

- ■ Treatment
  - • For tropical sprue: Folic acid, vitamin B_{12} replacement if necessary, tetracycline or trimethoprim-sulfamethoxazole for 1–6 months
  - • Strict elimination of gluten from diet (ie, wheat, rye, barley, and oat products) can be monitored using IgA antigliadin antibody; vitamin supplementation (especially vitamin B_{12} and calcium); steroids are used only in selected patients who may be having a fulminant reaction to reintroduction of dietary gluten

- ■ Pearl

Flat gut occurs where it comes into contact with gluten; if gluten is introduced past the upper small bowel by nasogastric tube, that part of the intestine will be spared.

Reference

Green PH, Jabri B: Coeliac disease. Lancet 2003;362:383. [PMID: 12907013]

Chronic Pancreatitis

- **Essentials of Diagnosis**
  - Persistent or recurrent abdominal pain
  - Pancreatic calcification by radiographic study
  - Pancreatic insufficiency with malabsorption and diabetes in one-third of patients
  - Causes: Alcoholism (most common), hereditary pancreatitis, untreated hyperparathyroidism, cystic fibrosis, or after abdominal trauma
  - Diagnostic studies include endoscopic retrograde cholangiopancreatography (beading of pancreatic duct with ectatic side branches), endoscopic ultrasound (stippling or stranding of parenchyma with ductal dilation or thickening), magnetic resonance cholangiopancreatography, and an abnormal secretin pancreatic stimulation test. Lipase and amylase usually normal

- **Differential Diagnosis**
  - Carcinoma of the pancreas
  - Diabetes mellitus
  - Malabsorption due to other causes
  - Intractable duodenal ulcer
  - Gallstones
  - Irritable bowel syndrome

- **Treatment**
  - Low-fat diet, pancreatic enzyme supplements, avoidance of alcohol
  - Pain management includes opioids and amitriptyline
  - Endoscopic sphincterotomy and pancreatic duct stenting as well as endoscopic ultrasound-guided celiac block for pain management have yielded disappointing results
  - Treatment of hyperlipidemia if present
  - Intravenous fluid and electrolyte replacement for acute exacerbations
  - Surgical therapy to restore free flow of bile or to treat intractable pain

- **Pearl**

Alcohol and trauma are the sole causes of chronic relapsing pancreatitis; as always, the history will tell the story.

Reference

Mitchell RM, Byrne MF, Baillie J: Pancreatitis. Lancet 2003;361:1447. [PMID: 12727412]

Clostridium difficile (Pseudomembranous) Colitis

- Essentials of Diagnosis
    - Profuse watery, green, foul-smelling, or bloody diarrhea
    - Cramping abdominal pain
    - Fecal leukocytes present in over half of patients
    - Fevers, marked abdominal tenderness, marked leukocytosis, hypovolemia, dehydration, and hypoalbuminemia are common
    - History of antibiotic use (especially penicillin family antibiotics and clindamycin), hospitalization or institutionalization
    - Many cases may be asymptomatic or associated with minimal symptoms
    - Diagnosis confirmed by positive stool antigen test or via sigmoidoscopy or colonoscopy

- Differential Diagnosis
    - Antibiotic-associated diarrhea (without *C difficile* or pseudomembranous colitis)
    - Other bacterial diarrheas
    - Inflammatory bowel disease
    - Parasitic (amebiasis) and viral (cytomegalovirus) causes of diarrhea and colitis

- Treatment
    - Discontinue offending antibiotic therapy
    - Replacement of fluid and electrolyte losses
    - Oral metronidazole, with vancomycin reserved for metronidazole-resistant cases or critically ill patients; treatment is for 10–14 days
    - Surgical therapy is needed rarely (1–3%) for severe cases with megacolon or impending perforation
    - Avoid opioids and antidiarrheal agents

- Pearl

The cause of the highest benign white count in all of medicine save pertussis.

Reference

Poutanen SM, Simor AE: *Clostridium difficile*-associated diarrhea in adults. CMAJ 2004;171:51. [PMID: 15238498]

Crohn's Disease

■ Essentials of Diagnosis

- Insidious onset, with intermittent bouts of diarrhea, low-grade fever, right lower quadrant pain; peripheral arthritis, spondylitis; rash less common but may be presenting symptom
- Complications include fistula formation, perianal disease with abscess, right lower quadrant mass and tenderness
- Anemia, leukocytosis, positive fecal occult blood
- Radiographic findings of thickened, stenotic bowel with ulceration, stricturing, or fistulas; characteristic skip areas
- Endoscopic biopsy with histologic demonstration of submucosal inflammation with fibrosis and granulomatous lesions
- Antibodies can be helpful in differentiating Crohn's from ulcerative colitis. In Crohn's, perinuclear anti-neutrophilic cytoplasmic antibodies (P-ANCA) are often negative and anti-*Saccharomyces cerevisiae* antibodies (ASCA) are often positive

■ Differential Diagnosis

- Ulcerative colitis
- Appendicitis
- Diverticulitis
- Intestinal tuberculosis
- Chronic infectious diarrhea
- Mesenteric adenitis
- Lymphoma, other tumors of small intestine
- Chronic intestinal ischemia
- Miscellaneous arthropathies and skin diseases

■ Treatment

- Low-residue and lactose-free diet during acute flares
- Antidiarrheals, antispasmodics, vitamin B_{12}, and calcium supplementation as needed
- Sulfasalazine or mesalamine for colonic disease
- Corticosteroids or 6-mercaptopurine for acute flares or extraintestinal complications
- Infliximab for refractory or fistulous disease, check for tuberculosis prior to treatment
- Surgery for refractory obstruction, fistula, or abscess

■ Pearl

Ileocecal disease is present in 40–50%, isolated small bowel disease in 30–40%, and isolated colonic disease in 20%.

Reference

Egan LJ, Sandborn WJ: Advances in the treatment of Crohn's disease. Gastroenterology 2004;126:1574. [PMID: 15168368]

Diffuse Esophageal Spasm

- **Essentials of Diagnosis**
  - Dysphagia, substernal pain, hypersalivation, reflux of recently ingested food
  - May be precipitated by ingestion of hot or cold foods
  - Endoscopic, radiographic, and manometric demonstration of non-propulsive hyperperistalsis; lower esophageal sphincter relaxes normally
  - "Nutcracker esophagus" variant with prolonged, high pressure (> 175 mm Hg) propulsive contractions

- **Differential Diagnosis**
  - Angina pectoris
  - Esophageal or mediastinal tumors
  - Aperistalsis
  - Achalasia
  - Psychiatric disease

- **Treatment**
  - Calcium channel blockers such as nifedipine or diltiazem in combination with nitrates often effective
  - Tricyclic antidepressants for substernal pain
  - Esophageal myotomy for refractory patients with severe disease, but may result in dysphagia

- **Pearl**

Like all painful esophageal motor disorders, consider myocardial ischemia as responsible until proved otherwise.

Reference

Richter JE: Oesophageal motility disorders. Lancet 2001;358:823. [PMID: 11564508]

Disaccharidase (Lactase) Deficiency

■ Essentials of Diagnosis

- Common in Asians and blacks, in whom lactase enzyme deficiency is nearly ubiquitous and begins in childhood; can also be acquired temporarily after gastroenteritis of other causes
- Symptoms vary from abdominal bloating, distention, cramps, and flatulence to explosive diarrhea in response to disaccharide ingestion
- Stool pH < 5.5; reducing substances present in stool
- Abnormal hydrogen breath test, resolution of symptoms on lactose-free diet or flat glucose response to disaccharide loading suggests the diagnosis

■ Differential Diagnosis

- Chronic mucosal malabsorptive disorders
- Irritable bowel syndrome
- Celiac sprue
- Small intestinal bacterial overgrowth
- Inflammatory bowel disease
- Pancreatic insufficiency
- Giardiasis
- Excess artificial sweetener use

■ Treatment

- Restriction of dietary lactose; usually happens by experience in affected minorities from early life
- Lactase enzyme supplementation
- Maintenance of adequate nutritional and calcium intake

■ Pearl

Consider this in undiagnosed diarrhea; the patient may not be aware of ingesting lactose-containing foods.

Reference

Swagerty DL Jr, Walling AD, Klein RM: Lactose intolerance. Am Fam Physician 2002;65:1845. [PMID: 12018807]

Duodenal Ulcer

3

- ■ Essentials of Diagnosis
  - • Epigastric pain 45–60 minutes following meals or nocturnal pain, both relieved by food or antacids, sometimes by vomiting; symptoms chronic and periodic; radiation to back common; patients may complain of weight gain
  - • Iron deficiency anemia, positive fecal occult blood; amylase elevated with posterior penetration
  - • Radiographic or endoscopic evaluation will demonstrate ulcer crater or deformity of duodenal bulb, and exclude other diagnoses such as malignancy
  - • Caused by *Helicobacter pylori* in 70% of cases, NSAIDs in 20–30%, Zollinger-Ellison syndrome in less than 1%; *H pylori* infection may be diagnosed serologically, with biopsy or by breath test
  - • Complications include hemorrhage, intractable pain, perforation, and obstruction

- ■ Differential Diagnosis
  - • Reflux esophagitis
  - • Gastritis
  - • Pancreatitis
  - • Cholecystitis
  - • Other peptic disease, eg, Zollinger-Ellison syndrome (1% of patients with peptic ulcer disease) or gastric ulcer

- ■ Treatment
  - • Eradicate *H pylori* when present
  - • Avoid tobacco, alcohol, xanthines, and ulcerogenic drugs, especially NSAIDs
  - • H_2 blockers, proton pump inhibitors, and sucralfate
  - • Surgery—now far less common—may be needed for ulcers refractory to medical management (rare) or for the management of complications (eg, perforation, uncontrolled bleeding); supraselective vagotomy preferred unless patient unstable or is obstructed

- ■ Pearl

Once an ulcer, always an ulcer; patients who develop a peptic ulcer have a lifetime increase in risk for recurrence.

Reference

Ford A, Delaney B, Forman D, Moayyedi P: Eradication therapy for peptic ulcer disease in *Helicobacter pylori* positive patients. Cochrane Database Syst Rev 2003;4:CD003840. [PMID: 14583996]

Emetogenic Esophageal Perforation (Boerhaave's Syndrome)

3

- ■ Essentials of Diagnosis
  - History of alcoholic binge drinking, excessive and rapid food intake, or both. May also occur after esophageal medical procedures
  - Violent vomiting or retching followed by sudden pain in chest or abdomen, odynophagia, dyspnea
  - Fever, shock, profound systemic toxicity, subcutaneous emphysema, mediastinal crunching sounds, rigid abdomen, tachypnea
  - Leukocytosis, salivary hyperamylasemia
  - Chest x-ray shows mediastinal widening, mediastinal emphysema, pleural effusion (often delayed)
  - Demonstration of rupture of lower esophagus by esophagogram with water-soluble opaque media or CT scan; no role for endoscopy

- ■ Differential Diagnosis
  - Myocardial infarction, pericarditis
  - Pulmonary embolism, pulmonary abscess
  - Aortic dissection
  - Ruptured viscus
  - Acute pancreatitis
  - Shock due to other causes
  - Caustic ingestion, pill esophagitis
  - Instrumental esophageal perforation

- ■ Treatment
  - Aggressive supportive measures with broad-spectrum antibiotics covering mouth organisms, nasogastric tube suctioning, and total parenteral nutrition
  - Surgical consultation with repair

- ■ Pearl

One of the few causes in medicine of hydrophobia.

Reference

Ochiai T, Hiranuma S, Takiguchi N, et al: Treatment strategy for Boerhaave's syndrome. Dis Esophagus 2004;17:98. [PMID: 15209751]

3

Esophageal Web

- Essentials of Diagnosis
  - Dysphagia, particularly for solids more than liquids
  - Plummer-Vinson syndrome if associated with iron deficiency anemia, glossitis, and spooning of nails; may be higher incidence of hypopharyngeal carcinoma
  - Can be associated with dermatologic diseases such as bullous pemphigoid, pemphigus vulgaris, or epidermolysis bullosa
  - Barium swallow (lateral view often required), esophagoscopy diagnostic (but often misses cervical esophageal webs)

- Differential Diagnosis
  - Esophageal ring (at gastroesophageal junction, may be due to acid reflux)
  - Achalasia
  - Esophageal diverticulum
  - Aperistalsis
  - Esophageal or mediastinal tumor
  - Esophageal stricture

- Treatment
  - Treat the iron deficiency after finding its cause—the web may resolve spontaneously
  - Esophagoscopy with disruption of webs adequate in most cases
  - Bougienage or endoscopic dilation required on occasion

- Pearl

Webs do not cause iron deficiency; the iron deficiency comes first, and the web is a connective tissue effect of the absence of the element iron.

Reference

Chung S, Roberts-Thomson IC: Gastrointestinal: upper oesophageal web. J Gastroenterol Hepatol 1999;14:611. No abstract available. [PMID: 10385074]

Foreign Bodies in the Esophagus

- ■ Essentials of Diagnosis
  - • Most common in children, edentulous older patients, and the severely mentally impaired
  - • Occurs at physiologic areas of narrowing (upper esophageal sphincter, the level of the aortic arch, or the diaphragmatic hiatus)
  - • Other predisposing factors favoring impaction include Zenker's diverticulum, webs, achalasia, peptic strictures, or malignancy
  - • Recent ingestion of food or foreign material (coins most commonly in children, meat bolus most common in adults), but the history may be missing
  - • Vague discomfort in chest or neck, dysphagia, inability to handle secretions, odynophagia, hypersalivation, and stridor or dyspnea in children
  - • Radiographic or endoscopic evidence of esophageal obstruction by foreign body

- ■ Differential Diagnosis
  - • Esophageal stricture
  - • Esophageal or mediastinal tumor
  - • Angina pectoris

- ■ Treatment
  - • Endoscopic removal with airway protection as needed and the use of an overtube if sharp objects are present
  - • Emergent endoscopy should be used for sharp objects, disk batteries (secondary to risk of perforation due to their caustic nature), or evidence of the inability to handle secretions; objects retained in the esophagus should be removed within 24 hours of ingestion
  - • Endoscopy is successful in over 90% of cases, avoid barium studies before endoscopy, as they impair visualization
  - • Observation and delayed endoscopy may be considered if the patient is without symptoms and radiologic studies are negative

- ■ Pearl

Treatment is ordinarily straightforward; diagnosis may not be.

Reference

Cerri RW, Liacouras CA: Evaluation and management of foreign bodies in the upper gastrointestinal tract. Pediatr Case Rev 2003;3:150. [PMID: 12865708]

3

Gastric Ulcer

■ Essentials of Diagnosis

- Epigastric pain unpredictably relieved by food or antacids; weight loss, anorexia, vomiting
- Iron deficiency anemia, fecal occult blood positive
- Ulcer demonstrated by barium study or endoscopy
- Caused by *Helicobacter pylori* (in 70% of cases), NSAIDs, gastric malignancy, or rarely, Zollinger-Ellison syndrome
- Endoscopic biopsy or documentation of complete healing necessary to exclude malignancy
- Complications include hemorrhage, perforation, and obstruction

■ Differential Diagnosis

- Other peptic ulcer disease
- Gastroesophageal reflux
- Gastric carcinoma
- Cholecystitis
- Esophagitis
- Gastritis
- Irritable or functional bowel disease such as dyspepsia

■ Treatment

- Eradicate *H pylori* when present
- Avoid tobacco, alcohol, xanthines, and ulcerogenic drugs, especially NSAIDs
- Proton pump inhibitors, sucralfate, H_2-receptor antagonists
- Surgery may be needed for ulcers refractory to medical management (rare, and must exclude cancer if ulcer not healing) or for the management of complications (eg, perforation, uncontrolled bleeding)

■ Pearl

Gastric ulcers lose weight; duodenal ulcers gain it.

Reference

Calam J, Baron JH: ABC of the upper gastrointestinal tract: Pathophysiology of duodenal and gastric ulcer and gastric cancer. BMJ 2001;323:980. [PMID: 11679389]

Gastritis

- **Essentials of Diagnosis**
  - May be acute (erosive) or indolent (atrophic); multiple varied causes
  - Symptoms often vague and include nausea, vomiting, anorexia, nondescript upper abdominal distress; significant hemorrhage may occur with or without symptoms
  - Mild epigastric tenderness to palpation; in some, physical signs absent
  - Iron deficiency anemia not unusual
  - Endoscopy with gastric biopsy for definitive diagnosis
  - Multiple associations include stress and diminished mucosal blood flow (burns, sepsis, critical illness), drugs (NSAIDs, salicylates), atrophic states (aging, pernicious anemia), previous surgery (gastrectomy, Billroth II), *Helicobacter pylori* infection, acute or chronic alcoholism

- **Differential Diagnosis**
  - Peptic ulcer
  - Hiatal hernia
  - Malignancy of stomach or pancreas
  - Cholecystitis
  - Ischemic cardiac disease

- **Treatment**
  - Avoidance of alcohol, caffeine, salicylates, tobacco, and NSAIDs
  - Investigate for presence of *Helicobacter pylori;* eradicate if present
  - Proton pump inhibitors in patients receiving oral feedings, H_2 inhibitors, or sucralfate
  - Prevention in high-risk patients (eg, intensive care setting) using these same agents

- **Pearl**

Ninety-five percent of gastroenterologists and a high proportion of other health care workers carry H pylori.

Reference

Genta RM: The gastritis connection: prevention and early detection of gastric neoplasms. J Clin Gastroenterol 2003;36(5 Suppl):S44; discussion S61. [PMID: 12702965]

Gastroesophageal Reflux Disease

3

- Essentials of Diagnosis
  - Substernal burning (pyrosis) or pressure, aggravated by recumbency and relieved with sitting; can cause chronic cough and occult blood loss
  - If suspected, H_2 blocker or proton pump inhibitor may be diagnostic and therapeutic; further testing when diagnosis unclear, symptoms refractory
  - Reflux, hiatal hernia may be found at barium study
  - Incompetent lower esophageal sphincter (LES); endoscopy with biopsy may be necessary to exclude other diagnoses
  - Esophageal pH helpful during symptoms
  - Diminished LES tone also seen in obesity, pregnancy, hiatal hernia, nasogastric tube

- Differential Diagnosis
  - Peptic ulcer disease
  - Angina pectoris
  - Achalasia, esophageal spasm, pill esophagitis

- Treatment
  - Weight loss, avoidance of late-night meals, elevation of head of bed
  - Avoid chocolate, caffeine, tobacco, alcohol
  - High-dose H_2 blockers or proton pump inhibitors
  - Motility stimulants (eg, metoclopramide) in selected patients
  - Surgical fundoplication for rare cases refractory to medical management

- Pearl

Eradication of Helicobacter pylori *may actually worsen GERD by increasing gastric acid secretion.*

Reference

Chang JT, Katzka DA: Gastroesophageal reflux disease, Barrett esophagus, and esophageal adenocarcinoma. Arch Intern Med 2004;164:1482. [PMID: 15277277]

Intestinal Tuberculosis

■ Essentials of Diagnosis

- Chronic abdominal pain, anorexia, bloating; weight loss, fever, diarrhea, new-onset ascites in many
- Mild right lower quadrant tenderness, as ileocecal area is the most commonly involved intestinal site; fistula-in-ano sometimes seen
- Barium study may reveal mucosal ulcerations or scarring and fibrosis with narrowing of the small or large intestine
- In peritonitis, ascitic fluid has high protein and mononuclear pleocytosis; peritoneal biopsy with granulomas is more sensitive than ascites AFB culture; high adenosine deaminase levels in ascitic fluid may suggest the diagnosis; TB peritonitis more common in those with immune compromise
- Complications include intestinal obstruction, hemorrhage, fistula formation, and bacterial overgrowth with malabsorption

■ Differential Diagnosis

- Carcinoma of the colon or small bowel
- Inflammatory bowel disease: Crohn's disease
- Ameboma or *Yersinia* infection
- Intestinal lymphoma or amyloidosis
- Ovarian or peritoneal carcinomatosis
- *Mycobacterium avium-intracellulare* infection

■ Treatment

- Standard therapy for tuberculosis, as infection heals the affected bowel may develop stricture

■ Pearl

Historically, many patients underwent exploratory laparotomy for suspected small bowel obstruction; improvement inevitably ensued without specific therapy.

Reference

Sheer TA, Coyle WJ: Gastrointestinal tuberculosis. Curr Gastroenterol Rep 2003;5:273. [PMID: 12864956]

Irritable Bowel Syndrome

3

- **Essentials of Diagnosis**
  - Chronic functional disorder characterized by abdominal pain, alteration in bowel habits, constipation and diarrhea (often alternating), dyspepsia, anxiety or depression
  - Variable abdominal tenderness
  - More common in women and if a history of physical abuse
  - Evaluation: History and physical exam, colonoscopy in patients over age 50; further testing as indicated for alarm symptoms or physical exam findings
  - Sigmoidoscopy may reveal spasm or mucus hypersecretion; other studies (such as CBC, ova and parasite, TSH) are normal.

- **Differential Diagnosis**
  - Inflammatory bowel disease
  - Celiac sprue or lactose intolerance
  - Chronic mesenteric ischemia
  - Diverticular disease
  - Peptic ulcer disease
  - Pancreatitis

- **Treatment**
  - Reassurance and explanation
  - High-fiber diet with or without fiber supplements; restricting dairy products may be helpful
  - Antispasmodic agents (eg, dicyclomine, hyoscyamine, propantheline), antidiarrheal or anticonstipation agents
  - Amitriptyline, selective serotonin reuptake inhibitors, and behavioral modification with relaxation techniques helpful for some patients
  - Tegaserod for women with constipation-predominant IBS (possible increase in gallbladder operations) or alosetron for women with diarrhea-predominant IBS (rare but serious increased risk for ischemic colitis)

- **Pearl**

Irritable bowel syndrome is the most common diagnosis resulting in office visits to a gastroenterologist; it ranks highly with primary care providers, too.

Reference

Mertz HR: Irritable bowel syndrome. N Engl J Med 2003;349:2136. [PMID: 14645642]

Mallory-Weiss Syndrome (Mucosal Laceration of the Gastroesophageal Junction)

3

- **Essentials of Diagnosis**
  - Hematemesis of bright red blood, often following prolonged or forceful vomiting or retching; majority lack this history
  - Because many patients are hypovolemic, portal pressure is low and bleeding unimpressive
  - More impressive in alcoholics with brisk bleeding because of associated coagulopathy and may involve esophageal varices
  - Endoscopic demonstration of vertical mucosal tear at cardioesophageal junction or proximal stomach
  - Hiatal hernia often associated

- **Differential Diagnosis**
  - Peptic ulcer
  - Esophageal varices
  - Gastritis
  - Reflux, infectious, or pill esophagitis

- **Treatment**
  - Usually none required; spontaneous resolution of bleeding unless concomitant varices present
  - Endoscopic hemostatic intervention with epinephrine injection or thermal coaptation for active bleeding; rarely, balloon tamponade, embolization, or surgery is required for uncontrolled bleeding

- **Pearl**

Hyperemesis of pregnancy is the most common cause, but bleeding is seldom reported by the patient since it is trivial due to dehydration and the absence of portal hypertension.

Reference

Younes Z, Johnson DA: The spectrum of spontaneous and iatrogenic esophageal injury: perforations, Mallory-Weiss tears, and hematomas. J Clin Gastroenterol 1999;29:306. [PMID: 10599632]

Polyps of the Colon & Rectum

■ Essentials of Diagnosis

- Discrete mass lesions arising from colonic epithelium and protruding into the intestinal lumen; polyps may be pedunculated or sessile
- Most patients asymptomatic; can be associated with chronic occult blood loss
- Family history may be present
- Diagnosed by sigmoidoscopy, colonoscopy, virtual colonoscopy or barium enema
- Removing polyps decreases the incidence of adenocarcinoma

■ Differential Diagnosis

- Adenocarcinoma
- Radiographic artifact
- Other luminal findings: Nonadenomatous (hyperplastic) polyps, lipomas, inverted diverticula

■ Treatment

- Surgical or endoscopic polypectomy in all cases with histologic review
- Colectomy for familial polyposis or Gardner's syndrome
- Surveillance colonoscopy every 3–5 years depending on number and histology of the polyps

■ Pearl

The incidence curves of adenomatous polyps and carcinoma by age are superimposable; the only place for a diagnosed polyp is in a jar.

Reference

Bond JH: Colon polyps and cancer. Endoscopy 2003;35:27. [PMID: 12510223]

Ulcerative Colitis

■ Essentials of Diagnosis

- Low-volume diarrhea, often bloody; tenesmus and cramping lower abdominal pain; associated with fever, weight loss, rash
- Mild abdominal tenderness, mucocutaneous lesions, erythema nodosum or pyoderma gangrenosum
- Anemia, accelerated sedimentation rate, hypoproteinemia, absent stool pathogens
- Ragged mucosa with loss of haustral markings on barium enema; colon involved contiguously from rectum, rectum nearly always involved
- Crypt abscesses on rectal mucosal biopsy
- Increased incidence of colonic adenocarcinoma with young age at onset, long-standing active disease, and pancolitis

■ Differential Diagnosis

- Bacterial, amebic, or ischemic colitis
- Diverticular disease
- Adenocarcinoma of the colon
- Benign colonic stricture
- Pseudomembranous colitis
- Granulomatous colitis or Crohn's disease
- Antibiotic-associated diarrhea
- Radiation colitis or collagenous colitis

■ Treatment

- Topical mesalamine or corticosteroids by enema or suppository
- Lactose-free diet during flares
- Sulfasalazine, mesalamine, or olsalazine for chronic therapy
- Mesalamine, corticosteroids, or cyclosporine for acute flares; some suggest obtaining amebic serologies before systemic steroids
- Fish oil, ciprofloxacin, nicotine may be of benefit in refractory disease
- Colectomy for toxic megacolon unresponsive to medical therapy, severe extracolonic manifestations, colonic malignancy or dysplasia, or (in selected patients with long-standing disease) for cancer prophylaxis
- Yearly colonoscopy after 8 years of pancolitis for dysplasia surveillance

■ Pearl

Four hepatobiliary complications: pericholangitis, chronic active hepatitis, sclerosing cholangitis, and cholangiocarcinoma; the first two parallel activity of colitis, the last two do not.

Reference

Hanauer SB: Medical therapy for ulcerative colitis 2004. Gastroenterology 2004;126:1582. [PMID: 15168369]

Whipple's Disease

3

■ Essentials of Diagnosis
  • Caused by infection with the bacillus *Tropheryma whippelii*
  • Rare disease, even more so in women and blacks
  • Insidious onset of fever, abdominal pain, malabsorption, arthralgias, weight loss, symptoms of steatorrhea, polyarthritis
  • Lymphadenopathy, arthritis, macular skin rash, various neurologic findings
  • Anemia, hypoalbuminemia, hypocarotenemia
  • Small bowel mucosal biopsy reveals characteristic foamy mononuclear cells filled with periodic acid-Schiff (PAS) staining material; electron microscopy shows bacilli in multiple affected organs

■ Differential Diagnosis
  • Celiac or tropical sprue
  • Inflammatory bowel disease, Crohn's disease
  • Ulcerative colitis
  • Intestinal lymphoma
  • Rheumatoid arthritis or HLA-B27 spondyloarthropathy
  • Hyperthyroidism
  • HIV infection

■ Treatment
  • Penicillin and streptomycin intravenously (ceftriaxone and streptomycin for central nervous system disease) for 10–14 days followed by trimethoprim-sulfamethoxazole (cefixime or doxycycline in sulfonamide-allergic patients)
  • Treatment for at least 1 year

■ Pearl

Oculomasticatory myorhythmia (continuous rhythmic motion of the eye muscles with mastication) or ocular-facial-skeletal myorhythmia is caused by Whipple's disease and nothing else.

Reference

Louis ED: Whipple disease. Curr Neurol Neurosci Rep 2003;3:470. [PMID: 14565900]

Zollinger-Ellison Syndrome (Gastrinoma)

■ Essentials of Diagnosis

- Severe, recurrent, intractable peptic ulcer disease, often associated with concomitant esophagitis; ulcers may be in atypical locations, like jejunum, but most occur in usual sites
- Eighty percent of cases are sporadic; the rest are associated with multiple endocrine neoplasia type 1 (MEN 1)
- Fasting serum gastrin > 150 pg/mL (often much higher) in the setting of a low gastric pH; elevated serum chromogranin A; renal insufficiency, proton pump inhibitors can also raise serum gastrin
- Diarrhea common, caused by inactivation of pancreatic enzymes; relieved by nasogastric tube suctioning immediately
- Gastrinomas may arise in pancreas, duodenum, or lymph nodes; over 50% are malignant but not usually aggressive
- Localization techniques include somatostatin receptor scintigraphy, thin-cut CT, MRI, endoscopic ultrasound, or intraoperative localization

■ Differential Diagnosis

- Peptic ulcer disease of other cause
- Esophagitis
- Gastritis
- Pancreatitis
- Cholecystitis
- Diarrhea or malabsorption from other causes

■ Treatment

- High-dose proton pump inhibitor (with goal of < 10 mEq/h of gastric acid secretion)
- Exploratory laparotomy for patients without preoperative evidence of unresectable metastatic disease
- Chemotherapy ineffective; interferon, octreotide, and hepatic artery embolization for metastatic disease
- Resection for localized disease
- Family counseling
- MEN 1–associated gastrinoma appears to have a lower incidence of hepatic metastases and a better long-term prognosis

■ Pearl

In Zollinger-Ellison syndrome, isolated gastric ulcer is never encountered.

Reference

Qureshi W, Rashid S: Zollinger-Ellison syndrome. Improved treatment options for this complex disorder. Postgrad Med 1998;104:155, 163. [PMID: 9676569]

Hepatobiliary Disorders

Acute Viral Hepatitis

- **Essentials of Diagnosis**
  - Jaundice, fever, chills; enlarged, tender liver
  - Anorexia, nausea, vomiting, malaise, symptoms of flu-like syndrome, arthralgias, and aversion to smoking
  - Normal to low white cell count; abnormal liver function studies (ALT > AST); serologic tests for hepatitis A (IgM antibody), hepatitis B (HBsAg), or hepatitis C (antibody) may be positive
  - Liver biopsy shows characteristic hepatocellular necrosis and mononuclear infiltrates
  - Hepatitis A: oral-fecal transmission, short incubation period; good prognosis, but rare cases of fulminant hepatic failure
  - Hepatitis B and hepatitis C: parenteral transmission, longer incubation period, progression to chronic disease more likely

- **Differential Diagnosis**
  - Alcoholic hepatitis
  - Cholestatic jaundice secondary to medications or herbals
  - Acetaminophen toxicity
  - Leptospirosis
  - Secondary syphilis
  - Q fever
  - Choledocholithiasis
  - Carcinoma of the pancreas
  - Hepatic vein thrombosis

- **Treatment**
  - Supportive care
  - Avoidance of hepatotoxins: Alcohol, acetaminophen
  - Treatment of acute hepatitis C is controversial

- **Pearl**

Hepatitis A is the only viral hepatitis characteristically causing spiking fevers.

Reference

Marsano LS: Hepatitis. Prim Care 2003;30:81. [PMID: 12825251]

Alcoholic Hepatitis

- ■ Essentials of Diagnosis
  - • Onset usually after years of alcohol intake; anorexia, nausea, abdominal pain
  - • Fever, jaundice, tender hepatomegaly, ascites, encephalopathy
  - • Macrocytic anemia, leukocytosis with left shift, thrombocytopenia, abnormal liver function tests (AST about double ALT, increased bilirubin, prolonged prothrombin time), hypergammaglobulinemia; AST rarely exceeds 300 U/L despite severity of illness
  - • Liver biopsy if diagnosis is in doubt

- ■ Differential Diagnosis
  - • Cholecystitis, cholelithiasis
  - • Cirrhosis due to other causes
  - • Non-alcoholic fatty liver
  - • Viral hepatitis
  - • Drug-induced hepatitis

- ■ Treatment
  - • General supportive measures, withdrawal of alcohol, avoidance of hepatotoxins (especially acetaminophen)
  - • Methylprednisolone (32 mg/d for 4 weeks) or pentoxifylline (400 mg three times a day for 4 weeks) may be beneficial in severe acute disease when discriminant function (4.6 [PT – control] + bilirubin [mg/dL]) is > 32; (study exclusion criteria: active GI bleeding, infection)

- ■ Pearl

Acute alcoholic hepatitis can be indistinguishable from acute cholecystitis with or without cholangitis; the abdominal ultrasound has saved many an unnecessary laparotomy.

Reference

Haber PS, Warner R, Seth D, Gorrell MD, McCaughan GW: Pathogenesis and management of alcoholic hepatitis. J Gastroenterol Hepatol 2003;18:1332. [PMID: 14675260]

Amebic Hepatic Abscess

4

- ■ Essentials of Diagnosis
  - Fever, right-sided abdominal pain, right pleuritic chest pain; preceding or concurrent diarrheal illness in minority
  - History of travel to or recent immigration from endemic region
  - Tender palpable liver ("punch" tenderness), localized intercostal tenderness
  - Anemia, leukocytosis with left shift, nonspecific liver test abnormalities
  - Positive serologic tests for *Entamoeba histolytica* in over 95% of patients, though may be negative early in infection
  - Increased right hemidiaphragm by radiography; ultrasound, CT scan, or liver scan demonstrates location and number of lesions

- ■ Differential Diagnosis
  - Pyogenic abscess
  - Acute hepatitis
  - Right lower lobe pneumonia
  - Cholelithiasis, cholecystitis
  - Appendicitis

- ■ Treatment
  - Metronidazole drug of choice; repeated courses occasionally necessary
  - Percutaneous needle aspiration for toxic patient
  - Oral course of luminal amebicides (iodoquinol, paromomycin sulfate) following acute therapy to eradicate intestinal cyst phase

- ■ Pearl

This is more a cyst than an abscess; thus, radionuclide WBC scans often miss it.

Reference

Wells CD, Arguedas M: Amebic liver abscess. South Med J 2004;97:673. [PMID: 15301125]

Ascites

- **Essentials of Diagnosis**

  - Usually associated with cirrhosis, but heart or kidney disease also causative
  - Evidence of shifting dullness, bulging flanks
  - Paracentesis for new-onset ascites or symptoms suggestive of spontaneous bacterial peritonitis
  - Fluid sent for cell count, protein; amylase, bacterial culture, cytology, and triglycerides as indicated
  - Serum–ascites albumin gradient ≥ 1.1 g/dL is virtually diagnostic of portal hypertension
  - > 250 neutrophils/µL with a percentage greater than 50% characteristic of infection

- **Differential Diagnosis**

  Due to portal hypertension:
  - Chronic liver disease (80–85% of all cases)
  - Cardiac failure (3%)

  Not due to portal hypertension:
  - Malignancy-related (10%) and tuberculosis

  Dialysis-related:
  - Pancreatic
  - Lymphatic tear (chylous)

- **Treatment**

  Treat as follows for ascites due to portal hypertension:
  - Sodium restriction (< 2 g/d)
  - Fluid restriction if serum sodium < 120 mmol/L
  - Diuretics: Usually spironolactone and furosemide in 100-mg to 40-mg ratio to address potassium balance
  - Large-volume paracentesis (4–6 L) for tense or refractory ascites with albumin replacement (6–10 g/L)
  - Transjugular intrahepatic portosystemic shunt (TIPS) or surgical shunting in refractory cases
  - Patients with spontaneous bacterial peritonitis treated for 5 days with a third-generation cephalosporin (eg, cefotaxime)
  - Spontaneous bacterial peritonitis prophylaxis (with norfloxacin or trimethoprim-sulfisoxazole) for patients with spontaneous bacterial peritonitis, gastrointestinal hemorrhage, or low-protein ascites (< 1.5 g/dL)

- **Pearl**

  Once spontaneous bacterial peritonitis occurs, liver transplant is the only intervention that prolongs life.

Reference

Gines P, Cardenas A, Arroyo V, Rodes J: Management of cirrhosis and ascites. N Engl J Med 2004;350:1646. [PMID: 15084697]

Autoimmune Hepatitis

- **Essentials of Diagnosis**
  - Insidious onset; usually affects young women
  - Fatigue, anorexia, arthralgias; dark urine; light stools in some
  - Jaundice, spider angiomas, hepatomegaly, acne, hirsutism
  - Abnormal liver function tests, most notably increased amino-transferases, polyclonal gammopathy
  - Associated with arthritis, thyroiditis, nephritis, Coombs-positive hemolytic anemia
  - Type 1: ANA or anti–smooth muscle antibody–positive; Type 2: Anti–liver/kidney microsomal antibody–positive
  - Patients may develop cirrhosis, predicted by biopsy features of chronic active hepatitis

- **Differential Diagnosis**
  - Chronic viral hepatitis
  - Non-alcoholic steatohepatitis (NASH)
  - Sclerosing cholangitis
  - Primary biliary cirrhosis
  - Wilson's disease
  - Hemochromatosis

- **Treatment**
  - General supportive measures (including exercise, calcium, and hormonal therapy to prevent osteoporosis)
  - In patients with elevated aminotransferases or gammaglobulins or for individual reasons: prednisone with or without azathioprine as a steroid-sparing agent
  - Liver transplantation for cirrhosis

- **Pearl**

Spider angiomas never occur below the waist.

Reference

Luxon BA: Autoimmune hepatitis. Making sense of all those antibodies. Postgrad Med 2003;114:79, 85. [PMID: 12875057]

Choledocholithiasis/Cholangitis

- **Essentials of Diagnosis**

  - Often a history of biliary tract disease; episodic attacks of right abdominal or epigastric pain that may radiate to the right scapula or shoulder; occasionally painless jaundice
  - Pain, fever, and jaundice (Charcot's triad); associated with nausea, vomiting, hypothermia, shock, and leukocytosis with a left shift
  - Elevated serum amylase and liver function tests, especially bilirubin and alkaline phosphatase
  - Abdominal imaging studies may reveal gallstones
  - Ultrasound or CT scan shows dilated biliary tree
  - Endoscopic retrograde cholangiopancreatography (ERCP) or magnetic resonance cholangiopancreatography (MRCP) localizes the degree and location of obstruction

- **Differential Diagnosis**

  - Carcinoma of the pancreas, ampulla of Vater, or common duct
  - Acute hepatitis
  - Acute cholecystitis or Mirizzi's syndrome
  - Biliary stricture
  - Drug-induced cholestatic jaundice
  - Pancreatitis
  - Other septic syndromes

- **Treatment**

  - Intravenous broad-spectrum antibiotics
  - Endoscopic papillotomy and stone extraction followed by laparoscopic or open cholecystectomy
  - A T tube may be placed in the common duct to decompress it for at least 7–8 postoperative days

- **Pearl**

Although choledocholithiasis is often asymptomatic, septic shock may occur with stunning rapidity; the sun should never set on this diagnosis.

Reference

Lahmann BE, Adrales G, Schwartz RW: Choledocholithiasis—principles of diagnosis and management. Curr Surg 2004;61:290. [PMID: 15165768]

Cholelithiasis (Gallstones)

- ■ Essentials of Diagnosis
    - • Frequently asymptomatic but may be associated with recurrent bouts of right-sided or midepigastric pain and nausea or vomiting after eating
    - • Ultrasound, CT scan, and plain films demonstrate stones within the gallbladder
    - • Increased incidence with female gender, chronic hemolysis, obesity, Native American origin, inflammatory bowel disease, diabetes mellitus, pregnancy, hypercholesterolemia

- ■ Differential Diagnosis
    - • Acute cholecystitis
    - • Acute pancreatitis
    - • Peptic ulcer disease
    - • Acute appendicitis
    - • Acute hepatitis
    - • Right lower lobe pneumonia
    - • Myocardial infarction
    - • Radicular pain in T6–T10 dermatome

- ■ Treatment
    - • Laparoscopic or open cholecystectomy for symptomatic patients only
    - • Bile salts (ursodeoxycholic acid) may cause dissolution of cholesterol stones
    - • Lithotripsy with concomitant bile salts administration may be successful

- ■ Pearl

In a patient with right upper quadrant densities on a plain film of the abdomen associated with hyperchromia and microcytosis, consider hereditary spherocytosis with premature cholelithiasis due to lifelong hemolysis.

Reference

Agrawal S, Jonnalagadda S: Gallstones, from gallbladder to gut. Management options for diverse complications. Postgrad Med 2000;108:143, 149. [PMID: 11004941]

Chronic Viral Hepatitis

■ **Essentials of Diagnosis**

- Fatigue, right upper quadrant discomfort, arthralgias, depression, nausea, anorexia
- In advanced cases (cirrhosis): jaundice, variceal bleeding, encephalopathy, ascites, spontaneous bacterial peritonitis, and hepatocellular carcinoma
- Persistent elevation in ALT (> 6 months)
- In hepatitis B, positive hepatitis B DNA with HBsAg present
- In hepatitis C, positive hepatitis C RNA

4

■ **Differential Diagnosis**

- Alcoholic cirrhosis
- Metabolic liver disorders (eg, non-alcoholic steatohepatitis), Wilson's disease, hemochromatosis
- Autoimmune hepatitis
- Cholestatic jaundice secondary to drugs

■ **Treatment**

- Avoidance of alcohol, acetaminophen
- Lamivudine or adefovir (interferon in selected cases) for patients with chronic active hepatitis B; pegylated interferon alfa and ribavirin for chronic hepatitis C
- Screening for hepatocellular cancer in all patients with chronic hepatitis B or hepatitis C with cirrhosis
- Vaccination against hepatitis A (and hepatitis B in patients with hepatitis C)
- Liver transplantation for advanced disease or hepatocellular carcinoma

■ **Pearl**

Hepatitis C is the most common cause worldwide of hepatocellular carcinoma.

Reference

Poynard T, Yuen MF, Ratziu V, Lai CL: Viral hepatitis C. Lancet 2003;362:2095. [PMID: 14697814]

Cirrhosis

■ Essentials of Diagnosis

- The outcome of many types of chronic hepatitis—viral, toxic, immune, and metabolic
- Insidious onset of malaise, weight loss, increasing abdominal girth, erectile dysfunction in men
- Spider angiomas, hepatosplenomegaly, palmar erythema, Dupuytren's contractures, gynecomastia, ascites, edema, asterixis
- Macrocytic anemia, thrombocytopenia, abnormal liver function (increased prothrombin time, hypoalbuminemia)
- Biopsy diagnostic with micro- or macronodular fibrosis
- Complications include gastrointestinal bleeding from esophageal or gastric varices, ascites and spontaneous bacterial peritonitis, hepatorenal syndrome

■ Differential Diagnosis

- Congestive heart failure
- Constrictive pericarditis
- Hemochromatosis
- Primary biliary cirrhosis
- Wilson's disease
- Schistosomiasis
- Nephrotic syndrome
- Hypothyroidism
- Budd-Chiari syndrome

■ Treatment

- Supportive care, abstinence from alcohol
- Beta-blockers or endoscopic eradication in patients with established varices
- Diuretics or large-volume paracenteses for ascites and edema
- Antibiotic treatment and secondary prophylaxis for spontaneous bacterial peritonitis; debatably, primary prophylaxis if ascites total protein is < 1.5 g/dL
- Lactulose for encephalopathy
- Transjugular intrahepatic portosystemic shunt for bleeding gastric varices, bleeding esophageal varices not controlled by endoscopic therapy, or refractory ascites
- Liver transplantation in selected cases

■ Pearl

Hepatitis A never causes cirrhosis.

Reference

Gines P, Cardenas A, Arroyo V, Rodes J: Management of cirrhosis and ascites. N Engl J Med 2004;350:1646. [PMID: 15084697]

Hepatic Encephalopathy

- ■ Essentials of Diagnosis
    - • Neurologic and psychiatric abnormalities resulting from liver dysfunction due to acute liver failure, cirrhosis, or major noncirrhotic portosystemic shunting
    - • Diagnosis requires history and physical examination suggestive of liver disease or portosystemic shunting
    - • Clinical manifestations range from mild confusion, personality changes, and sleep disturbances (stage I) to coma (stage IV)
    - • Asterixis, hyperreflexia, muscular rigidity, extensor plantar response, parkinsonian features, immobile facies, slow and monotonous speech
    - • Often triggered by gastrointestinal bleeding, infection, lactulose noncompliance, dietary protein overload, hypokalemia

- ■ Differential Diagnosis
    - • Systemic or central nervous system sepsis
    - • Hypoxia or hypercapnia
    - • Acidosis
    - • Uremia
    - • Use of sedatives or narcotics
    - • Postictal confusion
    - • Wernicke-Korsakoff syndrome
    - • Acute liver failure (cerebral edema or hypoglycemia)
    - • Delirium tremens
    - • Hyponatremia

- ■ Treatment
    - • Identify and treat precipitating factors listed above
    - • Lactulose, 30–60 mL by mouth or nasogastric tube (or rectally) every 2 hours until bowel movements occur; in resolving or chronic encephalopathy, titrate to maintain two or three loose stools per day
    - • If patients become hypernatremic, reduce lactulose dose or consider oral neomycin
    - • Flumazenil of temporary benefit
    - • Dietary protein restriction (< 70 g/d but > 40 g/d)
    - • Liver transplantation for chronic hepatic encephalopathy

- ■ Pearl

In a stable cirrhotic with new encephalopathy and none of the above precipitants, hepatocellular carcinoma is the most likely explanation.

Reference

Lizardi-Cervera J, Almeda P, Guevara L, Uribe M: Hepatic encephalopathy: a review. Ann Hepatol 2003;2:122. [PMID: 15115963]

Hepatic Vein Obstruction (Budd-Chiari Syndrome)

4

- **Essentials of Diagnosis**
    - Spectrum of disorders characterized by occlusion of the hepatic veins from a variety of causes, more common in women
    - Acute or chronic onset of tender, painful hepatic enlargement, jaundice, splenomegaly, and ascites
    - Doppler ultrasound or venography demonstrates occlusion of the hepatic veins; CT and MRI can also be helpful
    - Liver scintigraphy may show a prominent caudate lobe since its venous drainage may not be occluded; liver biopsy reveals characteristic central lobular congestion
    - Underlying causes include caval webs, polycythemia, right-sided heart failure, malignancy, "bush teas" (pyrrolizidine alkaloids), paroxysmal nocturnal hemoglobinuria, birth control pills, pregnancy, hypercoagulable states, Behçet's disease

- **Differential Diagnosis**
    - Cirrhosis
    - Constrictive pericarditis
    - Restrictive or dilated cardiomyopathy
    - Metastatic disease involving the liver
    - Granulomatous liver disease

- **Treatment**
    - Treatment of complications, eg, ascites, encephalopathy
    - Lifelong anticoagulation or treatment of underlying disease
    - Local thrombolysis in acute form of the disease
    - Portacaval, mesocaval, or mesoatrial shunt may be required
    - Transvenous intravascular portosystemic shunt may be considered in noncirrhotic patients
    - Liver transplantation for severe hepatocellular dysfunction

- **Pearl**

Inherited coagulopathies often cause abdominal venous thrombosis; not so in other venous diseases.

Reference

Menon KV, Shah V, Kamath PS: The Budd-Chiari syndrome. N Engl J Med 2004;350:578. [PMID: 14762185]

Hepatocellular Carcinoma

- ■ Essentials of Diagnosis
  - • One of the world's most common visceral tumors
  - • Hepatitis B, hepatitis C, alcoholic cirrhosis, hemochromatosis among the important risk factors
  - • Symptoms and physical exam findings may not help, as they are similar to those of underlying liver disease
  - • Decompensation (new ascites, hepatic encephalopathy, or jaundice) of previously stable cirrhosis may be the presenting symptom
  - • Edema due to inferior vena cava invasion or diarrhea are rare presenting symptoms
  - • Elevated (sometimes markedly) alpha-fetoprotein in some but not all; characteristic arterial phase helical CT scan

- ■ Differential Diagnosis
  - • Metastatic primary of other source
  - • Regenerating nodule

- ■ Treatment
  - • Surgical resection if adequate hepatic function and if tumor factors favorable (only one lobe involved and no extrahepatic spread)
  - • Transplant in highly selected patients
  - • If not transplant or resection candidates: Radiofrequency or alcohol ablation

- ■ Pearl

A normal hematocrit in cirrhosis suggests this diagnosis; the tumor may manufacture erythropoietin, and most cirrhotics are anemic.

Reference

Llovet JM, Burroughs A, Bruix J: Hepatocellular carcinoma. Lancet 2003; 362:1907. [PMID: 14667750]

Primary Biliary Cirrhosis

- ■ Essentials of Diagnosis
  - Usually affects women aged 40–60 with the insidious onset of pruritus, jaundice, fatigue, and hepatomegaly
  - Hepatomegaly in 70% with splenomegaly in 35%
  - Malabsorption, xanthomas, xanthomatous neuropathy, osteomalacia, and portal hypertension may be complications
  - Increased alkaline phosphatase and gamma glutamyl transpeptidase, cholesterol, bilirubin; positive antimitochondrial antibody in 95%
  - Liver biopsy reveals dense inflammatory infiltrate centered on bile duct

- ■ Differential Diagnosis
  - Chronic biliary tract obstruction, ie, cholelithiasis-related stricture
  - Bile duct carcinoma
  - Inflammatory bowel disease complicated by cholestatic liver disease
  - Sarcoidosis
  - Sclerosing cholangitis
  - Drug-induced cholestasis

- ■ Treatment
  - Cholestyramine, colestipol, or rifampin for pruritus
  - Calcium (high risk of osteoporosis, osteomalacia) and supplementation with vitamins A, D, E, and K
  - Ursodeoxycholic acid delays progression and extends survival; colchicine and methotrexate may be helpful
  - Liver transplant for refractory cirrhosis or hepatocellular cancer

- ■ Pearl

The perfect disease for cure by transplantation; no virus, no malignancy in explant.

Reference

Talwalkar JA, Lindor KD: Primary biliary cirrhosis. Lancet 2003;362:53. [PMID: 12853201]

Pyogenic Hepatic Abscess

- ■ Essentials of Diagnosis
  - Fever, jaundice, right upper quadrant tenderness, weight loss, pleuritic chest pain, cough, anorexia or nausea
  - Usually due to hematogenous or local spread of an intra-abdominal infection
  - Leukocytosis with left shift; nonspecific abnormalities of liver function studies
  - Most common organisms are *Escherichia coli, Proteus vulgaris, Enterobacter aerogenes,* and anaerobic species
  - Elevated right hemidiaphragm by radiography; ultrasound, CT scan, or liver scan demonstrates intrahepatic defect
  - Predisposing factors: Malignancy, recent endoscopy or surgery, diabetes, Crohn's disease, diverticulitis, appendicitis, recent trauma

- ■ Differential Diagnosis
  - Amebic hepatic abscess
  - Acute hepatitis
  - Right lower lobe pneumonia
  - Cholelithiasis, cholecystitis
  - Appendicitis

- ■ Treatment
  - Antibiotics with coverage of gram-negative organisms and anaerobes, antibiotics narrowed if specific organisms identified
  - Percutaneous or surgical drainage for cases refractory to medical management

- ■ Pearl

The classic triad of fever, jaundice, and hepatomegaly is not so classic; it is found in less than 10% of cases.

Reference

Johannsen EC, Sifri CD, Madoff LC: Pyogenic liver abscesses. Infect Dis Clin North Am 2000;14:547, vii. [PMID: 10987109]

Sclerosing Cholangitis

- Essentials of Diagnosis
  - Progressively obstructive jaundice, pruritus, malaise, anorexia, and indigestion, most common in young men aged 20–40 years
  - Two-thirds of cases have associated ulcerative colitis
  - Positive antineutrophil cytoplasmic antibody found in 70%; elevated total bilirubin and alkaline phosphatase common
  - Endoscopic retrograde cholangiopancreatography (ERCP) demonstrates thick or narrowed biliary ductal system
  - Absence of previous biliary stones, biliary surgery, congenital abnormalities, biliary cirrhosis, and cholangiocarcinoma necessary to make the diagnosis

- Differential Diagnosis
  - Choledocholithiasis
  - Drug-induced cholestasis
  - Carcinoma of pancreas or biliary tree
  - Hepatitis due to any cause
  - *Clonorchis sinensis* infection
  - AIDS cholangiopathy

- Treatment
  - At present, no specific medical therapy has been shown to have a major impact on the prevention of complications (cholangitis, obstruction, cholangiocarcinoma and hepatic failure) or survival
  - Ursodeoxycholic acid may improve liver function tests but does not alter natural history
  - Fat-soluble vitamin and calcium supplementation
  - Stenting or balloon dilation of dominant strictures by ERCP
  - Liver transplantation for decompensated disease

- Pearl

Most sclerosing cholangitis is seen in ulcerative colitis, but most ulcerative colitis is not complicated by sclerosing cholangitis.

Reference

Mendes FD, Lindor KD: Primary sclerosing cholangitis. Clin Liver Dis 2004;8:195. [PMID: 15062201]

Variceal Bleeding

- ■ Essentials of Diagnosis
  - • Sudden, painless large-volume episode of hematemesis with melena or hematochezia typical
  - • Antecedent history of liver disease and stigmas of liver disease or portal hypertension on physical examination
  - • Hepatic portal venous pressure gradient of ≥ 12 mm Hg is generally necessary for variceal bleeding
  - • Fifty percent of patients with alcoholic cirrhosis will present with esophageal varices within 2 years of diagnosis
  - • A 30–50% risk of death with each episode

- ■ Differential Diagnosis
  - • Peptic ulcer disease
  - • Mallory-Weiss tear
  - • Gastric varices
  - • Alcoholic gastritis
  - • Esophagitis
  - • Bleeding from portal hypertensive gastropathy
  - • Other less common sources: Dieulafoy's lesion, hemosuccus pancreaticus, aortoenteric fistulas

- ■ Treatment
  - • Appropriate resuscitation (intravenous resuscitation, correction of coagulopathy, blood transfusions, airway protection, antibiotic therapy for spontaneous bacterial peritonitis prophylaxis in patients with known ascites)
  - • Intravenous octreotide (100-μg bolus, 50-μg/h drip)
  - • Urgent endoscopic evaluation and treatment with band ligation or sclerotherapy; less successful in gastric varices
  - • Balloon tamponade (Minnesota-Sengstaken-Blakemore) as a temporizing measure or for endoscopic failures
  - • Transjugular intrahepatic portosystemic shunt (TIPS) or shunt surgery for gastric varices or refractory cases of esophageal varices
  - • Liver transplantation for appropriate candidates with recurrent bleeding episodes
  - • Prophylaxis of recurrent bleeding with endoscopic (band ligation) and pharmacologic therapy (propranolol, nadolol)

- ■ Pearl

In a patient with any possible exposure (eg, a person born in Puerto Rico with no other liver disease) consider schistosomiasis, even if there has been no visit to the endemic area for over 20 years.

Reference

Comar KM, Sanyal AJ: Portal hypertensive bleeding. Gastroenterol Clin North Am 2003;32:1079. [PMID: 14696298]

Hematologic Diseases

Acute Leukemia

- **Essentials of Diagnosis**
  - Rapid onset of fever, weakness, malaise, bleeding, bone or joint pain, infection
  - Pallor, fever, petechiae; lymphadenopathy, generally unimpressive; splenomegaly unusual
  - Pancytopenia with circulating leukemic blasts (rarely pancytopenia alone)
  - > 20% immature blasts in bone marrow
  - Abnormal cells either lymphoblasts (ALL) or myeloblasts (AML); immunohistochemistry and flow cytometry may separate; Auer rods (eosinophilic cytoplasmic inclusions) in blasts are diagnostic of AML

- **Differential Diagnosis**
  - Aplastic anemia
  - Severe B_{12} or folate deficiency
  - Severe infection, pertussis in particular
  - Chronic myelogenous leukemia/myeloproliferative disorders
  - Chronic lymphocytic leukemia
  - Infectious mononucleosis
  - Hodgkin's or non-Hodgkin's lymphoma
  - Metastatic malignancy to bone marrow
  - Miliary tuberculosis
  - Paroxysmal nocturnal hemoglobinuria

- **Treatment**
  - Aggressive combination chemotherapy with specific drugs dictated by cell type
  - Conventional-dose chemotherapy curative in minority of adults with acute leukemia; allogeneic and autologous bone marrow transplantation considered for appropriate patients

- **Pearl**

Remember that pain in expansile bone marrow can simulate mechanical back pain with bilateral leg radiation.

Reference

Pui CH, Relling MV, Downing JR: Acute lymphoblastic leukemia. N Engl J Med 2004;350:1535. [PMID: 15071128]

Agranulocytosis

- ■ Essentials of Diagnosis
  - Malaise of abrupt onset, chills, fever, sore throat
  - Mucosal ulceration
  - History of drug ingestion common (eg, trimethoprim-sulfamethoxazole, ganciclovir, propylthiouracil)
  - Profound granulocytopenia with relative lymphocytosis

- ■ Differential Diagnosis
  - Aplastic anemia
  - Myelodysplasia
  - Systemic lupus erythematosus (SLE)
  - Viral infection (HIV, CMV, hepatitis)
  - Acute leukemia
  - Felty's syndrome

- ■ Treatment
  - Stop offending drugs
  - Broad-spectrum antibiotics for fever
  - Trial of filgrastim (granulocyte colony-stimulating factor) for severe neutropenia
  - Allogeneic bone marrow transplant for appropriate refractory patients

- ■ Pearl

Sequential neutrophil counts are valueless in at-risk patients; a normal neutrophil count today may be agranulocytosis tomorrow.

Reference

Boxer L, Dale DC: Neutropenia: causes and consequences. Semin Hematol 2002;39:75. [PMID: 11957188]

Alpha-Thalassemia Trait

- ■ Essentials of Diagnosis
  - Commonly comes to attention because of CBC done for other reasons
  - Increased frequency in persons of African, Mediterranean, or southern Chinese ancestry
  - Microcytosis out of proportion to anemia; occasional target cells and acanthocytes on smear, but far less so than with beta-thalassemia; normal iron studies
  - Mentzer's index (MCV/RBC) < 13
  - No increase in hemoglobin A_2 or hemoglobin F
  - Diagnosis of exclusion in patient with modest anemia (definitive diagnosis depends on hemoglobin gene mapping)

- ■ Differential Diagnosis
  - Iron deficiency anemia
  - Other hemoglobinopathies
  - Sideroblastic anemia
  - Beta-thalassemia minor

- ■ Treatment
  - Oral folic acid supplementation
  - Avoidance of medicinal iron or oxidative agents
  - Red blood cell transfusions during pregnancy or stress (intercurrent illness) if hemoglobin falls below 9 g/dL

- ■ Pearl

Microcytosis without anemia or hyperchromia is with few exceptions alpha-thalassemia.

Reference

Gu X, Zeng Y: A review of the molecular diagnosis of thalassemia. Hematology 2002;7:203. [PMID: 14972782]

Anemia of Chronic Disease

- ■ Essentials of Diagnosis
  - Known chronic disease, particularly inflammatory; symptoms and signs usually those of responsible disease
  - Modest anemia (Hct ≥ 25%); red cells normal morphologically but may be slightly microcytic
  - Low serum iron with normal or low total iron-binding capacity, normal or high serum ferritin, normal or increased bone marrow iron stores, low soluble transferrin receptor and soluble transferrin receptor:log ferritin ratio

- ■ Differential Diagnosis
  - Iron deficiency anemia
  - Myelodysplasia
  - Sideroblastic anemia
  - Thalassemia

- ■ Treatment
  - None usually necessary
  - Red blood cell transfusions for symptomatic anemia
  - Recombinant erythropoietin (epoetin alfa)

- ■ Pearl

In anemia of chronic disease, the hemoglobin and hematocrit do not fall below 60% of baseline; if so, seek another cause of anemia.

Reference

Means RT Jr: Recent developments in the anemia of chronic disease. Curr Hematol Rep 2003;2:116. [PMID: 12901142]

Aplastic Anemia

- **Essentials of Diagnosis**
  - Lassitude, fatigue, malaise, other nonspecific symptoms
  - Pallor, purpura, mucosal bleeding, petechiae, signs of infection
  - Pancytopenia with normal cellular morphology; hypocellular bone marrow with fatty infiltration
  - Occasional history of exposure to an offending drug or radiation

- **Differential Diagnosis**
  - Bone marrow infiltrative process (tumor, some infections, granulomatous diseases)
  - Myelofibrosis
  - Acute leukemia
  - Hypersplenism
  - Viral infections including HIV, hepatitis
  - SLE
  - Hairy cell leukemia
  - Large granular lymphocyte disease

- **Treatment**
  - Allogeneic bone marrow transplantation for patients under age 30
  - Intensive immunosuppression with antithymocyte globulin, cyclosporine if transplant not feasible
  - Oral androgens may be of benefit
  - If SLE-associated, plasmapheresis and corticosteroids effective
  - Avoid transfusions if possible in patients who may be transplant candidates; otherwise, red blood cells and platelet transfusions, filgrastim (granulocyte colony-stimulating factor) or sargramostim (granulocyte-macrophage colony-stimulating factor) as necessary

- **Pearl**

The risk of aplastic anemia from chloramphenicol is one in 40,000 courses; one prescription per day statistically requires 100 years for a single case.

Reference

Keohane EM: Acquired aplastic anemia. Clin Lab Sci 2004;17:165. [PMID: 15314891]

Autoimmune Hemolytic Anemia

- ■ Essentials of Diagnosis
  - • Acquired anemia caused by IgG (warm) or IgM (cold) autoantibody
  - • Fatigue, malaise in many; occasional abdominal or back pain
  - • Pallor, jaundice, but palpable spleen uncommon
  - • Persistent anemia with microspherocytes and reticulocytosis; elevated indirect bilirubin and serum LDH
  - • Positive Coombs (direct antiglobulin) test
  - • Various drugs, underlying autoimmune or lymphoproliferative disorder may be causative

5

- ■ Differential Diagnosis
  - • Disseminated intravascular coagulation
  - • Hemoglobinopathy
  - • Hereditary spherocytosis
  - • Nonspherocytic hemolytic anemia
  - • Sideroblastic anemia
  - • Megaloblastic anemia

- ■ Treatment
  - • High-dosage steroids (warm antibody)
  - • Intravenous immune globulin (warm antibody)
  - • Plasmapheresis in severe cases (warm or cold antibody)
  - • Avoid cold, administer warmed blood/fluids (cold antibody)
  - • Splenectomy for refractory or recurrent cases (warm antibody)
  - • Immunosuppression (both warm and cold antibody)
  - • Cross-match difficult because of autoantibodies, so least incompatible blood used
  - • Splenectomy for refractory or recurrent cases
  - • More intensive immunosuppressive regimens available for refractory cases after splenectomy

- ■ Pearl

As in all cases of extravascular hemolysis, iron is recycled; multiple transfusions thus lead to iron overload.

Reference

Dhaliwal G, Cornett PA, Tierney LM Jr: Hemolytic anemia. Am Fam Physician 2004;69:2599. [PMID: 15202694]

Beta-Thalassemia Minor

■ Essentials of Diagnosis

- Symptoms variable depending on degree of anemia; no specific physical findings
- Mild and persistent anemia, hypochromia with microcytosis and target cells; red blood cell count normal or elevated
- Similar findings in one of patient's parents
- Patient often of Mediterranean, African, or southern Chinese ancestry
- Elevated hemoglobin A_2 and hemoglobin F
- Mentzer's index (MCV/RBC) < 13

■ Differential Diagnosis

- Iron deficiency anemia
- Other hemoglobinopathies, especially hemoglobin C disorders
- Sideroblastic anemia
- Alpha-thalassemia
- Anemia of chronic disease

■ Treatment

- Oral folic acid supplementation
- Avoidance of medicinal iron or oxidative agents
- Red blood cell transfusions during pregnancy or stress (intercurrent illness) if hemoglobin falls below 9 g/dL

■ Pearl

The hemoglobinopathies exhibit central red cell targeting; liver disease targeting tends to be eccentric.

Reference

Atweh GF, DeSimone J, Saunthararajah Y, et al: Hemoglobinopathies. Hematology (Am Soc Hematol Educ Program) 2003:14. [PMID: 14633775]

Chronic Lymphocytic Leukemia

- ### Essentials of Diagnosis
  - Fatigue in some; most asymptomatic; often discovered incidentally
  - Pallor, lymphadenopathy, splenomegaly common also
  - Sustained lymphocytosis > 5000/μL or higher, with some counts up to 1,000,000/μL; morphologically mature cells in most cases
  - Coombs-positive hemolytic anemia, immune thrombocytopenia, hypogammaglobulinemia late in course
  - Anemia, thrombocytopenia, bulky lymphadenopathy associated with poorer prognosis
  - Flow cytometry separates CLL from reactive lymphocytosis
  - May transform into high-grade lymphoid neoplasm (Richter's transformation)

- ### Differential Diagnosis
  - Infectious mononucleosis
  - Prolymphocytic leukemia
  - Pertussis
  - Mantle cell lymphoma
  - Hairy cell leukemia
  - Adult T cell leukemia/lymphoma
  - Other lymphoma with leukemic phase

- ### Treatment
  - Given the chronic, frequently indolent nature of the disease, chemotherapy is reserved for symptomatic patients or for young patients with advanced disease
  - Conventional chemotherapy has high response rate, but unlikely to be curative; much interest, however, in combinations of chemotherapy and immunotherapy
  - Allogeneic bone marrow transplantation potentially curative in selected patients
  - Steroids, immunoglobulin may help associated immune cytopenias

- ### Pearl

Smudge cells result from crushing of fragile leukemic cells during preparation of blood smear.

Reference

Shanafelt TD, Call TG: Current approach to diagnosis and management of chronic lymphocytic leukemia. Mayo Clin Proc 2004;79:388. [PMID: 15008611]

Chronic Myelogenous Leukemia

- ### Essentials of Diagnosis
  - Symptoms variable; often diagnosed by examination or blood count done for unrelated reasons
  - Splenomegaly in all cases; sternal tenderness in some
  - Leukocytosis, typically striking; immature white cells in peripheral blood and bone marrow; thrombocytosis, eosinophilia, basophilia common
  - Diagnosis relies on demonstration of Philadelphia chromosome t(9:22) by conventional cytogenetics, reverse transcriptase polymerase chain reaction (RT-PCR) of peripheral blood or bone marrow, or fluorescent in situ hybridization
  - Low leukocyte alkaline phosphatase level, markedly elevated serum vitamin B_{12} due to high B_{12} binding transcobalamins
  - Results in acute leukemia in 3–5 years without treatment

- ### Differential Diagnosis
  - Leukemoid reactions associated with infection, inflammation, or cancer
  - Other myeloproliferative disorders

- ### Treatment
  - Tyrosine kinase inhibitor (STI571; imatinib mesylate [Gleevec]) targeting specific molecular defect in CML cells is now first-line therapy
  - Combination of cytarabine (Ara-C) and interferon leads to cytogenetically complete remissions in a small minority of patients
  - Allogeneic bone marrow transplantation remains useful therapy for appropriate candidates

- ### Pearl

Pseudohypoglycemia and pseudohyperkalemia are in vitro artifacts resulting from continuing white cell metabolism of glucose and release of potassium into serum after clotting; consider this before inappropriate therapy is initiated.

Reference

Mughal TI, Goldman JM: Chronic myeloid leukemia: current status and controversies. Oncology (Huntingt) 2004;18:837, 847; discussion 847, 853. [PMID: 15255169]

Disseminated Intravascular Coagulation

- ▪ Essentials of Diagnosis
  - Evidence of abnormal bleeding or clotting, usually in a critically ill patient
  - Occurs as a result of activation and consumption of clotting and antithrombotic factors due to severe stressors such as sepsis, burns, massive hemorrhage
  - May occur in chronic, indolent form, usually associated with malignancy
  - Anemia, thrombocytopenia, elevated prothrombin time, and later, partial thromboplastin time, low fibrinogen, elevated fibrin degradation products and fibrin D-dimers

- ▪ Differential Diagnosis
  - Severe liver disease
  - Thrombotic thrombocytopenic purpura
  - Hemolytic-uremic syndrome
  - Vitamin K deficiency
  - Other microangiopathic hemolytic anemias (eg, prosthetic heart valve)
  - Sepsis-induced thrombocytopenia or anemia
  - Heparin-induced thrombocytopenia

- ▪ Treatment
  - Treat underlying disorder
  - Replacement of consumed blood factors with fresh frozen plasma, cryoprecipitate, and potentially antithrombin III
  - Heparin in selected cases, particularly acute promyelocytic leukemia
  - Antifibrinolytic therapy (aminocaproic acid or tranexamic acid) for refractory bleeding, but only in presence of heparin therapy

- ▪ Pearl

Remember that the fibrinogen and platelet count may be normal in chronic DIC.

Reference

Toh CH, Dennis M: Disseminated intravascular coagulation: old disease, new hope. BMJ 2003;327:974. [PMID: 14576251]

Drug-Induced Hemolytic Anemia

- ■ Essentials of Diagnosis
  - • Immune hemolytic anemia due to host antibody recognition of drug and red blood cell membrane
  - • Acute to subacute onset; elevated LDH, hyperbilirubinemia, reticulocytosis
  - • Rarely, fulminant presentation with laboratory abnormalities as noted plus hemoglobinemia-hemoglobinuria, renal failure, and hemodynamic instability
  - • Positive Coombs test with patient's blood; Coombs test using reagent red blood cells positive only in presence of offending drug

- ■ Differential Diagnosis
  - • Autoimmune hemolytic anemia
  - • Microangiopathic hemolytic anemia (eg, disseminated intravascular coagulation, thrombotic thrombocytopenic purpura)
  - • Delayed transfusion-related hemolysis
  - • Blood loss

- ■ Treatment
  - • Discontinue offending drug
  - • Plasmapheresis for severe cases, especially if drug has long serum half-life
  - • Intravenous immune globulin, steroids potentially of benefit

- ■ Pearl

An annoying prospect in an internal medicine patient; since many drugs can cause it and since typical patients are taking many drugs, the only way to be sure is to peel them off one by one until improvement is noted.

Reference

Dhaliwal G, Cornett PA, Tierney LM Jr: Hemolytic anemia. Am Fam Physician 2004;69:2599. [PMID: 15202694]

Essential Thrombocytosis

■ **Essentials of Diagnosis**

- Sustained elevated platelet count without other cause
- Painful burning of palms and soles (erythromelalgia) promptly and completely relieved with low-dose aspirin
- Arterial > venous thromboses
- Low likelihood of progression to fibrotic "spent" stage or acute leukemia
- May have mild elevations in white count and hematocrit; basophilia, eosinophilia, hypervitaminosis B_{12}

■ **Differential Diagnosis**

- Other myeloproliferative disorders (especially polycythemia vera)
- Chronic infection or autoimmune disease, visceral malignancy (reactive thrombocytosis)
- Iron deficiency

■ **Treatment**

- Platelet-lowering therapy for those with high risk of clotting (history of prior clotting, age > 60, established arterial vascular disease)
- Anagrelide and hydroxyurea most commonly used agents
- Low-dose aspirin for vasomotor symptoms

■ **Pearl**

It is the qualitative (not quantitative) platelet defect that results in clotting; reactive thrombocytosis is not a hypercoagulable state.

Reference

Schafer AI: Thrombocytosis. N Engl J Med 2004;350:1211. [PMID: 15028825]

Folic Acid Deficiency

■ Essentials of Diagnosis

- Nonspecific gastrointestinal symptoms, fatigue, dyspnea without neurologic complaints in a patient with malnutrition, often related to alcoholism
- Pallor, mild jaundice
- Pancytopenia, but counts not as low as in vitamin B_{12} deficiency; oval macrocytosis and hypersegmented neutrophils; megaloblastic marrow; normal vitamin B_{12} levels
- Red blood cell folate < 150 ng/mL diagnostic

■ Differential Diagnosis

- Vitamin B_{12} deficiency
- Myelodysplastic syndromes
- Infiltrative granulomatous or neoplastic bone marrow process
- Hypersplenism
- Paroxysmal nocturnal hemoglobinuria
- Acute leukemia

■ Treatment

- Exclude vitamin B_{12} deficiency prior to therapy
- Oral folic acid supplementation

■ Pearl

In countries such as England where vegetables may be overcooked, folate deficiency may occur in otherwise adequately nourished persons.

Reference

Allen LH: Folate and vitamin B_{12} status in the Americas. Nutr Rev 2004;62(6 Pt 2): S29; discussion S34. [PMID: 15298445]

Hairy Cell Leukemia

- ■ Essentials of Diagnosis
  - • Fatigue, abdominal pain, but often asymptomatic; susceptibility to bacterial infections
  - • Pallor, prominent splenomegaly, rare lymphadenopathy
  - • Pancytopenia, "hairy cell" morphology of leukocytes in periphery and marrow at high magnification
  - • "Dry tap" on bone marrow aspiration; diagnosis confirmed by flow cytometry; tartrate-resistant acid phosphatase (TRAP) stain also positive

5

- ■ Differential Diagnosis
  - • Myelofibrosis
  - • Chronic lymphocytic leukemia
  - • Waldenström's macroglobulinemia
  - • Non-Hodgkin's lymphoma
  - • Aplastic anemia
  - • Acute leukemia
  - • Infiltration of marrow by tumor or granuloma
  - • Paroxysmal nocturnal hemoglobinuria

- ■ Treatment
  - • Cladribine gives durable remissions in > 80% of patients
  - • Splenectomy for severe cytopenias or chemotherapy-resistant disease

- ■ Pearl
  Involved cells coexpress CD11c and CD22 on immunophenotyping.

Reference

Mey U, Strehl J, Gorschluter M, et al: Advances in the treatment of hairy-cell leukaemia. Lancet Oncol 2003;4:86. [PMID: 12573350]

Hemoglobin SC Disease

- **Essentials of Diagnosis**
  - Recurrent attacks of abdominal, joint, or bone pain
  - Splenomegaly, retinopathy (similar to diabetes)
  - Mild anemia, reticulocytosis, and few sickle cells on smear but many targets; 50% hemoglobin C, 50% hemoglobin S on electrophoresis
  - In situ thrombi of pulmonary artery and venous sinus of brain may simulate pulmonary emboli, may cause stroke

- **Differential Diagnosis**
  - Sickle cell anemia
  - Sickle thalassemia
  - Hemoglobin C disease
  - Cirrhosis
  - Pulmonary embolism
  - Beta thalassemia

- **Treatment**
  - No specific therapy for most patients
  - Otherwise treat as for SS hemoglobin

- **Pearl**

Unique among hemoglobinopathies, thrombotic complications are most severe during pregnancy, most notably in-situ pulmonary artery thrombi.

Reference

Nagel RL, Fabry ME, Steinberg MH: The paradox of hemoglobin SC disease. Blood Rev 2003;17:167. [PMID: 12818227]

Hemoglobin S–Thalassemia Disease

- Essentials of Diagnosis
  - Recurrent attacks of abdominal, joint, or bone pain
  - Splenomegaly
  - Mild to moderate anemia with low MCV; reticulocytosis; few sickle cells on smear with many target cells; increased hemoglobin A_2 by electrophoresis distinguishes from sickle cell disease, hemoglobin C

5

- Differential Diagnosis
  - Sickle cell anemia
  - Hemoglobin C disease
  - Hemoglobin SC disease
  - Cirrhosis

- Treatment
  - Chronic oral folic acid supplementation
  - Acute therapy as in sickle cell anemia

- Pearl

Like other sickle hemoglobin positives, complications tend to be less severe than in SC disease; targeting and sickling on the same smear tell the diagnostic story.

Reference

Clarke GM, Higgins TN: Laboratory investigation of hemoglobinopathies and thalassemias: review and update. Clin Chem 2000;46(8 Pt 2):1284. [PMID: 10926923]

Hemolytic Transfusion Reaction

■ Essentials of Diagnosis
- Chills and fever during blood transfusion
- Back, chest pain; dark urine
- Associated with vascular collapse, renal failure, and disseminated intravascular coagulation
- Hemolysis, hemoglobinuria, and severe anemia

5

■ Differential Diagnosis
- Leukoagglutination reaction
- IgA deficiency with anaphylactic transfusion reaction
- Myocardial infarction
- Acute abdomen due to other causes
- Pyelonephritis
- Bacteremia due to contaminated blood product

■ Treatment
- Stop transfusion immediately
- Hydration and intravenous mannitol to prevent renal failure

■ Pearl

Any adverse clinical event during transfusion should be considered and evaluated as a hemolytic reaction.

Reference

Janatpour K, Holland PV: Noninfectious serious hazards of transfusion. Curr Hematol Rep 2002;1:149. [PMID: 12901137]

Hemolytic-Uremic Syndrome

- ■ Essentials of Diagnosis
  - • Petechial rash, hypertension, acute-to-subacute renal failure
  - • Often preceded by gastroenteritis or exposure to offending medication
  - • Frequently associated with antecedent *Campylobacter* infection (may be very mild to occult)
  - • Laboratory reports notable for thrombocytopenia, anemia, renal failure, elevated LDH, normal prothrombin time and partial thromboplastin time as well as fibrin and fibrinogen degeneration products

- ■ Differential Diagnosis
  - • Disseminated intravascular coagulation
  - • Thrombotic thrombocytopenic purpura
  - • Catastrophic antiphospholipid antibody syndrome
  - • Pre-eclampsia–eclampsia
  - • Other microangiopathic hemolytic anemias

- ■ Treatment
  - • In children, disease is most often self-limited and managed with supportive care
  - • In adults, stop potentially offending drugs
  - • Plasmapheresis for refractory cases

- ■ Pearl

In childhood cases, E coli *O157:H7 infection is the typical precipitant.*

Reference

Blackall DP, Marques MB: Hemolytic uremic syndrome revisited: Shiga toxin, factor H, and fibrin generation. Am J Clin Pathol 2004;121(Suppl):S81. [PMID: 15298153]

Hemophilia A & B

- **Essentials of Diagnosis**
  - Lifelong history of bleeding in a male
  - Slow, prolonged bleeding after minor injury or surgery; spontaneous hemarthroses common
  - Prolonged partial thromboplastin time corrected by mixing patient's plasma with a normal specimen
  - Low factor VIII coagulant activity (hemophilia A) or factor IX coagulant activity (hemophilia B)

- **Differential Diagnosis**
  - von Willebrand's disease
  - Disseminated intravascular coagulation
  - Afibrinogenemia and dysfibrinogenemia
  - Heparin administration
  - Acquired factor deficiencies or inhibitors (eg, paraproteins with anti-VIII or anti-IX activity)

- **Treatment**
  - Avoidance of aspirin
  - Factor replacement for any bleeding with factor VIII concentrates (hemophilia A) or factor IX complex (hemophilia B) or during invasive procedures
  - Increased factor dosing, steroids, or immunosuppressants if factor inhibitor develops
  - Desmopressin acetate before surgical procedures for hemophilia A may benefit selected patients

- **Pearl**

Christmas disease (factor IX deficiency) is the index patient's name, not the holiday.

Reference

Rick ME, Walsh CE, Key NS: Congenital bleeding disorders. Hematology (Am Soc Hematol Educ Program) 2003:559. [PMID: 14633799]

Heparin-Induced Thrombocytopenia (HIT)

■ Essentials of Diagnosis

- Moderate thrombocytopenia developing 4–14 days after institution of heparin (type 2); may be sooner if previously exposed to heparin (type 1)
- Venous and arterial thromboses, skin necrosis rarely
- Positive serotonin release assay, heparin-induced platelet aggregation, or ELISA for antiheparin-platelet factor 4 antibodies
- Rapid recovery of platelet count following discontinuation of heparin

■ Differential Diagnosis

- DIC
- Drug-induced thrombocytopenia
- Sepsis
- Idiopathic thrombocytopenic purpura

■ Treatment

- Immediate discontinuation of all exposure to heparin (including IV heparin flushes)
- Anticoagulation with direct thrombin inhibitors (lepirudin or argatroban) or danaparoid

■ Pearl

Absolutely not dose-related; even hep-locks and line flushes can do it.

Reference

Warkentin TE: Heparin-induced thrombocytopenia: pathogenesis and management. Br J Haematol 2003;121:535. [PMID: 12752095]

Hereditary Spherocytosis

■ Essentials of Diagnosis

- Chronic hemolytic anemia of variable severity, often with exacerbations during coincident illnesses
- Malaise, abdominal discomfort in symptomatic patients
- Jaundice, splenomegaly in severely affected patients
- Variable anemia with spherocytosis and reticulocytosis; elevated MCHC; increased osmotic fragility test and increased red cell fragility as measured with ektacytometry (ie, measurement of the shear stress a red blood cell can withstand before lysing)
- Negative Coombs test
- Family history of anemia, jaundice, splenectomy

■ Differential Diagnosis

- Autoimmune hemolytic anemia
- Hemoglobin C disease
- Iron deficiency anemia
- Alcoholism
- Burns

■ Treatment

- Oral folic acid supplementation
- Pneumococcal vaccination if splenectomy contemplated
- Splenectomy for symptomatic patients

■ Pearl

The only condition in medicine causing a hyperchromic, microcytic anemia.

Reference

Bolton-Maggs PH, Stevens RF, Dodd NJ, et al; General Haematology Task Force of the British Committee for Standards in Haematology: Guidelines for the diagnosis and management of hereditary spherocytosis. Br J Haematol 2004;126:455. [PMID: 15287938]

Hodgkin's Disease

- ■ Essentials of Diagnosis
  - In most cases the disorder starts in one node group and spreads in an orderly, contiguous fashion
  - Regionally enlarged, rubbery, painless lymphadenopathy (often cervical); hepatosplenomegaly variable
  - Reed-Sternberg cells (or variants) in lymph node or bone marrow biopsy diagnostic
  - Diagnosis often requires excisional lymph node biopsy, fine-needle aspirates often nondiagnostic; patients considered stage A if no constitutional symptoms are present and stage B if they have fevers, night sweats, or significant weight loss
  - Younger patients tend to have supradiaphragmatic disease with favorable histology; older individuals tend toward more aggressive pathology, infradiaphragmatic involvement

- ■ Differential Diagnosis
  - Non-Hodgkin's lymphoma
  - Lymphadenitis secondary to infections (tuberculosis and cat-scratch disease)
  - Pseudolymphoma caused by phenytoin
  - Lymphomatoid granulomatosis
  - Sarcoidosis
  - HIV disease
  - SLE

- ■ Treatment
  - Staging (I–IV) with chest x-ray, CT scans of chest, abdomen, and pelvis, gallium or PET scan, and bone marrow biopsy; laparotomy (if results would alter therapy) now infrequently necessary
  - Radiation therapy for localized disease or short course of combination chemotherapy with less extensive radiation
  - Combination chemotherapy for disseminated disease with or without radiation to bulky areas of disease

- ■ Pearl

When a patient develops pain in a lymph node soon after drinking alcohol, think Hodgkin's.

Reference

Diehl V, Thomas RK, Re D: Part II: Hodgkin's lymphoma—diagnosis and treatment. Lancet Oncol 2004;5:19. [PMID: 14700605]

Idiopathic Thrombocytopenic Purpura

- ■ Essentials of Diagnosis
  - • Mucosal bleeding, easy bruising and bleeding
  - • Petechiae, ecchymoses; splenomegaly rare
  - • Severe thrombocytopenia, prolonged bleeding time; elevated platelet-associated IgG in 95%, though nonspecific; bone marrow with normal to increased megakaryocytes
  - • May be associated with autoimmune diseases (eg, SLE), HIV infection, lymphoproliferative disorders, or with Coombs-positive hemolytic anemia (Evans' syndrome)

- ■ Differential Diagnosis
  - • Acute leukemia
  - • Myelodysplastic syndrome
  - • Thrombotic thrombocytopenic purpura
  - • Disseminated intravascular coagulation
  - • Chronic lymphocytic leukemia
  - • Aplastic anemia
  - • Alcohol abuse
  - • Drug toxicity (eg, quinidine, digoxin)
  - • AIDS
  - • SLE

- ■ Treatment
  - • Prednisone, intravenous immune globulin, or anti Rh-D immune globulin (WinRho) in Rh-positive patients all have high rates of success acutely
  - • Splenectomy if no response to initial therapy, for relapsed disease, or for patients requiring high doses of steroids to maintain an acceptable platelet count
  - • Danazol, vincristine, vinblastine, azathioprine, cyclophosphamide, cyclosporine, and rituximab for refractory cases; plasma immuno-adsorption may also be successful in some refractory cases
  - • Reserve platelet transfusion for life-threatening hemorrhages; bleeding sometimes stops even as the platelet count rises slightly if at all

- ■ Pearl

The order of platelet bleeding as the count falls: first skin, then mucous membrane, finally viscera; thus, absence of cutaneous petechiae means a low likelihood of intracranial hemorrhage.

Reference

Stasi R, Provan D: Management of immune thrombocytopenic purpura in adults. Mayo Clin Proc 2004;79:504. [PMID: 15065616]

Iron Deficiency Anemia

- ■ Essentials of Diagnosis
  - Lassitude; in children under age 2, poor muscle tone, delayed motor development
  - Pallor, cheilosis, and koilonychia
  - Hypochromic microcytic red cells late in disease; indices normal early, occasional thrombocytosis
  - Serum iron low, total iron-binding capacity increased; absent marrow iron; serum ferritin < 15 ng/mL classically, but concomitant illness may elevate it
  - Newer tests include increased serum soluble transferrin receptor and transferrin receptor:log ferritin ratio
  - Occult blood loss invariably causative in adults; malabsorption or dietary insufficiency rarely causes deficiency

- ■ Differential Diagnosis
  - Anemia of chronic disease
  - Myelodysplasia
  - Thalassemia
  - Sideroblastic anemias, including lead intoxication

- ■ Treatment
  - Oral ferrous sulfate or ferrous gluconate three times daily for 6–12 months
  - Parenteral iron for selected patients with severe, clinically significant iron deficiency with continuing chronic blood loss
  - Evaluation for occult blood loss

- ■ Pearl

Remember iron deficiency as a treatable cause of obesity; ice cream craving is one of many associated picas.

Reference

Beutler E, Hoffbrand AV, Cook JD: Iron deficiency and overload. Hematology (Am Soc Hematol Educ Program) 2003:40. [PMID: 14633776]

Multiple Myeloma

- **Essentials of Diagnosis**
  - Weakness, weight loss, recurrent infection, bone (especially back) pain, often resulting in pathologic fractures
  - Pallor, bony tenderness; spleen is not enlarged
  - Anemia; accelerated sedimentation rate; elevated serum calcium, renal insufficiency; normal alkaline phosphatase; elevated B_2 microglobulin; narrowed anion gap in most
  - Nephrotic syndrome (with associated amyloidosis causing albuminuria or by light chains in urine)
  - Elevated serum globulin with monoclonal spike on serum or urine protein electrophoresis
  - Infiltration of bone marrow with clonal proliferation of plasma cells
  - Lytic bone lesions with negative bone scan

- **Differential Diagnosis**
  - Benign monoclonal gammopathy of undetermined significance (MGUS)
  - Metastatic cancer
  - Lymphoproliferative disorder with associated monoclonal spike
  - Hyperparathyroidism
  - Primary amyloidosis

- **Treatment**
  - Pamidronate or zoledronic acid for patients with extensive bone disease or hypercalcemia
  - Autologous bone marrow transplant now standard for disease palliation, though unlikely to be curative
  - Combination chemotherapy with alkylating agents (eg, melphalan), steroids, and vincristine used frequently pretransplant, or for patients not able to undergo transplantation
  - Radiation therapy for local bone pain or pathologic fractures
  - Novel therapies such as thalidomide, revamid, and bortezomib offer significant response rates with minimal side effects even in heavily pretreated, refractory patients

- **Pearl**

The counterintuitive three no's of myeloma: no fever, no increased alkaline phosphatase, no splenomegaly.

Reference

Sirohi B, Powles R: Multiple myeloma. Lancet 2004;363:875. [PMID: 15031034]

Myelodysplastic Syndromes

- **Essentials of Diagnosis**
  - Clonal hematopoietic disorder characterized by ineffective hematopoiesis leading to bone marrow hypercellularity with a variable presence of blasts and peripheral blood cytopenias
  - Subtypes include: Refractory anemia (RA), refractory anemia with ringed sideroblasts (RARS), refractory anemia with excess blasts (RAEB), and chronic myelomonocytic leukemia (CMML)
  - Evolution to acute leukemia may occur within months (RAEB) to many years (RA, RARS)
  - Morphologic dysplasia frequently seen in cells of myeloid lineage (eg, Pelger-Huët anomaly, hypogranular-hypolobulated neutrophils, giant platelets, macrocytosis, and acanthocytosis)
  - Previous chemotherapy predisposes (especially alkylating agents such as cyclophosphamide and topoisomerase II inhibitors such as etoposide)

- **Differential Diagnosis**
  - Acute myeloid leukemia
  - Aplastic anemia
  - Anemia of chronic disease
  - Alcohol-induced sideroblastic anemia
  - Other causes of specific cytopenias
  - Other causes of macrocytic anemias

- **Treatment**
  - Supportive care with red cell or platelet transfusions
  - Erythropoietin (epoetin alfa), filgrastim (G-CSF), and CC-5013 (Revlimid) may benefit selected patients
  - Low-dose DNA hypomethylating agents (azacitidine, decitabine) may improve blood counts and delay onset of AML
  - Allogeneic bone marrow transplantation for appropriate patients

- **Pearl**

Consider myelodysplastic syndrome in older patients with hematocrits less than 60% of lifetime high and no other obvious cause.

Reference

Hofmann WK, Lubbert M, Hoelzer D, Phillip Koeffler H: Myelodysplastic syndromes. Hematol J 2004;5:1. [PMID: 14745424]

Myelofibrosis

- **Essentials of Diagnosis**
  - Fatigue, abdominal discomfort, bleeding, bone pain
  - Massive splenomegaly, variable hepatomegaly
  - Anemia, leukocytosis or leukopenia; leukoerythroblastic peripheral smear with marked poikilocytosis, giant platelets, left-shifted myeloid series
  - Dry tap on bone marrow aspiration

- **Differential Diagnosis**
  - Chronic myelocytic leukemia
  - Other myeloproliferative disorders
  - Hemolytic anemias
  - Lymphoma
  - Metastatic cancer involving bone marrow
  - Hairy cell leukemia

- **Treatment**
  - Red blood cell transfusion support
  - Androgenic steroids, thalidomide ± prednisone, and interferon alfa may decrease transfusion requirements and reduce spleen size
  - Erythropoietin may be of benefit in selected patients
  - Splenectomy for painful splenomegaly, severe thrombocytopenia, or extraordinary red blood cell requirements
  - Autologous or allogeneic bone marrow transplantation in select patients

- **Pearl**

With hilar adenopathy, transverse myelitis, or any mass lesion complicating myelofibrosis, extramedullary hematopoiesis may be responsible.

Reference

Barosi G: Myelofibrosis with myeloid metaplasia. Hematol Oncol Clin North Am 2003;17:1211. [PMID: 14560783]

Non-Hodgkin's Lymphoma

- **Essentials of Diagnosis**
  - Many symptom-free and come to attention because of lymphadenopathy
  - Fever, night sweats, weight loss in many
  - Common in HIV infection, where isolated central nervous system lymphoma and other extranodal involvement are typical
  - Behaves as though origin is multicentric
  - Variable hepatosplenomegaly; rubbery enlargement of lymph nodes
  - Lymphatic and extranodal masses on imaging; elevated LDH in many, bone marrow positive in one-third
  - Lymph node or involved extranodal tissue biopsies diagnostic; most useful clinical classification separates non-Hodgkin's lymphomas into low, intermediate, and aggressive groups based on immunophenotype, cell morphology, nodal architecture, and cytogenetics

- **Differential Diagnosis**
  - Hodgkin's disease
  - Metastatic cancer
  - Infectious mononucleosis
  - Cat-scratch disease
  - Pseudolymphoma caused by phenytoin
  - Sarcoidosis
  - Primary HIV infection

- **Treatment**
  - Staging with CT scans of the chest, abdomen, and pelvis; gallium or PET scan (for aggressive disease); bone marrow biopsy and lumbar puncture in selected cases
  - Treatment individualized depending on histology and prognostic factors: Age, stage, serum LDH, extranodal disease, performance status
  - With indolent disease, local radiation therapy; chemotherapy for symptomatic, more aggressive advanced disease; monoclonal antibody therapy useful in relapses
  - Autologous bone marrow transplantation effective in relapsed intermediate and highly aggressive lymphoma and perhaps for high-risk primary lymphoma

- **Pearl**

A single intracranial lesion in an AIDS patient is lymphoma; multiple lesions is toxoplasmosis until proved otherwise.

Reference

Hennessy BT, Hanrahan EO, Daly PA: Non-Hodgkin lymphoma: an update. Lancet Oncol 2004;5:341. [PMID: 15172354]

Paroxysmal Nocturnal Hemoglobinuria

■ Essentials of Diagnosis

- Episodic red-brown urine, especially on first morning specimen
- Variable anemia with or without leukopenia, thrombocytopenia; reticulocytosis; positive urine hemosiderin, elevated serum LDH
- Flow cytometry of red cells negative for CD55 or CD59, positive sucrose hemolysis test or Ham's test
- Iron deficiency often concurrent
- Intra-abdominal venous thrombosis in some patients

■ Differential Diagnosis

- Hemolytic anemia
- DIC or hypercoagulable state
- Myelodysplasia
- Aplastic anemia

■ Treatment

- Prednisone for moderate to severe cases
- Oral iron replacement if iron-deficient
- Allogeneic bone marrow transplantation for severe cases
- Long-term anticoagulation for thrombotic events

■ Pearl

One of the few intravascular hemolytic anemias, which leads to iron deficiency; most hemolysis occurs extravascularly with its conservation.

Reference

Smith LJ: Paroxysmal nocturnal hemoglobinuria. Clin Lab Sci 2004;17:172. [PMID: 15314892]

Polycythemia Vera

■ Essentials of Diagnosis

• Acquired myeloproliferative disorder with overproduction of all three hematopoietic cell lines; dominated by erythrocytosis
• Pruritus (especially following a hot shower), tinnitus, blurred vision in some
• Venous thromboses, often in uncommon sites (eg, splenic or portal vein thromboses); plethora, splenomegaly
• Erythrocytosis; eosinophilia, basophilia, thrombocytosis common; elevated total red blood cell mass, normal P_{O_2}
• Increased serum vitamin B_{12}, leukocyte alkaline phosphatase levels usually elevated; hyperuricemia
• Increased incidence of leukemia late in course; higher incidence of peptic ulcer

■ Differential Diagnosis

• Hypoxemia (pulmonary or cardiac disease, high altitude)
• Carboxyhemoglobin (tobacco use)
• Certain hemoglobinopathies characterized by tight O_2 binding
• Congenital erythrocytosis (activating mutations of Epo receptor or VHL gene)
• Erythropoietin-secreting tumors
• Cystic renal disease
• Spurious erythrocytosis with decreased plasma volume and high normal red cell mass (Gaisböck's syndrome)
• Other myeloproliferative disorders

■ Treatment

• Phlebotomy to Hct < 45%
• Hydroxyurea if elevated WBC and platelet count or if patient cannot tolerate phlebotomy
• Myelosuppressive therapy with radiophosphorus (^{32}P) or alkylating agents only for patients with high phlebotomy requirements, intractable pruritus, or marked thrombocytosis
• Avoidance of medicinal iron; low-iron diet
• Aspirin 81–100 mg a day safe and effective in reducing thrombotic risk in all patients without substantially increasing risk of bleeding
• Deep venous thrombosis prophylaxis for any surgical procedure or prolonged period of immobilization

■ Pearl

Do not give iron to a patient with anemia from a bleeding ulcer and a palpable spleen—the hemorrhage may be concealing this disease.

Reference

Stuart BJ, Viera AJ: Polycythemia vera. Am Fam Physician 2004;69:2139. [PMID: 15152961]

Pure Red Cell Aplasia

5

- **Essentials of Diagnosis**
  - Autoimmune disease in which IgG antibody attacks erythroid precursors
  - Lassitude, malaise; nonspecific examination except for pallor
  - Severe anemia with normal red blood cell morphology; myeloid and platelet lines unaffected; low or absent reticulocyte count
  - Reduced or absent erythroid precursors in normocellular marrow
  - Rare associations with systemic lupus erythematosus, chronic lymphocytic leukemia, non-Hodgkin's lymphoma and thymoma

- **Differential Diagnosis**
  - Aplastic anemia
  - Myelodysplastic syndromes
  - Drug-induced red cell aplasia
  - Parvovirus B19 infection

- **Treatment**
  - Evaluate for underlying disease
  - Immunosuppressive therapy with prednisone, cyclophosphamide, antithymocyte globulin, tacrolimus/cyclosporine
  - High-dose intravenous immune globulin in selected patients
  - Thymectomy in patients with thymoma may be beneficial

- **Pearl**

In patients with red cell aplasia and arthritis absent features of systemic lupus erythematosus, parvovirus B19 infection is the diagnosis.

Reference

Djaldetti M, Blay A, Bergman M, Salman H, Bessler H: Pure red cell aplasia— a rare disease with multiple causes. Biomed Pharmacother 2003;57:326. [PMID: 14568226]

Sickle Cell Anemia

- Essentials of Diagnosis
  - Caused by substitution of valine for glutamine in the sixth position on the beta chain
  - Recurrent episodes of fever with pain in arms, legs, or abdomen starting in early childhood
  - Splenomegaly in early childhood *only;* jaundice, pallor; adults are functionally asplenic
  - Anemia and elevated reticulocyte count with irreversibly sickled cells on peripheral smear; elevated indirect bilirubin, LDH; positive sickling test; hemoglobin S and F on electrophoresis
  - Complications include *Salmonella* osteomyelitis, remarkably high incidence of encapsulated infections, and ischemic complications in any sluggish or hypoxic part of the circulation (eg, medullary interstitium of kidney)
  - Five types of crises: Pain, aplastic, megaloblastic, sequestration, hemolytic
  - Positive family history and lifelong history of hemolytic anemia

- Differential Diagnosis
  - Other hemoglobinopathies
  - Acute rheumatic fever
  - Osteomyelitis
  - Acute abdomen due to any cause
  - If hematuria present, renal stone or tumor

- Treatment
  - Chronic oral folic acid supplementation
  - Hydration and analgesics
  - Hydroxyurea for patients with frequent crises
  - Partial exchange transfusions for intractable vaso-occlusive crises, acute chest syndrome, stroke or transient ischemic attack, priapism
  - Transfusion for hemolytic or aplastic crises and during third trimester of pregnancy
  - Pneumonia vaccination
  - Genetic counseling

- Pearl

In regard to sickle cell anemia: anything disease can do, so may trait.

Reference

Claster S, Vichinsky EP: Managing sickle cell disease. BMJ 2003;327:1151. [PMID: 14615343]

Sideroblastic Anemia

- ■ Essentials of Diagnosis
  - Dimorphic (ie, normal and hypochromic) red blood cell population on smear
  - Hematocrit may reach 20%
  - Most often result of clonal stem cell disorder, though rarely may be drugs, lead, or alcohol; may be a megaloblastic component
  - Elevated serum iron with high percentage saturation; marrow is diagnostic with abnormal ringed sideroblasts (iron deposits encircling red blood cell precursor nuclei)
  - Minority progress to acute leukemia

- ■ Differential Diagnosis
  - Iron deficiency anemia
  - Post-transfusion state
  - Anemia of chronic disease
  - Thalassemia

- ■ Treatment
  - Remove offending toxin if present
  - Chelation therapy for lead toxicity
  - Pyridoxine 200 mg/d occasionally helpful
  - Does not respond to erythropoietin (epoetin alfa)

- ■ Pearl

In the anemic alcoholic patient who is not bleeding, sideroblastic anemia may be the diagnosis; reticulocytosis 3 days after discontinuation of ethanol is characteristic, with the serum iron plummeting.

Reference

Alcindor T, Bridges KR: Sideroblastic anaemias. Br J Haematol 2002;116:733. [PMID: 11886376]

Thalassemia Major

- ■ Essentials of Diagnosis
  - • Severe anemia from infancy; positive family history
  - • Massive splenomegaly
  - • Hypochromic, microcytic red cells with severe poikilocytosis, target cells, acanthocytes, and basophilic stippling on smear
  - • Mentzer's index (MCV/RBC) < 13
  - • Greatly elevated hemoglobin F level

- ■ Differential Diagnosis
  - • Other hemoglobinopathies
  - • Congenital nonspherocytic hemolytic anemia

- ■ Treatment
  - • Regular red blood cell transfusions
  - • Oral folic acid supplementation
  - • Splenectomy for secondary hemolysis due to hypersplenism
  - • Deferoxamine to avoid iron overload
  - • Allogeneic bone marrow transplantation in selected cases

- ■ Pearl

With low-MCV anemia in a patient of Mediterranean origin, thalassemia is the presumptive diagnosis until proved otherwise.

Reference

Rund D, Rachmilewitz E: New trends in the treatment of beta-thalassemia. Crit Rev Oncol Hematol 2000;33:105. [PMID: 10737372]

Thrombotic Thrombocytopenic Purpura (TTP)

■ Essentials of Diagnosis
- Petechial rash, mucosal bleeding, fever, altered mental status, renal failure; many cases in HIV infection
- Laboratory reports are notable for anemia, dramatically elevated LDH, normal prothrombin and partial thromboplastin times, fibrin degradation products, and thrombocytopenia
- Most cases probably related to acquired inhibitor of von Willebrand factor–cleaving protease; may also be secondary to drugs, chemotherapy, or cancer
- Demonstrating decreased activity of vWF-cleaving protease inhibitor (ADAMTS13) may be diagnostic, but tests not commonly available

■ Differential Diagnosis
- Disseminated intravascular coagulation
- Preeclampsia-eclampsia
- Other microangiopathic hemolytic anemias
- Catastrophic antiphospholipid antibody syndrome
- Hemolytic-uremic syndrome

■ Treatment
- Immediate plasmapheresis
- Fresh frozen plasma infusions help if plasmapheresis not readily available
- Splenectomy and immunosuppressive or cytotoxic medications for refractory cases

■ Pearl

A previously rare disease which has doubled in incidence during the AIDS epidemic.

Reference

Lammle B, George JN: Thrombotic thrombocytopenic purpura: advances in pathophysiology, diagnosis, and treatment—introduction. Semin Hematol 2004;41:1. [PMID: 14727253]

Vitamin B₁₂ Deficiency

- ■ Essentials of Diagnosis
  - • Dyspnea on exertion, nonspecific gastrointestinal symptoms
  - • Constant symmetric numbness and tingling of the feet; later, poor balance and dementia manifest
  - • Pallor, mild jaundice, decreased vibratory and position sense
  - • Pancytopenia with oval macrocytes and hypersegmented neutrophils, increased MCV, megaloblastic bone marrow; low serum vitamin B_{12}; positive Schilling test
  - • Neurologic manifestations occur without anemia in rare cases, including dementia
  - • Hematologic response to pharmacologic doses of folic acid
  - • History of total gastrectomy, bowel resection, bacterial overgrowth, fish tapeworm, Crohn's disease, or autoimmune endocrinopathies (eg, diabetes mellitus, hypothyroidism)

- ■ Differential Diagnosis
  - • Folic acid deficiency
  - • Myelodysplastic syndromes
  - • Occasional hemolytic anemias with megaloblastic red cell precursors in marrow
  - • Infiltrative granulomatous or malignant processes causing pancytopenia
  - • Hypersplenism
  - • Paroxysmal nocturnal hemoglobinuria
  - • Acute leukemia

- ■ Treatment
  - • Vitamin B_{12} 100 μg intramuscularly daily during first week, then weekly for 1 month
  - • Lifelong B_{12} 100 μg intramuscularly every month thereafter
  - • Hypokalemia may complicate early therapy

- ■ Pearl

An arrest in reticulocytosis shortly after institution of therapy means concealed iron deficiency until proved otherwise.

Reference

Andres E, Loukili NH, Noel E, et al: Vitamin B_{12} (cobalamin) deficiency in elderly patients. CMAJ 2004;171:251. [PMID: 15289425]

Von Willebrand's Disease

- ■ Essentials of Diagnosis
  - • History of lifelong excessive bruising and mucosal bleeding; excessive bleeding during previous surgery, dental extraction, or childbirth
  - • Usually prolonged bleeding time, especially after aspirin, but platelet count normal
  - • Variable abnormalities in factor VIII level, von Willebrand factor, or ristocetin cofactor activity
  - • Prolonged partial thromboplastin time when factor VIII levels decreased

- ■ Differential Diagnosis
  - • Qualitative platelet disorders
  - • Waldenström's macroglobulinemia
  - • Aspirin ingestion
  - • Hemophilias
  - • Dysfibrinogenemia

- ■ Treatment
  - • Avoid aspirin
  - • vWF and factor VIII concentrates for severe bleeding or for surgical procedures in most cases
  - • Desmopressin acetate in type I disease may be sufficient to raise vWF and factor VIII to acceptable levels
  - • Tranexamic acid for bleeding not responsive to other interventions

- ■ Pearl

Remember von Willebrand's disease in patients who have a past surgical history of erratic bleeding patterns; aspirin may have been given in the bleeding instances, other analgesics when hemostasis was more easily achieved.

Reference
Lee JW: von Willebrand disease, hemophilia A and B, and other factor deficiencies. Int Anesthesiol Clin 2004;42:59. [PMID: 15205640]

Waldenström's Macroglobulinemia

■ Essentials of Diagnosis

- Fatigue, symptoms of hyperviscosity (altered mental status, bleeding, or thrombosis)
- Variable hepatosplenomegaly and lymphadenopathy; boxcar retinal vein engorgement
- Anemia with rouleau formation; monoclonal IgM paraprotein; increased serum viscosity; narrowed anion gap
- Lymphoplasmacytoid infiltrate in marrow
- Absence of bone lesions

■ Differential Diagnosis

- Benign monoclonal gammopathy
- Chronic lymphocytic leukemia with M spike
- Multiple myeloma
- Lymphoma

■ Treatment

- Plasmapheresis for severe hyperviscosity (stupor or coma)
- Chemotherapy including chlorambucil, cyclophosphamide, fludarabine, cladribine
- Monoclonal antibody therapy (rituximab) may be effective

■ Pearl

There's rouleaux and then there's rouleaux; some can be found on any blood smear, but they are in every field in Waldenström's and myeloma.

Reference

Ghobrial IM, Gertz MA, Fonseca R: Waldenström macroglobulinaemia. Lancet Oncol 2003;4:679. [PMID: 14602248]

6

Rheumatologic & Autoimmune Disorders

Adult Still's Disease

■ **Essentials of Diagnosis**

- Occurs in younger adults with some cases over fifty
- Fevers > 39°C, daily peak with return to normal temperature, may antedate seronegative arthritis by months; occasional cases entirely nonarticular; sore throat common
- Proximal interphalangeal and metacarpophalangeal joints, wrists, knees, hips, and shoulders are most commonly involved
- Evanescent, salmon-colored maculopapular rash involving the trunk and extremities during fever spikes; may be elicited by mechanical irritation
- Additional findings include hepatosplenomegaly, hepatitis, lymphadenopathy, pleuropericarditis, leukocytosis, thrombocytosis, anemia, and elevations of the erythrocyte sedimentation rate, C-reactive protein level, and ferritin

■ **Differential Diagnosis**

- Leukemia or lymphoma
- Arthritis associated with inflammatory bowel disease or psoriasis
- Acute, early rheumatoid arthritis
- Viral syndrome such as acute HIV
- Chronic infection (eg, culture-negative endocarditis)
- Systemic vasculitis; SLE
- Lyme disease
- Granulomatous diseases (eg, sarcoidosis, Crohn's disease)

■ **Treatment**

- Aspirin often dramatically lyses fever
- NSAIDs (eg, ibuprofen, 800 mg three times daily)
- Corticosteroids, hydroxychloroquine, methotrexate, azathioprine, and other immunosuppressive agents are used as second-line agents

■ **Pearl**

One of three diseases in all of medicine with biquotidian fever spikes; kala azar and gonococcal endocarditis are the others.

Reference

Kadar J, Petrovicz E: Adult-onset Still's disease. Best Pract Res Clin Rheumatol 2004;18:663. [PMID: 15454125]

Amyloidosis

- **Essentials of Diagnosis**
  - A group of disorders characterized by deposition in tissues of ordinarily soluble peptides; can be systemic or localized
  - Four groups when systemic: AL, AA, AB_2M, and genetic
  - AL derived from immunoglobulin light chain associated with plasma cell dyscrasias; peripheral neuropathy, postural hypotension, nephrotic syndrome, cardiomyopathy, gut hypomotility, hepatosplenomegaly, malabsorption, carpal tunnel syndrome, macroglossia, arthropathy, and cutaneous lesions
  - AA derived from serum amyloid A; seen in chronic inflammatory disorders; renal, hepatic involvement common
  - AB_2M derived from B_2 microglobulin that is not filtered in dialysis patients; carpal tunnel syndrome common
  - Genetic amyloid derived from numerous mutant proteins rendered insoluble; many syndromes
  - Beta amyloid protein found in Alzheimer's plaques
  - Green birefringence under polarizing microscope after Congo red staining seen in all tissues infiltrated by amyloid; biopsy of same thus diagnostic

- **Differential Diagnosis**
  - Hemochromatosis
  - Subacute bacterial endocarditis
  - Chronic infection
  - Sarcoidosis
  - Waldenström's macroglobulinemia
  - Metastatic neoplasm
  - Other causes of nephrotic syndrome

- **Treatment**
  - Preventive colchicine in familial Mediterranean fever to prevent AA deposits
  - Melphalan, prednisone, marrow transplant in some
  - Treat underlying disease if present

- **Pearl**

The combination of nephrotic syndrome and hepatosplenomegaly in a middle-aged patient is amyloidosis; only rarely can other single processes cause it.

Reference

Buxbaum JN: The systemic amyloidoses. Curr Opin Rheumatol 2004;16:67. [PMID: 14673392]

Ankylosing Spondylitis

■ Essentials of Diagnosis

- Gradual onset of backache in adults under age 40 with progressive limitation of back motion and chest expansion
- Diminished anterior flexion of lumbar spine, loss of lumbar lordosis, inflammation at tendon insertions
- Peripheral arthritis and anterior uveitis in many
- Aortic insufficiency with cardiac conduction defects in some
- Cauda equina syndrome, apical pulmonary fibrosis are late complications
- HLA-B27 histocompatibility antigen present in over 90% of patients; rheumatoid factor absent
- Radiographic evidence of bilateral sacroiliac joint sclerosis; demineralization and squaring of the vertebral bodies with calcification of the anterior and lateral spinal ligaments (bamboo spine)

■ Differential Diagnosis

- Rheumatoid arthritis
- Osteoporosis
- Reactive arthritis
- Arthritis associated with inflammatory bowel disease
- Psoriatic arthritis
- Diffuse idiopathic skeletal hyperostosis (DISH)
- Synovitis-acne-pustulosis-hyperostosis-osteitis (SAPHO) syndrome

■ Treatment

- Physical therapy to maintain posture and mobility
- NSAIDs (eg, indomethacin 50 mg three times daily) often marginally effective
- Sulfasalazine reported effective in some patients
- Intra-articular corticosteroids for synovitis; ophthalmic corticosteroids for uveitis
- Institute methotrexate in those with persistent arthritis; if symptoms progress or are debilitating initiate anti-tumor necrosis factor agents
- Surgery for severely affected joints

■ Pearl

In a patient with burned-out ankylosing spondylitis and symptomatic benign prostatic hyperplasia, test the cauda equina distribution neurologically before undertaking prostatectomy.

Reference

Kataria RK, Brent LH: Spondyloarthropathies. Am Fam Physician 2004;69:2853. [PMID: 15222650]

Arthritis Associated with Inflammatory Bowel Disease

- ■ Essentials of Diagnosis
  - Peripheral arthritis: Asymmetric oligoarthritis that typically involves the knees, ankles, and occasionally the upper extremities; in some patients with ulcerative colitis, severity of findings can parallel bowel disease activity
  - Spondylitis: Clinically identical to ankylosing spondylitis; also with bilateral sacroiliitis; HLA-B27 antigen present in most patients in a male:female ratio of 4:1
  - Articular features may precede intestinal symptoms, especially in Crohn's disease
  - Extra-articular manifestations may also occur in Crohn's disease (erythema nodosum) and in ulcerative colitis (pyoderma gangrenosum)

- ■ Differential Diagnosis
  - Reactive arthritis
  - Ankylosing spondylitis
  - Psoriatic arthritis
  - Rheumatoid arthritis

- ■ Treatment
  - Treat underlying intestinal inflammation
  - Aspirin, other NSAIDs (eg, indomethacin, 50 mg three times daily)
  - Physical therapy for spondylitis

- ■ Pearl

The younger the patient, the less the gastrointestinal complaints; thus, arthritis in adolescence should prompt a search for inflammatory bowel disease despite absence of symptoms.

Reference

Holden W, Orchard T, Wordsworth P: Enteropathic arthritis. Rheum Dis Clin North Am 2003;29:513, viii. [PMID: 12951865]

Behçet's Syndrome

- **Essentials of Diagnosis**
  - Usually occurs in young adults from Mediterranean countries or Japan; incidence decreases if patient's descendants emigrate elsewhere
  - Most common: Recurrent painful oral aphthous ulcerations (99%) and genital ulcers (80%), ocular lesions in half (uveitis, hypopyon, iritis, keratitis, optic neuritis), and skin lesions (erythema nodosum, superficial thrombophlebitis, cutaneous hypersensitivity, folliculitis)
  - Less common: Gastrointestinal erosions, epididymitis, glomerulonephritis, cranial nerve palsies, aseptic meningitis, and focal neurologic lesions
  - Pathergy test—a papule or a pustule forms 24–48 hours after simple trauma such as a needle prick
  - Diagnosis is clinical
  - HLA-B5 histocompatibility antigen often present

- **Differential Diagnosis**
  - HLA-B27 spondyloarthropathies
  - Oral aphthous ulcers
  - Herpes simplex infection
  - Erythema multiforme
  - SLE
  - HIV infection
  - Infective endocarditis
  - Inflammatory bowel disease

- **Treatment**
  - Local mydriatics in all patients with eye findings to prevent synechiae from forming; close follow-up by experienced ophthalmologist critical
  - Corticosteroids
  - Colchicine (for erythema nodosum and arthralgia)
  - Chlorambucil, azathioprine commonly used; cyclosporine occasionally successful in those with eye disease

- **Pearl**

Stroke in a young native Japanese woman is Behçet's syndrome unless proven otherwise.

Reference

Yurdakul S, Hamuryudan V, Yazici H: Behçet syndrome. Curr Opin Rheumatol 2004;16:38. [PMID: 14673387]

Carpal Tunnel Syndrome

- ■ Essentials of Diagnosis
  - The most common entrapment neuropathy, caused by compression of the median nerve (which innervates the flexor muscles of the wrist and fingers)
  - Middle aged women and those with a history of repetitive use of the hands commonly affected
  - Pain classically worse at night (sleep with hands curled into the body) and exacerbated by hand movement
  - Initial symptoms of pain or paresthesias in thumb, index, middle, and lateral part of ring finger; progression to thenar eminence wasting
  - Pain radiation to forearm, shoulder, neck, chest, or other fingers of the hand not uncommon
  - Positive Tinel's sign
  - Usually idiopathic; in bilateral onset consider secondary causes including rheumatoid arthritis, amyloidosis, sarcoidosis, hypothyroidism, diabetes, pregnancy, acromegaly, gout
  - Diagnosis is primarily clinical; detection of deficits by electrodiagnostic testing (assessing nerve conduction velocity) very helpful to guide referral for surgical release

- ■ Differential Diagnosis
  - C6 or C7 cervical radiculopathy
  - Thoracic outlet syndrome leading to brachial plexus neuropathy
  - Mononeuritis multiplex
  - Syringomyelia
  - Multiple sclerosis
  - Angina pectoris, especially when left-sided

- ■ Treatment
  - Conservative measures initially, including hand rest, splinting, anti-inflammatory medications
  - Steroid injection into the carpal tunnel occasionally
  - Surgical decompression in a few; best done prior to development of thenar atrophy

- ■ Pearl

When obtaining a history of arm pain, remember that carpal tunnel syndrome affects the radial three and one-half fingers and myocardial ischemia the ulnar one and one-half—and hope it's the right arm.

Reference

Katz JN, Simmons BP: Clinical practice. Carpal tunnel syndrome. N Engl J Med 2002;346:1807. [PMID: 12050342]

Chondrocalcinosis & Pseudogout
(Calcium Pyrophosphate Dihydrate Deposition Disease)

- ■ Essentials of Diagnosis
  - • Subacute, recurrent, and underappreciated cause of chronic arthritis, usually involving large joints (especially knees, shoulders, and wrists) and almost always accompanied by chondrocalcinosis of the affected joints
  - • May be hereditary, idiopathic, or associated with metabolic disorders, including hemochromatosis, hypoparathyroidism, osteoarthritis, ochronosis, diabetes mellitus, hypothyroidism, Wilson's disease, and gout
  - • Identification of calcium pyrophosphate rhomboidal crystals (strong positive birefringence) in the joint fluid is diagnostic
  - • Radiographs may reveal chondrocalcinosis or signs of degenerative joint disease at the following sites: Knee (medial meniscus), fibrocartilaginous portion of the symphysis pubica, and articular disk of the wrist with calcium in the triangular ligament

- ■ Differential Diagnosis
  - • Gout
  - • Calcium phosphate disease (hydroxyapatite arthropathy)
  - • Calcium oxalate deposition disease
  - • Degenerative joint disease
  - • Rheumatoid arthritis

- ■ Treatment
  - • Treat underlying disease if present
  - • Aspirin, other NSAIDs (eg, indomethacin, 50 mg three times daily)
  - • Intra-articular injection of corticosteroids (eg, triamcinolone, 10–40 mg)
  - • Colchicine, 0.6 mg twice daily, occasionally useful for prophylaxis

- ■ Pearl

Pseudogout is the clinical syndrome, chondrocalcinosis the radiologic finding; finding the latter does not diagnose the former.

Reference

Ea HK, Liote F: Calcium pyrophosphate dihydrate and basic calcium phosphate crystal-induced arthropathies: update on pathogenesis, clinical features, and therapy. Curr Rheumatol Rep 2004;6:221. [PMID: 15134602]

6

Churg-Strauss Vasculitis
(Allergic Granulomatosis & Angiitis)

- ### Essentials of Diagnosis
  - Granulomatous vasculitis of small- and medium-sized blood vessels
  - Four of the following have a sensitivity of 85% and specificity of 100% for diagnosis: Asthma; allergic rhinitis; transient pulmonary infiltrates; palpable purpura or extravascular eosinophils; mononeuritis multiplex; and peripheral blood eosinophilia

- ### Differential Diagnosis
  - Wegener's granulomatosis
  - Eosinophilic pneumonia
  - Polyarteritis nodosa (often overlaps)
  - Hypersensitivity vasculitis

- ### Treatment
  - Corticosteroids
  - Cyclophosphamide in addition probably has better outcome

- ### Pearl

Leukotriene inhibitors such as montelukast, given for asthma, have been implicated as causing some cases of Churg-Strauss syndrome.

Reference

Noth I, Strek ME, Leff AR: Churg-Strauss syndrome. Lancet 2003;361:587. [PMID: 12598156]

Cryoglobulinemia

- ■ Essentials of Diagnosis
  - • Refers to any globulin precipitable at lower than body temperature
  - • Any elevation of globulin may be associated
  - • Monoclonal gammopathies, reactive hypergammaglobulinemia, cryoprecipitable immune complexes are associated with acral cold symptoms because of higher titers of cryoproteins
  - • Essential mixed cryoglobulinemia occurs in patients serologically positive for hepatitis C
  - • Symptoms and signs depend upon type; most common are palpable purpura, arthralgias, and nephritis
  - • Low erythrocyte sedimentation rate

- ■ Differential Diagnosis
  - • Multiple myeloma, Waldenström's macroglobulinemia
  - • Chronic inflammatory diseases such as endocarditis, sarcoidosis, rheumatoid arthritis, Sjögren's syndrome

- ■ Treatment
  - • Entirely dependent on cause

- ■ Pearl

In a patient with back pain whose blood "clots" per the laboratory despite heparinization of the specimen, the diagnosis is myeloma with a cryoprecipitable M-spike.

Reference

Ferri C, Zignego AL, Pileri SA: Cryoglobulins. J Clin Pathol 2002;55:4. [PMID: 11825916]

Degenerative Joint Disease (Osteoarthritis)

- ■ Essentials of Diagnosis
  - Progressive degeneration of articular cartilage and hypertrophy of bone at the articular margin
  - Affects almost all joints, especially weight-bearing and frequently used joints; hips, knees, shoulders, and first carpometacarpal joint (thumb on dominant hand) most common
  - Primary degenerative joint disease most commonly affects the terminal interphalangeal joints (Heberden's nodes), hips, and first carpometacarpal joints
  - Morning stiffness brief; pain worse with use
  - Radiographs reveal narrowing of the joint spaces, osteophytes, subchondral sclerosis and cyst formation

- ■ Differential Diagnosis
  - Rheumatoid arthritis
  - Seronegative spondyloarthropathies
  - Crystal-induced arthritides
  - Hyperparathyroidism
  - Multiple myeloma
  - Hemochromatosis

- ■ Treatment
  - Weight reduction; exercise to strengthen periarticular muscle
  - NSAIDs or acetaminophen
  - Glucosamine and chondroitin sulfate possibly effective
  - Topical capsaicin cream on large affected joints may help some
  - Intra-articular corticosteroid injection (eg, triamcinolone, 10–40 mg) in selected patients (up to 3 times yearly)
  - Surgery for severely affected joints, especially hip and knee; timing dictated by debilitating pain

- ■ Pearl

Morning stiffness lasts an hour in rheumatoid arthritis, fifteen minutes in degenerative joint disease.

Reference

Haq I, Murphy E, Dacre J: Osteoarthritis. Postgrad Med J 2003;79:377. [PMID: 12897215]

Eosinophilic Fasciitis

- ■ Essentials of Diagnosis
    - • Occurs predominantly in men
    - • Pain, swelling, stiffness, and tenderness of the hands, forearms, feet, or legs, evolving to woody induration and retraction of subcutaneous tissue within days to weeks
    - • Associated with peripheral eosinophilia, polyarthralgias, arthritis, carpal tunnel syndrome; no Raynaud's phenomenon
    - • Biopsy of deep fascia is diagnostic
    - • Association with aplastic anemia, thrombocytopenia

6

- ■ Differential Diagnosis
    - • Systemic sclerosis
    - • Eosinophilia myalgia syndrome
    - • Hypothyroidism
    - • Trichinosis
    - • Mixed connective tissue disease

- ■ Treatment
    - • NSAIDs
    - • Short course of corticosteroids
    - • Antimalarials

- ■ Pearl

Perhaps the only systemic disease in medicine confined strictly to the fascia.

Reference

Pope JE: Scleroderma overlap syndromes. Curr Opin Rheumatol 2002;14:704. [PMID: 12410095]

Fibrositis (Fibromyalgia)

- ■ Essentials of Diagnosis
  - • Most frequent in women ages 20–50
  - • Chronic aching pain and stiffness of trunk and extremities, especially around the neck, shoulder, low back, and hips
  - • Elicit pain with mild palpation (enough pressure to blanch your fingernail) at 11 of 18 bilateral tender points: Occiput, low cervical, trapezius, supraspinatus, second rib at costochondral junction, lateral epicondyle, gluteal region, greater trochanter, and medial fat pad of the knee
  - • Associated with fatigue, headaches, subjective numbness, irritable bowel symptoms; often occurs following a physically or emotionally traumatic event
  - • Nearly universal description of non-restful sleep
  - • Absence of objective signs of inflammation; normal laboratory studies, including erythrocyte sedimentation rate
  - • A diagnosis of exclusion after you work through the following differential diagnosis

- ■ Differential Diagnosis
  - • Chronic fatigue syndrome
  - • Hypothyroidism
  - • Hypocalcemia
  - • Lymphoma
  - • Paraneoplastic syndrome
  - • Rheumatoid arthritis
  - • SLE
  - • Depression
  - • Polymyalgia rheumatica
  - • HIV disease

- ■ Treatment
  - • Reassure patient that that you have ruled out cancer or chronic infection; despite the pain, this is a nonlethal disease
  - • Patients who improve are those who identify some physical activity they enjoy and can do without exertion
  - • Aspirin, other NSAIDs
  - • Tricyclics offer transient relief related to anti-insomniac effect; cyclobenzaprine, chlorpromazine
  - • Injection of trigger points with corticosteroids works for some

- ■ Pearl

Consider the diagnosis in patients who exhibit the "wince reflex": they wince each time you touch them during your exam.

Reference

Bennett RM: The rational management of fibromyalgia patients. Rheum Dis Clin North Am 2002;28:181, v. [PMID: 12122913]

Gonococcal Arthritis

■ Essentials of Diagnosis

- Two clinical scenarios: (1) Septic joint with mono- or oligoartic-ular involvement and no skin changes; or (2) a systemic process with oligoarticular arthritis, tenosynovitis, and characteristic purpuric skin lesions on the distal extremities
- Septic joint variant: White cell count in synovial fluid 20,000–50,000/μL; synovial fluid Gram's stain and culture more likely to be positive
- Systemic presentation variant: Lower synovial cell counts, negative Gram's stain and culture of joint fluid since signs secondary to inflammation due to bacterial debris, not direct infection
- Urethral, cervical, throat, skin lesion, and rectal cultures on chocolate or Thayer-Martin agar for *Neisseria gonorrhoeae* have higher yield, may be positive in the absence of symptoms
- Recurrent disseminated gonococcal infection seen with congenital complement component deficiencies

■ Differential Diagnosis

- Nongonococcal bacterial arthritis
- Reactive arthritis
- Lyme disease
- Sarcoidosis
- Infective endocarditis
- Meningococcemia with arthritis
- Seronegative spondyloarthropathy
- Acute viral hepatitis

■ Treatment

- Obtain VDRL, consider HIV testing
- Intravenous ceftriaxone or ceftizoxime for 7 days followed by oral cefixime or ciprofloxacin
- Daily reaspiration of the synovial fluid if it reaccumulates

■ Pearl

A negative sexual exposure history does not rule out the diagnosis; get all the cultures.

Reference

Bardin T: Gonococcal arthritis. Best Pract Res Clin Rheumatol 2003;17:201. [PMID: 12787521]

Gout

- ■ Essentials of Diagnosis
  - Especially common among native Pacific Islanders
  - Broad spectrum of disease, including recurrent arthritic attacks, tophi, interstitial nephropathy, and uric acid nephrolithiasis
  - First attack typically nocturnal and usually monarticular, with pain "worsened by the weight of the bedsheet"; may become polyarticular with repeated attacks
  - Affects in descending order of frequency: The first metatarsophalangeal joint (podagra), mid foot, ankle, knee, wrist, elbow; hips and shoulders typically spared
  - Hyperuricemia may be primary (caused by overproduction [10%] or underexcretion [90%] of uric acid) or secondary to diuretic use, cytotoxic drugs (especially cyclosporine), myeloproliferative disorders, multiple myeloma, chronic renal disease
  - After long periods of untreated gout, tophi (monosodium urate deposits with an associated foreign body reaction) develop in subcutaneous tissues, cartilage, ears, and other tissues
  - Identification of weakly negatively birefringent, needlelike sodium urate crystals in joint fluid or tophi is diagnostic

- ■ Differential Diagnosis
  - Cellulitis
  - Septic arthritis
  - Pseudogout
  - Rheumatoid arthritis
  - Chronic lead intoxication (saturnine gout)

- ■ Treatment
  - Treat the acute arthritis first and the hyperuricemia later
  - For acute attacks: Dramatic therapeutic response to NSAIDs (eg, indomethacin, 50 mg three times daily), intra-articular or systemic corticosteroids
  - For chronic prophylaxis in patients with frequent acute attacks, tophaceous deposits, or renal damage: Allopurinol and probenecid (uricosuric agent) with concomitant oral colchicine
  - Avoid thiazides and loop diuretics

- ■ Pearl

Long-standing "rheumatoid arthritis" sparing the shoulders and hips is most likely gout.

Reference

Terkeltaub RA: Clinical practice. Gout. N Engl J Med 2003;349:1647. [PMID: 14573737]

Hypersensitivity Vasculitis

- **Essentials of Diagnosis**
  - Necrotizing vasculitis of small blood vessels
  - Palpable purpura of lower extremities the predominant feature; skin biopsy yields findings of leukocytoclastic vasculitis
  - Most commonly occurs in response to a new antigen: Numerous medications, neoplasms, serum sickness, viral or bacterial infection, or congenital complement deficiency
  - On occasion associated with fever, arthralgias, abdominal pain with or without gastrointestinal bleeding, pulmonary infiltrates, kidney involvement with hematuria

- **Differential Diagnosis**
  - Polyarteritis nodosa
  - Henoch-Schönlein purpura
  - Essential mixed cryoglobulinemia
  - ANCA-associated vasculitides (Wegener's, MPAN)
  - Meningococcemia
  - Gonococcemia

- **Treatment**
  - Treat underlying disease if present
  - Discontinue offending drug
  - Corticosteroids in severe cases

- **Pearl**

The palpable purpura of hypersensitivity vasculitis is dependent, and thus is scattered across the legs of the ambulatory patient but prominent on the sacrum and hamstrings of the bedfast patient.

Reference

Cuellar ML: Drug-induced vasculitis. Curr Rheumatol Rep 2002;4:55. [PMID: 11798983]

Infectious Osteomyelitis

■ Essentials of Diagnosis

- Infection usually occurs via hematogenous seeding of the bone; metaphyses of long bones and vertebrae most frequently involved
- Subacute vague pain and tenderness of affected bone or back with little or no fever in adults; more acute presentation in children
- Organisms include *Staphylococcus aureus,* coagulase-negative staphylococci, group A streptococci, gram-negative rods, anaerobic and polymicrobial infections, tuberculosis, brucellosis, histoplasmosis, coccidioidomycosis, blastomycosis
- Blood cultures may be negative; biopsy of bone is diagnostic
- Radiographs early in the course are often negative, but periostitis may be detected 2–3 weeks into the course, followed by periarticular demineralization and erosion of bone
- Radionuclide bone scan is 90% sensitive and may be positive within 2 days after onset of symptoms, though offers no information as to pathogen

■ Differential Diagnosis

- Acute bacterial arthritis
- Rheumatic fever
- Cellulitis
- Multiple myeloma
- Ewing's sarcoma
- Metastatic neoplasia

■ Treatment

- Intravenous antibiotics after appropriate cultures have been obtained
- Oral ciprofloxacin, 750 mg twice daily for 6–8 weeks, may be effective in limited osteomyelitis
- In older patients, treat with broad-spectrum antibiotics as for a gram-negative bacteremia as a consequence of urinary, biliary, intestinal, and lower respiratory infections
- Débridement if response to antibiotics is poor

■ Pearl

In chronic osteomyelitis: once an osteo, always an osteo.

Reference

Lew DP, Waldvogel FA: Osteomyelitis. Lancet 2004;364:369. [PMID: 15276398]

Microscopic Polyangiitis (MPAN)

■ Essentials of Diagnosis
- Necrotizing vasculitis affecting arterioles, capillaries, and venules
- Presents with rapidly progressive glomerular nephritis (RPGN), often with palpable purpura; diffuse alveolar hemorrhage in some
- 80% of cases ANCA-associated, most often in the P-ANCA pattern with anti-myeloperoxidase antibodies; like all ANCA-associated vasculitides, affects men and women equally with predilection for whites more than blacks
- Diagnosis most often made on renal biopsy showing pauci-immune RPGN

■ Differential Diagnosis
- Polyarteritis nodosa
- Wegener's granulomatosis
- Churg-Strauss vasculitis
- Goodpasture's syndrome
- Cryoglobulinemic vasculitis

■ Treatment
- Institute intravenous steroids acutely with cytotoxic agents such as cyclophosphamide
- Maintenance therapy can include steroids, with cyclophosphamide or azathioprine

■ Pearl

The abnormal ANCA alone is insufficient to make this diagnosis: tissue is the issue.

Reference

Seo P, Stone JH: The antineutrophil cytoplasmic antibody-associated vasculitides. Am J Med 2004;117:39. [PMID: 15210387]

Polyarteritis Nodosa

- ■ **Essentials of Diagnosis**
  - Systemic illness causing inflammation and necrosis of medium-sized arteries
  - Distribution of affected arteries dictates clinical manifestations which include: Fever, hypertension, abdominal pain, arthralgias, myalgias, cotton-wool spots and microaneurysms in fundus, pericarditis, myocarditis, palpable purpura, mononeuritis multiplex, livedo reticularis, ischemic bowel, and nonglomerulonephritic renal failure
  - Acceleration of sedimentation rate in most; serologic evidence of hepatitis B or hepatitis C in 30–50%
  - P-ANCA positive in less than 20% of cases
  - Diagnosis confirmed by biopsy or visceral angiography

- ■ **Differential Diagnosis**
  - Wegener's granulomatosis
  - Churg-Strauss vasculitis
  - Hypersensitivity vasculitis
  - Subacute endocarditis
  - Essential mixed cryoglobulinemia
  - Microscopic polyangiitis (MPAN)
  - Cholesterol atheroembolic disease

- ■ **Treatment**
  - Corticosteroids with cyclophosphamide for systemic vasculitis; azathioprine is used as a maintenance immunosuppressant

- ■ **Pearl**

PAN seldom causes glomerulonephritis; if you observe hematuria with RBC casts or dysmorphic reds, consider an alternative diagnosis.

Reference

Herbert CR, Russo GG: Polyarteritis nodosa and cutaneous polyarteritis nodosa. Skin Med 2003;2:277; quiz 284. [PMID: 14673260]

Polymyalgia Rheumatica & Giant Cell Arteritis

- **Essentials of Diagnosis**
  - Patients usually over age 50
  - Polymyalgia rheumatica characterized by pain and stiffness (often morning stiffness), not weakness, of the shoulder and pelvic girdle lasting 1 month or more without evidence of infection or malignancy
  - Associated with fever, little if any joint swelling, sedimentation rate > 40 mm/h, and dramatic response to prednisone 15 mg/d
  - Giant cell (temporal) arteritis frequently coexists with polymyalgia rheumatica; headache, jaw claudication, temporal artery tenderness
  - Monocular vision changes represent medical emergencies; blindness is permanent
  - Diagnosis confirmation by 5 cm temporal artery biopsy remains reliable for 1–2 weeks after starting steroids

- **Differential Diagnosis**
  - Multiple myeloma
  - Chronic infection, eg, endocarditis, visceral abscess
  - Neoplasm
  - Rheumatoid arthritis
  - Depression
  - Myxedema
  - Carotid plaque with embolic amaurosis fugax
  - Carotid Takayasu's arteritis

- **Treatment**
  - Prednisone 10–20 mg/d for polymyalgia rheumatica
  - Prednisone 60 mg/d immediately on suspicion of temporal arteritis; treat for at least 4 months depending on response of symptoms—not sedimentation rate
  - Methotrexate or azathioprine spares steroids in some patients with side effects on high doses

- **Pearl**

Instruct patients with polymyalgia rheumatica to keep 60 mg of prednisone with them at all times; they should take it and seek care immediately if visual symptoms develop.

Reference

Weyand CM, Goronzy JJ: Giant-cell arteritis and polymyalgia rheumatica. Ann Intern Med 2003;139:505. [PMID: 13679329]

Polymyositis-Dermatomyositis

- **Essentials of Diagnosis**
  - Bilateral proximal muscle weakness for both entities
  - Dermatomyositis characterized by true weakness and skin changes: Periorbital edema and a purplish (heliotrope) rash over the upper eyelids in many; violaceous, occasionally scaly papules overlying the dorsal surface of the interphalangeal joints of the hands (Gottron's papules)
  - Serum CK and aldolase elevated; ANA uncommonly positive save in overlap syndromes; anti-Jo-1 antibodies in the subset of patients who have associated interstitial lung disease; anti-Mi-2 is more specific for dermatomyositis but is insensitive
  - Muscle biopsy and characteristic electromyographic pattern are diagnostic
  - May be associated with rheumatoid arthritis, SLE, scleroderma, or mixed connective tissue disease, in which case it is called overlap syndrome
  - Dermatomyositis associated with increased incidence of malignancy; may precede or follow detection of cancer

- **Differential Diagnosis**
  - Endocrine myopathies (eg, hyperthyroidism, Cushing's)
  - Polymyalgia rheumatica
  - Myasthenia gravis; Eaton-Lambert syndrome
  - Muscular dystrophy
  - Rhabdomyolysis
  - Parasitic myositis
  - Drug-induced myopathies (eg, corticosteroids, alcohol, colchicine, statins, zidovudine, hydroxychloroquine)
  - Adult glycogen storage disease
  - Mitochondrial myopathy

- **Treatment**
  - Corticosteroids are cornerstone initially
  - Methotrexate or azathioprine spares steroids, start early in therapy
  - Intravenous immune globulin for some cases of dermatomyositis
  - Search for malignancy should encompass age-appropriate cancer screening and follow-up on abnormalities detected on physical exam or basic laboratory evaluation

- **Pearl**

Biopsy at the site of a previous EMG will show inflammation; pick the same muscle on the other side.

Reference

Dalakas MC, Hohlfeld R: Polymyositis and dermatomyositis. Lancet 2003; 362:971. [PMID: 14511932]

Psoriatic Arthritis

- **Essentials of Diagnosis**
  - Classically a destructive arthritis of distal interphalangeal joints; many patients also have peripheral arthritis involving shoulders, elbows, wrists, knees, and ankles, often asymmetrically
  - Sacroiliitis (unilateral) in B27-positive patients
  - Occurs in 15–20% of patients with psoriasis; small number experience inflammatory arthritis absent characteristic skin changes
  - Psoriatic arthritis associated with nail pitting, onycholysis, sausage digits, arthritis mutilans (severe deforming arthritis)
  - Rheumatoid factor negative; serum uric acid may be elevated
  - Radiographs may reveal irregular destruction of joint spaces and bone, pencil-in-cup deformity of the phalanges, sacroiliitis

- **Differential Diagnosis**
  - Rheumatoid arthritis
  - Ankylosing spondylitis
  - Arthritis associated with inflammatory bowel disease
  - Reactive arthritis
  - Juvenile spondyloarthropathy

- **Treatment**
  - NSAIDs (eg, ibuprofen, 800 mg three times daily)
  - Sulfasalazine reportedly effective in patients with symmetric polyarthritis
  - Intra-articular corticosteroid injection; sterilize skin carefully as psoriatic lesions are colonized with staphylococci and streptococci
  - Methotrexate useful, institute early
  - Anti-TNF agents very effective
  - Treatment of psoriasis helpful in many but not in sacroiliitis

- **Pearl**

In an inflammatory arthritis of uncertain cause, look for early signs of psoriasis in the intergluteal folds, the umbilicus, and along the hairline.

Reference

Mease PJ: Current treatment of psoriatic arthritis. Rheum Dis Clin North Am 2003;29:495. [PMID: 12951864]

Reactive Arthritis

- ■ Essentials of Diagnosis
  - Predominantly diagnosed in young men but also occurs in women (painless vaginal mucosal lesions often not appreciated)
  - Triad of urethritis, conjunctivitis (or uveitis), and arthritis, occur synchronously in 10% of cases (Reiter's syndrome); conjunctivitis may be subtle and evanescent
  - Follows invasive dysenteric infection (with *Shigella, Salmonella, Yersinia, Campylobacter*) or sexually transmitted infection (with *Chlamydia*)
  - Asymmetric, oligoarticular arthritis typically involving the knees and ankles; look for tendinitis and plantar fasciitis
  - Associated with fever, mucocutaneous lesions, stomatitis, optic neuritis, circinate balanitis, prostatitis, keratoderma blenorrhagicum (nearly indistinguishable from psoriatic lesions), pericarditis, and aortic regurgitation
  - HLA-B27 histocompatibility antigen in most

- ■ Differential Diagnosis
  - Gonococcal arthritis
  - Rheumatoid arthritis
  - Ankylosing spondylitis
  - Psoriatic arthritis
  - Arthritis associated with inflammatory bowel disease
  - Juvenile spondyloarthropathy

- ■ Treatment
  - NSAIDs (eg, indomethacin, 50 mg three times daily); often ineffective
  - Tetracycline for associated *Chlamydia trachomatis* infection; obtain VDRL, consider HIV testing
  - Azathioprine, methotrexate when NSAIDs insufficient to control inflammation
  - Sulfasalazine may help in some patients
  - Intra-articular corticosteroids for arthritis, ophthalmic corticosteroids for uveitis

- ■ Pearl

Synovial fluid occasionally shows characteristic cells: large mononuclear cell with ingested polymorphonuclear leukocytes which may have inclusion bodies.

Reference

Flores D, Marquez J, Garza M, Espinoza LR: Reactive arthritis: newer developments. Rheum Dis Clin North Am 2003;29:37, vi. [PMID: 12635499]

Reflex Sympathetic Dystrophy

- **Essentials of Diagnosis**
  - Severe pain and tenderness, most commonly of the hand or foot, associated with vasomotor instability, skin atrophy, edema and hyperhidrosis; atrophic, nonfunctional hand or foot seen late in disease
  - Usually follows direct trauma to the hand, foot, or knee, stroke, peripheral nerve injury, or arthroscopic knee surgery
  - Shoulder-hand variant with restricted ipsilateral shoulder movement common after neck or shoulder injuries or following myocardial infarction
  - Characteristic disparity between degree of injury (usually modest) and degree of pain (debilitating)
  - Triple phase bone scan reveals increased uptake in the early phases of the disease; radiographs show severe osteopenia (Sudeck's atrophy) late in the course

- **Differential Diagnosis**
  - Rheumatoid arthritis
  - Polymyositis
  - Scleroderma
  - Gout, pseudogout
  - Acromegaly
  - Multiple myeloma
  - Osteoporosis due to other causes

- **Treatment**
  - Supportive care
  - Physical therapy is critical to salvage extremity function; active and passive exercises combined with benzodiazepines
  - Stellate ganglion or lumbar sympathetic block
  - Short course of corticosteroids given early in course

- **Pearl**

Exquisite pain in the asymmetrically swollen distal extremity, consider RSD.

Reference

Schott GD: Reflex sympathetic dystrophy. J Neurol Neurosurg Psychiatry 2001;71:291. No abstract available. [PMID: 11511699]

Rheumatoid Arthritis

■ Essentials of Diagnosis

- A disease of younger women, though may occur in both genders
- Symmetric, inflammatory, destructive polyarthritis of peripheral joints, often involving wrists and hands
- Symptoms of stiffness worse with disuse (eg, morning stiffness)
- Chronic, persistent synovitis with formation of pannus that erodes cartilage, bone, ligaments, and tendons
- Joint deformities may develop; ulnar deviation common
- IgM rheumatoid factor present in up to 85%; 20% of seropositive patients have subcutaneous nodules
- Extra-articular manifestations, most common among strongly seropositive patients with nodules, include systemic vasculitis, pleural exudative effusion (low in glucose), scleritis, sicca symptoms, Felty's syndrome
- Radiographic findings include juxta-articular and sometimes generalized osteopenia, narrowing of the joint spaces, and bony erosions, particularly of the MCPs and ulnar styloid

■ Differential Diagnosis

- SLE
- Degenerative joint disease
- Polymyalgia rheumatica
- Polyarticular gout or pseudogout
- Lyme disease
- Serum sickness
- Inflammatory osteoarthritis
- Parvovirus B19 infection

■ Treatment

- Pharmacologic doses of aspirin, other NSAIDs
- Disease-modifying anti-rheumatic drugs (DMARDs), including methotrexate, sulfasalazine, hydroxychloroquine, azathioprine, and leflunomide (alone or in combination) in patients with moderate disease activity
- Refractory disease and the presence of poor prognostic features may be treated with anti-TNF therapy (infliximab or etanercept, after assessing risk of tuberculosis and other infections)
- Surgery for severely affected joints

■ Pearl

A flare of a single joint in a patient with established rheumatoid arthritis is a septic joint until proved otherwise.

Reference

O'Dell JR: Therapeutic strategies for rheumatoid arthritis. N Engl J Med 2004;350:2591. [PMID: 15201416]

Septic Arthritis
(Nongonococcal Acute Bacterial Arthritis)

- ■ Essentials of Diagnosis
  - Acute pain, swelling, erythema, warmth, and limited movement of joints
  - Typically monarticular; knee, hip, wrist, shoulder, or ankle most often involved
  - Infection usually occurs via hematogenous seeding of the synovium
  - Previous joint damage (eg, DJD, erosive arthritis) and intravenous drug abuse predispose
  - Most common organisms: *Staphylococcus aureus,* group A streptococci, *Escherichia coli,* and *Pseudomonas aeruginosa; Haemophilus influenzae* in children under 5 years of age; *Staphylococcus epidermidis* following arthroscopy or joint surgery
  - White cell count in synovial fluid > 50,000/μL; synovial fluid culture positive in 50–75%, blood culture in 50%

- ■ Differential Diagnosis
  - Gonococcal arthritis
  - Microcrystalline synovitis
  - Rheumatoid arthritis
  - Still's disease
  - Infective endocarditis (may be associated)

- ■ Treatment
  - Intravenous antibiotics should be administered empirically
  - Joint will require serial draining procedures either by needle aspiration or in the operating room if joint involved is inaccessible at the bedside (eg, shoulder, hip)
  - Rest, immobilization, and elevation
  - Removal of prosthetic joint or other foreign implants to prevent development of osteomyelitis

- ■ Pearl

Pneumococcal arthritis in the absence of pneumonia or endocarditis means multiple myeloma until proved otherwise.

Reference

Nade S: Septic arthritis. Best Pract Res Clin Rheumatol 2003;17:183. [PMID: 12787520]

Sjögren's Syndrome

- **Essentials of Diagnosis**
  - Destruction of exocrine glands, leading to mucosal and conjunctival dryness secondary to inflammatory infiltrate
  - Dry mouth (xerostomia) and dry eyes (keratoconjunctivitis sicca), decreased tear production, parotid enlargement, severe dental caries, loss of taste and smell
  - Occasionally associated with glomerulonephritis, renal tubular acidosis, biliary cirrhosis, pancreatitis, neuropsychiatric dysfunction, polyneuropathy, interstitial pneumonitis, thyroiditis, cardiac conduction defects
  - Over 50% have cytoplasmic antibodies, anti-Ro (SS-A), and anti-La (SS-B)
  - Decreased lacrimation measured by Schirmer's filter paper test; biopsy of minor salivary glands of lower lip confirms diagnosis
  - Secondary form may also be observed in patients with rheumatoid arthritis, SLE, systemic sclerosis, polymyositis, or polyarteritis

- **Differential Diagnosis**
  - Sarcoidosis
  - Sialolithiasis
  - Tuberculosis
  - Lymphoma
  - Waldenström's macroglobulinemia
  - Anticholinergic medications
  - Chronic irritation from smoking

- **Treatment**
  - Symptomatic relief of dryness with artificial tears, chewing gum, sialagogues
  - Cholinergic drugs such as pilocarpine
  - Meticulous care of teeth and avoidance of sugar-containing candies
  - Corticosteroids or azathioprine; cyclophosphamide for peripheral neuropathy, interstitial pneumonitis, glomerulonephritis, and vasculitis

- **Pearl**

Consider sarcoidosis or parotitis before making the diagnosis of Sjögren's syndrome.

Reference

Kassan SS, Moutsopoulos HM: Clinical manifestations and early diagnosis of Sjögren syndrome. Arch Intern Med 2004;164:1275. [PMID: 15226160]

Systemic Lupus Erythematosus

■ Essentials of Diagnosis

- Multisystem inflammatory autoimmune disorder with periods of exacerbation and remission, principally in young women
- Four or more of the following 11 criteria must be present: malar and discoid rashes; photosensitivity; oral ulcers; arthritis; serositis; renal and neurologic disease; immune hematologic disorders (eg, Coombs-positive hemolytic anemia and thrombocytopenia); positive antinuclear antibody or other immunopathies (eg, antibody to native double-stranded DNA or Sm antigen, false-positive RPR)
- Also associated with fever, myositis, alopecia, myocarditis, vasculitis, lymphadenopathy, conjunctivitis, antiphospholipid antibodies with hypercoagulability and miscarriages
- Renal involvement includes crescentic, mesangial, and less commonly, membranous glomerulonephritis
- Syndrome may be drug-induced (eg, procainamide, hydralazine), primarily serosal and cutaneous, not renal or neurological

■ Differential Diagnosis

- Rheumatoid arthritis
- Vasculitis
- Sjögren's syndrome
- Systemic sclerosis
- Endocarditis
- Lymphoma
- Glomerulonephritis due to other cause

■ Treatment

- Mild disease (ie, arthralgias with dermatologic findings) often responds to hydroxychloroquine and NSAIDs
- Moderate disease activity (ie, refractory to antimalarials): Corticosteroids and azathioprine, methotrexate, or mycophenolate mofetil
- Corticosteroids and cyclophosphamide for lupus cerebritis and lupus nephritis
- Avoid sun exposure

■ Pearl

The so-called lupus anticoagulant is in fact associated with hypercoagulability; the name refers to an in-vitro phenomenon prolonging the PTT.

Reference

Dall'Era M, Davis JC: SLE. How to manage, when to refer. Postgrad Med 2003;114:31, 40. [PMID: 14650091]

Systemic Sclerosis (Scleroderma)

- ■ Essentials of Diagnosis
  - • Diffuse systemic sclerosis (20%): Proximal skin thickening; interstitial lung disease; greater risk of hypertensive renal crisis
  - • Limited disease (80%) or CREST syndrome (calcinosis cutis, Raynaud's phenomenon, esophageal hypomotility, sclerodactyly, and telangiectasia): Skin tightening in distal extremities and feet; lower risk of renal disease; more commonly develop pulmonary hypertension and biliary cirrhosis
  - • For both forms, Raynaud's phenomenon typical; if severe can lead to acral ulceration; may be associated with intestinal hypomotility, myocarditis, pericarditis, hypertension
  - • ANA frequently useful in systemic sclerosis; anticentromere antibody positive in 1% of patients with diffuse scleroderma and 50% of those with limited form; antitopoisomerase I (Scl-70) in one-third of patients with diffuse systemic sclerosis and 20% of those with limited form, and a poor prognostic factor

- ■ Differential Diagnosis
  - • Eosinophilic fasciitis
  - • Overlap syndromes with scleroderma
  - • Graft-versus-host disease
  - • Amyloidosis
  - • Raynaud's disease
  - • Cryoglobulinemia

- ■ Treatment
  - • Focus is on symptomatic relief since no effective disease modifiers exist
  - • Angiotensin-converting enzyme blockers to treat hypertensive crisis occasionally seen in patients with diffuse systemic sclerosis
  - • Corticosteroids not helpful and may even precipitate renal crisis; penicillamine also not helpful
  - • Cyclophosphamide may provide benefit in those with interstitial lung disease
  - • Warm clothing, smoking cessation, and extended-release calcium channel blockers for Raynaud's phenomenon; intravenous iloprost may be helpful for digital ulcers
  - • H_2-receptor antagonists or omeprazole for esophageal reflux

- ■ Pearl

Malabsorption in systemic sclerosis is due not to intestinal fibrosis but to bacterial overgrowth from hypomotility.

Reference

Valentini G, Black C: Systemic sclerosis. Best Pract Res Clin Rheumatol 2002;16:807. [PMID: 12473275]

Takayasu's Arteritis ("Pulseless Disease")

- ■ Essentials of Diagnosis
  - Large-vessel vasculitis involving the aortic arch and its major branches
  - Seen most commonly in the third to fifth decade of life with predominance in women
  - Associated most commonly with absent peripheral pulses; may see myalgias, arthralgias, headaches, angina, claudication, erythema nodosum–like lesions, hypertension, bruits, cerebrovascular insufficiency, aortic insufficiency
  - Angiography reveals narrowing, stenosis, and aneurysms of the aortic arch and its major branches
  - Bruits may be heard over the subclavian arteries or aorta in up to 40% of patients; additionally, there may be a >10 mm Hg difference in systolic blood pressure in the two arms
  - Rich collateral flow visible in the shoulder, chest, and neck areas

- ■ Differential Diagnosis
  - Giant cell arteritis
  - Syphilitic aortitis
  - Severe atherosclerosis

- ■ Treatment
  - Corticosteroids
  - Cyclophosphamide or methotrexate added for severe disease
  - Surgical bypass or reconstruction of affected vessels

- ■ Pearl

Clinically and pathologically identical to giant cell arteritis except in the strikingly disparate epidemiology.

Reference

Johnston SL, Lock RJ, Gompels MM: Takayasu arteritis: a review. J Clin Pathol 2002;55:481. [PMID: 12101189]

Thromboangiitis Obliterans (Buerger's Disease)

- **Essentials of Diagnosis**
  - Inflammatory disease involving small- and medium-sized arteries and veins of the distal upper and lower extremities
  - Described first in young men who were heavy cigarette smokers, but since observed in men and women alike of any age
  - Associated with migratory superficial segmental thrombophlebitis of superficial veins, absent peripheral pulses, claudication, numbness, paresthesias, Raynaud's phenomenon, ulceration and gangrene of fingertips and toes
  - Angiography reveals multiple occluded segments in the small- and medium-sized arteries of the arms and legs

6

- **Differential Diagnosis**
  - Atherosclerosis
  - Raynaud's disease
  - Livedo reticularis due to other cause
  - Antiphospholipid antibody syndrome
  - Cholesterol atheroembolic disease
  - Limited systemic sclerosis

- **Treatment**
  - Smoking cessation is essential
  - Warm clothing, nifedipine for Raynaud's phenomenon
  - Surgical sympathectomy of some value
  - Amputation required in some, though surgery often begets more surgery as wounds heal poorly with diminished perfusion

- **Pearl**

The addiction to nicotine is fierce; patients continue to smoke even with limb prostheses.

Reference

Olin JW: Thromboangiitis obliterans (Buerger's disease). N Engl J Med 2000;343:864. [PMID: 10995867]

Wegener's Granulomatosis

■ **Essentials of Diagnosis**

- Vasculitis associated with glomerulonephritis and necrotizing granulomas of upper and lower respiratory tracts
- Slight male predominance with peak incidence in fourth and fifth decades
- Ninety percent present with upper or lower respiratory tract symptoms, including perforation of nasal septum, chronic sinusitis, otitis media, mastoiditis, cough, dyspnea, hemoptysis
- Proptosis, scleritis, arthritis, purpura, or neuropathy (mononeuritis multiplex) may also be present
- C-ANCA in 90% correlates with anti–proteinase 3 antibodies
- Biopsy in the correct clinical setting yields the diagnosis: Sinus, nonspecific; lung, granulomatous necrotizing vasculitis; renal, focal glomerulonephritis
- Eosinophilia not a feature
- Chest film may reveal large nodular densities; urinalysis may show hematuria, red cell casts; CT scans of sinuses may reveal bony erosion

■ **Differential Diagnosis**

- Polyarteritis nodosa
- Churg-Strauss vasculitis
- Goodpasture's syndrome
- Takayasu's arteritis
- Microscopic polyarteritis
- Lymphomatoid granulomatosis
- Lymphoproliferative disorders (especially angiocentric T-cell lymphoma)

■ **Treatment**

- Corticosteroids
- Primarily oral cyclophosphamide or methotrexate; chronic cyclophosphamide therapy predisposes to bladder cancer, therefore significant fluid intake during therapy to irrigate the bladder is important
- Trimethoprim-sulfamethoxazole effective in mild disease; given to all patients not allergic to sulfonamides

■ **Pearl**

In 10% of renal biopsies, pathognomonic granulomatous vasculitis is seen in renal arterioles.

Reference

Lamprecht P, Gross WL: Wegener's granulomatosis. Herz 2004;29:47. [PMID: 14968341]

Endocrine Disorders

Acromegaly

- **Essentials of Diagnosis**
  - Excessive growth of hands (increased glove size), feet (increased shoe size), jaw (protrusion), face, tongue; visual field loss, coarse facial features, deep voice
  - Amenorrhea, headaches, excessive sweating
  - Hyperglycemia, hypogonadotropic hypogonadism
  - Elevated serum insulin-like growth factor-1 (IGF-1)
  - Elevated serum growth hormone with failure to suppress after an oral glucose load
  - Enlarged sella, thickened skull, and terminal phalanx tufting; MRI pituitary tumor in 90% by MRI

- **Differential Diagnosis**
  - Physiologic growth spurt
  - Familial coarse features
  - Myxedema

- **Treatment**
  - Transsphenoidal resection of adenoma is successful in many patients; medical therapy is necessary for those with residual disease
  - The majority of patients respond to treatment with somatostatin analogues (eg, octreotide) or growth hormone receptor antagonist (eg, pegvisomant)
  - Pituitary irradiation may be necessary if patients are not cured by surgical and medical therapy
  - Hormone replacement for residual panhypopituitarism

- **Pearl**

The wallet biopsy: compare the present appearance of the patient with an older photograph on the driver's license and you make the diagnosis . . . noninvasively.

Reference

Melmed S et al: Guidelines for acromegaly management. J Clin Endocrinol Metab 2002;87:4054. [PMID: 12213843]

Adult Hypothyroidism & Myxedema

- ■ Essentials of Diagnosis
  - Cold intolerance, constipation, weight gain, hoarseness, altered mentation, depression, hypermenorrhea
  - Hypothermia, bradycardia, dry skin with yellow tone (carotenemia); nonpitting edema; macroglossia; delayed relaxation of deep tendon reflexes
  - Low serum FT_4; TSH elevated in primary hypothyroidism; macrocytic anemia
  - Myxedema coma may be associated with obtundation, profound hypothermia, hypoventilation, hypotension, striking bradycardia; pleural and pericardial effusions
  - Associated with other autoimmune endocrinopathies

- ■ Differential Diagnosis
  - Chronic fatigue syndrome
  - Congestive heart failure
  - Primary amyloidosis
  - Depression
  - Exposure hypothermia
  - Parkinson's disease

- ■ Treatment
  - Levothyroxine replacement starting with low doses and increasing gradually until euthyroid
  - Treat myxedema coma with intravenous levothyroxine; if adrenal insufficiency is suspected, add intravenous hydrocortisone

- ■ Pearl

Treating myxedema may precipitate addisonian crisis because of subclinical concomitant adrenal insufficiency; add steroids to thyroid hormone until adrenocortical insufficiency has been ruled out.

Reference

Roberts CG et al: Hypothyroidism. Lancet 2004;363:793. [PMID 15016491]

Diabetes Insipidus

- **Essentials of Diagnosis**
  - Polyuria with volumes of 2–20 L/d; polydipsia, intense thirst
  - Serum osmolality > urine osmolality
  - Urine specific gravity usually < 1.006 during ad libitum fluid intake
  - Inability to concentrate urine with fluid restriction, resulting in hypernatremia
  - Central diabetes insipidus (vasopressin-deficient) caused by hypothalamic or pituitary disease
  - Nephrogenic diabetes insipidus (vasopressin-resistant) may be familial or caused by lithium, chronic renal disease, hypokalemia, hypercalcemia, demeclocycline
  - Vasopressin challenge establishes central cause

7

- **Differential Diagnosis**
  - Psychogenic polydipsia
  - Osmotic diuresis
  - Diabetes mellitus
  - Beer potomania

- **Treatment**
  - Ensure adequate free water intake
  - Intranasal desmopressin acetate for central diabetes insipidus
  - Hydrochlorothiazide or indomethacin for nephrogenic diabetes insipidus

- **Pearl**

Demeclocycline and other tetracyclines can cause nephrogenic diabetes insipidus; be sure to inquire about prior medications during evaluation of diabetes insipidus.

Reference

Robertson GL: Antidiuretic hormone. Normal and disordered function. Endocrinol Metab Clin North Am 2001;30:671. [PMID 11571936]

Diabetic Ketoacidosis

- **Essentials of Diagnosis**
  - Acute polyuria and polydipsia, marked fatigue, nausea and vomiting, coma
  - Fruity breath; dehydration, hypotension if severe volume depletion occurs; Kussmaul respirations
  - Hyperglycemia > 250 mg/dL, ketonemia, acidemia with blood pH < 7.3 and serum bicarbonate < 15 mEq/L, elevated anion gap; glycosuria and ketonuria; total body potassium depleted despite elevation in serum potassium
  - Due to insulin deficiency or increased insulin requirements in a type 1 diabetic (eg, in association with myocardial ischemia, surgery, infection, gastroenteritis, intra-abdominal disease, or medical noncompliance)

- **Differential Diagnosis**
  - Alcoholic ketoacidosis
  - Uremia
  - Lactic acidosis
  - Sepsis

- **Treatment**
  - Intravenous regular insulin replacement with careful laboratory monitoring
  - Aggressive volume resuscitation with saline; dextrose should be added to intravenous fluids once glucose reaches 250–300 mg/dL
  - Potassium, magnesium, and phosphate replacement
  - Identify and treat precipitating cause

- **Pearl**

Very low pH and severe hyperkalemia look bad, but not as bad as they appear; osmolality determines the outcome.

Reference

American Diabetes Association: Hyperglycemic crises in patients with diabetes. Diabetes Care 2001;24:154. [PMID: 11221603]

Gynecomastia

- ■ Essentials of Diagnosis
    - • Glandular enlargement of the male breast
    - • Often asymmetric or unilateral and may be tender
    - • Common in puberty and among elderly men
    - • In questionable cases, gynecomastia can be confirmed by mammography or ultrasound
    - • Multiple causes include obesity, chronic liver disease, hypogonadism, Klinefelter's syndrome, androgen resistance, adrenal tumors, testicular tumors and those producing β-hCG, hyperthyroidism, and drugs (eg, estrogens, phytoestrogens, spironolactone, flutamide, ketoconazole, cimetidine, diazepam, digoxin, tricyclic antidepressants, isoniazid, alcohol, marijuana, heroin)

- ■ Differential Diagnosis
    - • Associations noted above
    - • Benign or malignant tumors of the breast

- ■ Treatment
    - • Careful testicular examination; measurement of liver function as well as β-hCG, LH, testosterone, and estradiol to determine underlying disorder
    - • Remove offending drug or treat underlying condition; reassurance if idiopathic
    - • Consider needle biopsy of suspicious areas of breast enlargement
    - • Consider surgical correction for severe cases

- ■ Pearl
One percent of breast carcinoma occurs in men; although its biologic traits are the same as in women, a poorer prognosis relates to delay in diagnosis.

Reference

Mather R et al. Gynecomastia: pathomechanisms and treatment strategies. Horm Res 1997;48:95. [PMID: 11546925]

Hirsutism & Virilizing Diseases of Women

- **Essentials of Diagnosis**
  - Menstrual disorders, hirsutism, acne
  - Virilization may occur; increased muscularity, balding, deepening of the voice, enlargement of the clitoris
  - Occasionally a pelvic mass is palpable if due to tumor
  - Serum testosterone and androstenedione often elevated; serum dehydroepiandrosterone sulfate (DHEAS) elevated in adrenal disorders
  - May be due to polycystic ovary syndrome, congenital adrenal hyperplasia, ovarian or adrenal tumors, ACTH-dependent Cushing's syndrome

- **Differential Diagnosis**
  - Familial, idiopathic, or drug-related hirsutism
  - Cushing's syndrome
  - Exogenous androgen ingestion

- **Treatment**
  - Surgical removal of ovarian or adrenal tumor if present
  - Oral contraceptives to suppress ovarian androgen excess and normalize menses
  - Glucocorticoids for congenital adrenal hyperplasia
  - Spironolactone and cyproterone acetate to ameliorate hirsutism; finasteride and flutamide may help in refractory cases
  - Consider metformin for women with polycystic ovary syndrome

- **Pearl**

Check the drug history in hirsutism; it's more likely to be causative than the above syndromes.

Reference

Rittmaster RS: Hirsutism. Lancet 1997;349:191. [PMID: 9111556]

Hypercortisolism (Cushing's Syndrome)

- ■ Essentials of Diagnosis
  - Weakness, muscle wasting, weight gain, central obesity, psychosis, hirsutism, acne, menstrual irregularity, hypogonadism
  - Moon facies, buffalo hump, thin skin, easy bruisability, purple striae, poor wound healing, hypertension, osteoporosis
  - Hyperglycemia, glycosuria, leukocytosis, lymphocytopenia; may have hypokalemia with ectopic ACTH secretion
  - Elevated plasma cortisol and urinary free cortisol; failure to suppress plasma cortisol with exogenous dexamethasone (overnight low-dose dexamethasone test)
  - A normal or high ACTH level indicates ACTH-dependent Cushing's disease (pituitary adenoma or ectopic ACTH syndrome); a low ACTH level indicates adrenal tumor; imaging studies should be targeted accordingly
  - Adrenal CT will reveal adrenal tumor if present
  - Obtain pituitary MRI for ACTH-dependent Cushing's, followed by petrosal sinus sampling for ACTH if MRI is negative or equivocal

- ■ Differential Diagnosis
  - Chronic alcoholism
  - Depression
  - Diabetes mellitus
  - Exogenous glucocorticoid administration
  - Severe obesity

- ■ Treatment
  - Transsphenoidal resection of pituitary adenoma if present; radiation therapy for residual disease
  - Resection of adrenal tumor if present
  - Resection of ectopic ACTH-producing tumor if able to localize (eg, carcinoid, small-cell carcinoma of the lung)
  - Ketoconazole or metyrapone to suppress cortisol in unresectable cases
  - Bilateral adrenalectomy for adrenal hyperplasia in refractory cases of ACTH-dependent Cushing's syndrome

- ■ Pearl

If you see the above clinical picture in a man, the elevated cortisol isn't likely due to classic Cushing's disease; this is a rare disease with a 10:1 female-to-male ratio.

Reference

Arnaldi G et al: Diagnosis and complications of Cushing's syndrome: a consensus statement. J Clin Endocrinol Metab 2003;88:5593. [PMID: 14671138]

Hyperosmotic Nonketotic Diabetic Coma

- **Essentials of Diagnosis**
  - Gradual onset of polyuria, polydipsia, dehydration, and weakness; in severe cases, may progress to obtundation and coma
  - Occurs in patients with type 2 diabetes, typically in elderly patients with reduced fluid intake
  - Profound hyperglycemia (> 600 mg/dL), hyperosmolality (> 310 mOsm/kg); pH > 7.3, serum bicarbonate > 15 mEq/L; ketosis and acidosis are usually absent

- **Differential Diagnosis**
  - Cerebrovascular accident or head trauma
  - Diabetes insipidus
  - Hypoglycemia
  - Hyperglycemia

- **Treatment**
  - Aggressive volume resuscitation with normal saline until patient euvolemic, then with hypotonic saline
  - Regular insulin 15 units intravenously plus 15 units subcutaneously initially is usually effective, followed by subcutaneous insulin every 4 hours
  - Careful monitoring of serum sodium, osmolality, and glucose
  - Dextrose-containing fluids when glucose is 250–300 mg/dL
  - Potassium and phosphate replacement as needed

- **Pearl**

As for diabetic ketoacidosis, osmolality determines the outcome; it's the reason this condition's prognosis is worse than that of ketoacidosis, in which osmolality is usually normal.

Reference

Trence DL et al: Hyperglycemic crises in diabetes mellitus type 2. Endocrinol Metab Clin North Am 2001;30:817. [PMID 11727401]

Hyperprolactinemia

- ## Essentials of Diagnosis
  - Women: Menstrual disturbance (oligomenorrhea, amenorrhea), galactorrhea, infertility
  - Men: Hypogonadism; decreased libido and erectile dysfunction; galactorrhea; infertility
  - Serum prolactin usually > 100 ng/mL for prolactin-secreting pituitary adenomas
  - May be caused by primary hypothyroidism
  - Pituitary adenoma often demonstrated by MRI

- ## Differential Diagnosis
  - Primary hypothyroidism
  - Use of prolactin-stimulating drugs
  - Pregnancy or lactation
  - Hypothalamic disease
  - Cirrhosis; renal failure
  - Chronic nipple stimulation; chest wall injury

- ## Treatment
  - Dopamine agonists (eg, bromocriptine or cabergoline) usually shrink pituitary adenoma and restore fertility
  - Transsphenoidal resection for large pituitary tumors and for those causing visual compromise or refractory to dopamine agonists

- ## Pearl

Be certain a patient with a suspected prolactinoma does not have a psychiatric history; most psychotropics cause hyperprolactinemia.

Reference

Molitch ME: Disorders of prolactin secretion. Endocrinol Metab Clin North Am 2001;30:585. [PMID 11571932]

Hyperthyroidism

- ■ Essentials of Diagnosis
  - • Sweating, weight loss, heat intolerance, irritability, weakness, increased number of bowel movements, menstrual irregularity
  - • Sinus tachycardia or atrial fibrillation, tremor, warm moist skin, eye findings (stare, lid lag); diffuse goiter, thyroid bruit and exophthalmos in Graves' disease
  - • Serum FT_4 and FT_3 increased; TSH low or undetectable
  - • Radioiodine uptake scan will differentiate Graves' disease, toxic nodule, and thyroiditis; may also be useful in identifying rare ectopic thyroid tissue (ovarian teratoma)
  - • Thyroid-stimulating immunoglobulin and thyroid autoantibodies are often positive in Graves' disease

- ■ Differential Diagnosis
  - • Anxiety, neurosis, or mania
  - • Pheochromocytoma
  - • Exogenous thyroid administration
  - • Catabolic illness
  - • Chronic alcoholism

- ■ Treatment
  - • Supportive care for patients with thyroiditis
  - • Propranolol for symptomatic relief of catecholamine-mediated symptoms
  - • Antithyroid drugs (methimazole or propylthiouracil) for patients with Graves' disease; chance of remission greater for milder cases/smaller goiters while more severe cases may eventually require radioactive iodine treatment
  - • Radioactive iodine ablation provides definitive therapy and is indicated for refractory Graves' disease and in patients with toxic nodular disease; in older patients or those with severe hyperthyroidism, treat first with antithyroid drugs
  - • Subtotal thyroidectomy for failure of medical therapy if radioactive iodine is contraindicated (eg, pregnancy) or for very large nodular goiters; euthyroid state should be achieved medically before surgery

- ■ Pearl

In patients over 60, when you think it's hyperthyroidism it's hypo-, and when you think it's hypo- it's hyper-; the diseases become increasingly atypical with age.

Reference

Cooper DS: Hyperthyroidism. Lancet 2003;362:459. [PMID: 12927435]

Hypoglycemia in the Adult

- ■ Essentials of Diagnosis
  - • Blurred vision, diplopia, headache, slurred speech, weakness, sweating, palpitations, tremulousness, altered mentation; focal neurologic signs common
  - • Plasma glucose < 40 mg/dL
  - • Causes include alcoholism, postprandial hypoglycemia (eg, post-gastrectomy), insulinoma, medications (insulin, sulfonylureas, pentamidine), adrenal insufficiency

- ■ Differential Diagnosis
  - • Central nervous system disease
  - • Hypoxia
  - • Psychoneurosis
  - • Pheochromocytoma

- ■ Treatment
  - • Intravenous glucose (oral glucose for patients who are conscious and able to swallow)
  - • Intramuscular glucagon if no intravenous access available
  - • Treatment of underlying disease or removal of offending agent (eg, alcohol, pentamidine, sulfonylureas)
  - • For patients with postprandial (reactive) hypoglycemia, eating small frequent meals with reduced proportion of carbohydrates may help

- ■ Pearl

In a hypothermic patient with altered mental status, treatment of hypoglycemia precedes all other diagnostic and therapeutic measures.

Reference

Service FJ: Hypoglycemic disorders. N Engl J Med 1995;332:1144. [PMID: 7700289]

Hypoparathyroidism

- **Essentials of Diagnosis**
  - Tetany, carpopedal spasms, tingling of lips and hands; altered mentation
  - Positive Chvostek's sign (facial muscle contraction on tapping the facial nerve) and Trousseau's phenomenon (carpal spasm after application of arm cuff); dry skin and brittle nails; cataracts
  - Serum calcium low; serum phosphate high; serum parathyroid hormone low to absent
  - Long ST segment resulting in long QT interval on ECG
  - History of previous thyroidectomy or neck surgery in patients with surgical hypoparathyroidism

- **Differential Diagnosis**
  - Pseudohypoparathyroidism
  - Vitamin D deficiency syndromes
  - Acute pancreatitis
  - Hypomagnesemia
  - Chronic renal failure
  - Hypoalbuminemia

- **Treatment**
  - For acute tetany, intravenous calcium gluconate, followed by oral calcium carbonate and vitamin D derivatives
  - Correct concurrent hypomagnesemia
  - Chronic therapy includes high-calcium diet in addition to calcium and vitamin D supplements
  - Avoid phenothiazines (prolonged QT interval) and furosemide (increases symptoms of hypocalcemia)

- **Pearl**

Radiotherapy causes hypothyroidism but never hypoparathyroidism; the parathyroids are among the most resistant tissues in the body to radiation.

Reference

Rude RK: Hypocalcemia and hypoparathyroidism. Curr Ther Endocrinol Metab 1997;6:546. [PMID: 9174804]

Male Hypogonadism

- **Essentials of Diagnosis**
  - Diminished libido and impotence
  - Sparse growth of male body hair
  - Testes may be small or normal in size; serum testosterone is usually decreased
  - Serum gonadotropins (LH and FSH) are decreased in hypogonadotropic hypogonadism; they are increased in primary testicular failure (hypergonadotropic hypogonadism)
  - Causes of hypogonadotropic hypogonadism include chronic illness, malnutrition, drugs, pituitary tumor, Cushing's syndrome, hyperprolactinemia, congenital syndromes (eg, Kallman's syndrome)
  - Causes of hypergonadotropic hypogonadism include Klinefelter's syndrome, anorchia or cryptorchidism, testicular trauma, orchitis, myotonic dystrophy, hemochromatosis, gonadal dysgenesis, and defects in testosterone biosynthesis

- **Differential Diagnosis**
  - Conditions noted above
  - Androgen insensitivity
  - Neurogenic or vascular erectile dysfunction
  - Hypothyroidism

- **Treatment**
  - Evaluate and treat underlying disorder
  - Testosterone replacement (intramuscular or transdermal)

- **Pearl**

One of the reasons to check the first cranial nerve: anosmia is a feature of Kallman's syndrome.

Reference

Hayes FJ et al: Hypogonadotropic hypogonadism. Endocrinol Metab Clin North Am 1998;27:739. [PMID: 9922906]

Osteoporosis

- ■ Essentials of Diagnosis
  - • Asymptomatic or associated with back pain from vertebral fractures; loss of height; kyphosis
  - • Demineralization of spine, hip, and pelvis by radiograph; vertebral compression fractures; spontaneous fractures often discovered incidentally
  - • Bone mineral density more than 2.5 SD below the average value for a young adult

- ■ Differential Diagnosis
  - • Osteomalacia
  - • Multiple myeloma
  - • Metastatic carcinoma
  - • Hypophosphatemic disorders
  - • Osteogenesis imperfecta
  - • Secondary osteoporosis due to glucocorticoids, hyperthyroidism, hypogonadism, alcoholism, renal or liver disease

- ■ Treatment
  - • Diet adequate in calcium and vitamin D with supplements to achieve 1000–1500 mg elemental calcium and 400 IU vitamin D daily
  - • Regular exercise
  - • Fall prevention strategies
  - • Effective antiresorptive therapies include bisphosphonates (eg, alendronate, risedronate), selective estrogen receptor modulators (SERMS; eg, raloxifene), estrogen replacement therapy, and calcitonin
  - • Effective anabolic therapy includes recombinant parathyroid hormone (eg, teriparatide)
  - • Men with hypogonadism are treated with testosterone

- ■ Pearl

Easily the most debilitating nonmalignant disease of bone.

Reference

Brown SA et al: Osteoporosis. Med Clin North Am 2003;87:1039. [PMID 14621330]

Paget's Disease (Osteitis Deformans)

- ■ Essentials of Diagnosis
  - Often asymptomatic or associated with bone pain, fractures, and bone deformity (bowing, kyphosis)
  - Serum calcium and phosphate normal; alkaline phosphatase elevated; urinary hydroxyproline elevated
  - Dense, expanded bones on x-ray resulting from accelerated bone turnover and disruption of normal architecture; osteolytic lesions in the skull and extremities; vertebral fractures; fissure fractures in the long bones
  - May have neurologic sequelae due to nerve compression as pagetic bones enlarge (eg, deafness)

- ■ Differential Diagnosis
  - Osteogenic sarcoma
  - Multiple myeloma
  - Fibrous dysplasia
  - Metastatic carcinoma
  - Osteitis fibrosa cystica (hyperparathyroidism)

- ■ Treatment
  - No treatment for asymptomatic patients
  - Treat symptomatic disease with inhibitors of osteoclastic resorption (bisphosphonates or calcitonin)
  - The role of prophylactic treatment to prevent bone deformities or neurologic sequelae is not well established

- ■ Pearl

Was Paget's disease the cause of Beethoven's deafness? Only his pictures suggest it, as no alkaline phosphatase determinations were available between 1770 and 1828.

Reference

Delmas PD et al: The management of Paget's disease of bone. N Engl J Med 1997;336:558. [PMID: 9023094]

Panhypopituitarism

- ■ Essentials of Diagnosis
  - • Sexual dysfunction, weakness, easy fatigability; poor resistance to stress, cold, or fasting; axillary and pubic hair loss
  - • Hypotension, often orthostatic; visual field defects if pituitary tumor present
  - • Deficient cortisol response to ACTH; low serum T_4 with low or low-normal TSH; serum prolactin level may be elevated
  - • Low serum testosterone in men; amenorrhea; FSH and LH are low or low-normal
  - • MRI may reveal a pituitary or hypothalamic lesion

7

- ■ Differential Diagnosis
  - • Anorexia nervosa or severe malnutrition
  - • Hypothyroidism
  - • Addison's disease
  - • Cachexia due to other causes (eg, carcinoma or tuberculosis)
  - • Empty sella syndrome

- ■ Treatment
  - • Surgical removal of pituitary tumor if present; pituitary irradiation may be necessary for residual tumor but increases likelihood of permanent hypopituitarism
  - • Lifelong endocrine replacement therapy with corticosteroids, thyroid hormone, sex hormones, and if indicated, growth hormone

- ■ Pearl

In a woman with suspected panhypopituitarism, ask about a previous pregnancy with postpartum bleeding; it could be Sheehan's syndrome.

Reference

Vance ML: Hypopituitarism. N Engl J Med 1994;330:1651. [PMID: 8043090] Erratum published in: N Engl J Med 1994;331:487.

Pheochromocytoma

- **Essentials of Diagnosis**
  - Paroxysmal or sustained hypertension; postural hypotension
  - Episodes of palpitations, perspiration, and headache; anxiety, nausea, chest or abdominal pain
  - Pallor is the most reliable physical sign
  - Hypermetabolism with normal thyroid tests; mild hyperglycemia may be present
  - Elevated urinary catecholamines, metanephrines, and vanillylmandelic acid are diagnostic; elevated plasma free metanephrines helpful in identifying patients with genetic subtypes
  - CT or MRI can confirm and localize pheochromocytoma; ^{123}I-MIBG scan may help to localize tumors

- **Differential Diagnosis**
  - Essential hypertension
  - Thyrotoxicosis
  - Panic attacks
  - Preeclampsia-eclampsia
  - Acute intermittent porphyria

- **Treatment**
  - Surgical removal of tumor or tumors
  - Alpha blockade with phenoxybenzamine prior to surgery
  - Beta-adrenergic receptor blockade can be added after effective alpha blockade to help control tachycardia
  - Adequate volume replenishment mandatory prior to surgery
  - Oral phenoxybenzamine or metyrosine for symptomatic treatment in patients with inoperable tumors; metastatic pheochromocytoma may be treated with chemotherapy or ^{131}I-MIBG

- **Pearl**

Rule of tens: 10% bilateral, 10% malignant, 10% extra-adrenal, 10% familial, and 10% normotensive.

Reference

Kudva YC et al. Clinical review 164: The laboratory diagnosis of adrenal pheochromocytoma: the Mayo Clinic Experience. J Clin Endocrinol Metab 2003;88:4533. [PMID: 14557417]

Primary Adrenal Insufficiency (Addison's Disease)

- ■ Essentials of Diagnosis
  - • Weakness, anorexia, weight loss, abdominal pain, nausea and vomiting; increased skin pigmentation
  - • Hypotension, dehydration; postural symptoms
  - • Hyponatremia, hyperkalemia, hypoglycemia, lymphocytosis, and eosinophilia; increased serum urea nitrogen and calcium may be present
  - • Serum cortisol levels low to absent and ACTH elevated; cortisol level fails to rise after cosyntropin (ACTH) stimulation
  - • Often associated with other autoimmune endocrinopathies; may also be due to trauma, infection (especially tuberculosis, histoplasmosis), adrenal hemorrhage, or adrenoleukodystrophy

- ■ Differential Diagnosis
  - • Secondary adrenal insufficiency
  - • Anorexia nervosa
  - • Malignancy
  - • Infection
  - • Salt-wasting nephropathy
  - • Hemochromatosis

- ■ Treatment
  - • In acute adrenal crisis, treat immediately with intravenous hydrocortisone (100 mg intravenously every 8 hours) once the diagnosis is suspected; provide appropriate volume resuscitation and blood pressure support; consider empiric antibiotics
  - • In chronic adrenal insufficiency, maintenance therapy includes glucocorticoids (hydrocortisone) and mineralocorticoids (fludrocortisone)
  - • Increase glucocorticoid dose for trauma, surgery, infection, or stress

- ■ Pearl

If the systolic blood pressure is over 100 mm Hg without orthostatic findings, it is not classic Addison's.

Reference

Oelkers W: Adrenal insufficiency. N Engl J Med 1996;335:1206. [PMID: 8815944]

Primary Aldosteronism

- **Essentials of Diagnosis**
  - Hypertension, polyuria, fatigue, and weakness
  - Hypokalemia, metabolic alkalosis
  - Elevated plasma and urine aldosterone levels with suppressed plasma renin activity level
  - May be associated with adrenocortical adenoma or bilateral adrenocortical hyperplasia
  - Rarely due to glucocorticoid-remediable aldosteronism
  - Adrenal mass often demonstrated by CT

- **Differential Diagnosis**
  - Essential hypertension
  - Periodic paralysis
  - Congenital adrenal hyperplasia (11- or 17-hydroxylase deficiency)
  - Pseudohyperaldosteronism: Licorice ingestion, Liddle's syndrome
  - Chronic diuretic use or laxative abuse
  - Unilateral renovascular disease
  - Cushing's syndrome

- **Treatment**
  - Surgical resection of unilateral adenoma secreting aldosterone (Conn's syndrome)
  - Mineralocorticoid antagonist therapy (spironolactone or eplerenone) for bilateral adrenal hyperplasia; surgery does not cure hypertension in these cases and is not generally recommended
  - Dexamethasone for glucocorticoid-remediable aldosteronism
  - Antihypertensive therapy as necessary

- **Pearl**

If the sodium is less than 140 mg/dL and a spot urine potassium less than 40 mg/dL, the hypertension is likely to have another etiology.

Reference

Young WF Jr: Minireview: primary aldosteronism—changing concepts in diagnosis and treatment. Endocrinology 2003;144:2208. [PMID: 12746276]

Primary Hyperparathyroidism

- **Essentials of Diagnosis**
  - Renal stones, bone pain, mental status changes, constipation ("stones, bones, moans, and abdominal groans"), polyuria; many patients are asymptomatic
  - Serum and urine calcium elevated; low-normal to low serum phosphate; high-normal or elevated serum parathyroid hormone level; alkaline phosphatase often elevated
  - Bone radiographs show cystic bone lesions (brown tumors) and subperiosteal resorption of cortical bone, especially the phalanges (osteitis fibrosa cystica); may have osteoporosis and pathologic fractures
  - History of renal stones, nephrocalcinosis, recurrent peptic ulcer disease, or recurrent pancreatitis may be present

- **Differential Diagnosis**
  - Familial hypocalciuric hypercalcemia
  - Hypercalcemia of malignancy
  - Renal failure
  - Vitamin D intoxication or milk-alkali syndrome
  - Sarcoidosis, granulomatous disorders
  - Hyperthyroidism
  - Multiple myeloma

- **Treatment**
  - Parathyroidectomy for patients with symptomatic disease, markedly elevated calcium level, hypercalciuria, kidney stones, or bone disease
  - Bisphosphonates (eg, pamidronate) for acute treatment of severe hypercalcemia while preparing for surgery
  - For patients with mild asymptomatic disease: Maintain adequate fluid intake and avoid immobilization, thiazide diuretics, and calcium-containing antacids; follow for disease progression

- **Pearl**

The natural history of untreated asymptomatic hyperparathyroidism is generally benign, but long-term monitoring is necessary in those who do not receive surgery.

Reference

Bilezikian JP et al: Summary statement from a workshop on asymptomatic primary hyperparathyroidism: a perspective for the 21st century. J Clin Endocrinol Metab 2002;87:5353. [PMID 12466320]

Simple & Nodular Goiter

- **Essentials of Diagnosis**
  - Single or multiple thyroid nodules found on thyroid palpation
  - Large multinodular goiters may be associated with compressive symptoms (dysphagia, cough, stridor)
  - Measurement of free thyroxine (FT_4) and TSH; radioiodine uptake scan helpful in selected cases for distinguishing cold from hot nodules

- **Differential Diagnosis**
  - Graves' disease (diffuse toxic goiter)
  - Autoimmune thyroiditis
  - Carcinoma of the thyroid

- **Treatment**
  - Fine-needle biopsy for solitary or dominant nodules; carcinomas or suspicious cold lesions require surgery
  - Levothyroxine treatment may suppress growth and cause regression in benign nodules or multinodular goiter; contraindicated if TSH is low
  - Surgery for severe compressive symptoms

- **Pearl**

Pharmacologic amounts of iodine, as in contrast-enhanced radiographic studies, may result in hyperthyroidism via the Jod-Basedow phenomenon; inquire about diagnostic studies previously performed for other reasons in a newly hyperthyroid patient.

Reference

Hegedus L et al: Management of simple nodular goiter: current status and future perspectives. Endocr Rev 2003;24:102. [PMID 12588812]

Thyroiditis

- **Essentials of Diagnosis**
  - Painful enlarged thyroid gland in acute and subacute forms; painless enlargement in chronic form
  - Generally classified as chronic lymphocytic (Hashimoto's) thyroiditis and subacute (granulomatous) thyroiditis; suppurative thyroiditis and Riedel's thyroiditis are uncommon
  - Thyroid function tests variable, with serum T_4 and T_3 levels often high in acute forms and low in chronic disease
  - Elevated erythrocyte sedimentation rate and reduced radioiodine uptake in subacute thyroiditis
  - Thyroid autoantibodies positive in Hashimoto's thyroiditis

7

- **Differential Diagnosis**
  - Endemic goiter
  - Graves' disease (diffuse toxic goiter)
  - Carcinoma of the thyroid
  - Pyogenic infections of the neck

- **Treatment**
  - Antibiotics for suppurative thyroiditis
  - Nonsteroidal anti-inflammatory drugs for subacute thyroiditis; prednisone in severe cases; symptomatic treatment with propranolol
  - Levothyroxine replacement for Hashimoto's thyroiditis
  - Partial thyroidectomy for local severe pressure or adhesions in Riedel's thyroiditis

- **Pearl**

The patient can be hyper-, hypo-, or euthyroid depending on the course of the disease at the time of testing.

Reference

Pearce EN et al: Thyroiditis. N Engl J Med 2003;348:2646. [PMID 12826640] Erratum published in: N Engl J Med 2003;349:620.

Type 1 Diabetes Mellitus

- **Essentials of Diagnosis**
    - Crisp onset, no family history
    - Polyuria, polydipsia, weight loss
    - Fasting plasma glucose > 126 mg/dL; random plasma glucose > 200 mg/dL with symptoms; glycosuria
    - Associated with ketosis in untreated state; may present as medical emergency (diabetic ketoacidosis)
    - Long-term risks include retinopathy, nephropathy, neuropathy, and cardiovascular disease

- **Differential Diagnosis**
    - Nondiabetic glycosuria (eg, Fanconi's syndrome)
    - Diabetes insipidus
    - Acromegaly
    - Cushing's disease or syndrome
    - Pheochromocytoma
    - Medications (eg, glucocorticoids, niacin)

- **Treatment**
    - Insulin treatment is required
    - Patient education is crucial, emphasizing dietary management, intensive insulin therapy, self-monitoring of blood glucose, hypoglycemia awareness, foot and eye care

- **Pearl**

The prognosis of diabetic ketoacidosis is better than that of a nonketotic hyperosmolar state: hyperosmolality is the most important prognostic factor in both.

Reference

Havas S: Educational guidelines for achieving tight control and minimizing complications of type 1 diabetes. Am Fam Physician 1999;60:1985. [PMID: 10569502]

Type 2 Diabetes Mellitus

- ■ Essentials of Diagnosis
  - Most patients are older and tend to be obese
  - Gradual onset of polyuria, polydipsia; often asymptomatic
  - Candidal vaginitis in women, chronic skin infection, generalized pruritus, blurred vision
  - Fasting plasma glucose > 126 mg/dL; random plasma glucose > 200 mg/dL with symptoms; glycosuria; elevated glycosylated hemoglobin (A_{1c}); ketosis rare
  - Family history often present; frequently associated with hypertension, hyperlipidemia, and atherosclerosis
  - May present as a medical emergency (especially in the elderly) as nonketotic hyperosmolar coma
  - Long-term risks include retinopathy, nephropathy, neuropathy, and cardiovascular disease

- ■ Differential Diagnosis
  - Nondiabetic glycosuria (eg, Fanconi's syndrome)
  - Diabetes insipidus
  - Acromegaly
  - Cushing's disease or syndrome
  - Pheochromocytoma
  - Medications (eg, glucocorticoids, niacin)
  - Severe insulin resistance syndromes
  - Altered mental status due to other cause

- ■ Treatment
  - Patient education is important, emphasizing dietary management, exercise, weight loss, self-monitoring of blood glucose, hypoglycemia awareness, foot and eye care
  - Mild cases may be controlled initially with diet, exercise, and weight loss
  - Oral hypoglycemic agents if diet is ineffective; insulin may be required if combination oral agents fail

- ■ Pearl

The cause of the most profound involuntary weight loss in medicine with a normal physical examination.

Reference

DeFronzo RA: Pharmacologic therapy for type 2 diabetes mellitus. Ann Intern Med 1999;131:281. [PMID: 10454950]

8

Infectious Diseases

BACTERIAL INFECTIONS

Actinomycosis

- **Essentials of Diagnosis**
  - Due to anaerobic gram-positive rod (*Actinomyces* species) part of the normal mouth flora; becomes pathogenic when introduced into traumatized tissue
  - Chronic suppurative lesion of the skin (cervicofacial in 60%) with sinus tract formation; thoracic or abdominal abscesses seen; pelvic disease associated with intrauterine devices
  - Accelerated sedimentation rate; anemia, thrombocytosis
  - Isolation of *Actinomyces* species or sulfur granule from pus by anaerobic culture
  - Sulfur granules show gram-positive hyphae on smear

- **Differential Diagnosis**
  - Lung cancer
  - Other causes of cervical adenitis
  - Scrofula
  - Nocardiosis
  - Crohn's disease
  - Pelvic inflammatory disease of other cause

- **Treatment**
  - Long-term penicillin
  - Surgical drainage necessary in selected cases

- **Pearl**

Poor dental hygiene in the face of the above clinical scenario noted necessitates consideration of actinomycosis.

Reference

Smego RA Jr, Foglia G: Actinomycosis. Clin Infect Dis 1998;26:1255; quiz 1262. [PMID: 9636842]

Anthrax (*Bacillus anthracis*)

- **Essentials of Diagnosis**
  - History of industrial or agricultural exposure (farmer, veterinarian, tannery or wool worker); a potential agent in biological warfare and bioterrorism
  - Persistent necrotic ulcer on exposed surface
  - Regional adenopathy, fever, malaise, headache, nausea and vomiting
  - Inhalation of spores causes severe tracheobronchitis and pneumonia with dyspnea and cough, mediastinal and hilar lymphadenopathy
  - Hematologic spread with profound toxic and cardiovascular collapse may complicate either cutaneous or pulmonary form
  - Confirmation of diagnosis by culture or specific fluorescent antibody test, but clinical picture highly suggestive

- **Differential Diagnosis**
  - Skin lesions: staphylococcal or streptococcal infection
  - Pulmonary disease: tuberculosis, sarcoidosis, lymphoma with mediastinal adenopathy, plague, tularemia

- **Treatment**
  - Therapy for postexposure prophylaxis is oral doxycycline or oral ciprofloxacin
  - Optimal therapy for confirmed disease due to a susceptible strain is oral or intravenous ciprofloxacin or oral doxycycline
  - Mortality rate is high despite proper therapy, especially in pulmonary disease

- **Pearl**

A rare infectious disease in which the patient "dies sterile"—all organisms are eliminated, but the toxicity is lethal.

Reference

Wenner KA, Kenner JR: Anthrax. Dermatol Clin 2004;22:247, v. [PMID: 15207306]

Bacillary Dysentery (Shigellosis)

- **Essentials of Diagnosis**
  - Fever, malaise, toxicity, diarrhea (typically bloody), cramping, abdominal pain
  - Positive fecal leukocytes; organism isolated in stool; in immuno-suppressed patients, blood culture often positive, but—not so in others

- **Differential Diagnosis**
  - *Campylobacter* and *Salmonella* infection
  - Amebiasis
  - Ulcerative colitis
  - Viral gastroenteritis
  - Food poisoning

- **Treatment**
  - Supportive care
  - Antibiotics determined based on sensitivities of local *Shigella* species; trimethoprim-sulfamethoxazole and ciprofloxacin are the usual drugs of choice, although resistance to these agents is increasing

- **Pearl**

The first organism associated with reactive arthritis.

Reference

Jennison AV, Verma NK: *Shigella flexneri* infection: pathogenesis and vaccine development. FEMS Microbiol Rev 2004;28:43. [PMID: 14975529]

Botulism (*Clostridium botulinum*)

■ Essentials of Diagnosis
  • History of recent ingestion of home-canned, smoked, or vacuum-packed foods; intravenous drug users also at risk (see below)
  • Sudden onset of cranial nerve paralysis, diplopia, dry mouth, dysphagia, dysphonia, and progressive muscle weakness
  • Fixed and dilated pupils in 50%
  • In infants: irritability, weakness, and hypotonicity
  • Demonstration of toxin in serum or food

■ Differential Diagnosis
  • Bulbar poliomyelitis
  • Myasthenia gravis
  • Posterior cerebral circulation ischemia
  • Tick paralysis
  • Guillain-Barré syndrome or variant
  • Inorganic phosphorus poisoning

■ Treatment
  • Removal of unabsorbed toxin from gut
  • Specific antitoxin
  • Vigilant support, including attention to respiratory function
  • Penicillin

■ Pearl

In intravenous drug users with cranial nerve findings, this picture is classic for wound botulism caused by black tar heroin.

Reference

Cherington M: Botulism: update and review. Semin Neurol 2004;24:155. [PMID: 15257512]

Brucellosis (*Brucella* Species)

- ■ Essentials of Diagnosis
  - Invariable history of animal exposure (veterinarian, slaughter-house) or ingestion of unpasteurized milk or cheese
  - Vectors are cattle, hogs, and goats
  - Insidious onset of fever, diaphoresis, anorexia, fatigue, headache, back pain
  - Cervical and axillary lymphadenopathy, hepatosplenomegaly
  - Lymphocytosis with normal total white cell count; positive blood, cerebrospinal fluid, or bone marrow culture after days to weeks; serologic tests positive in second week of illness
  - Osteomyelitis, epididymitis, meningitis, and endocarditis may complicate

- ■ Differential Diagnosis
  - Lymphoma
  - Infective endocarditis
  - Tuberculosis
  - Q fever
  - Typhoid fever
  - Tularemia
  - Malaria
  - Other causes of osteomyelitis

- ■ Treatment
  - Rifampin and doxycycline required for 21 days

- ■ Pearl

In clinically typical brucellosis, dilution of previously negative serum sample is ordered to exclude a prozone effect; dramatically high titers are falsely negative unless diluted.

Reference

Sarinas PS, Chitkara RK: Brucellosis. Semin Respir Infect 2003;18:168. [PMID: 14505279]

Campylobacter Enteritis (*Campylobacter jejuni*)

- ■ Essentials of Diagnosis
  - • Outbreaks associated with consumption of raw milk
  - • Fever, vomiting, abdominal pain, bloody diarrhea
  - • Fecal leukocytes present; presumptive diagnosis by darkfield or phase contrast microscopy of stool wet mount
  - • Definitive diagnosis by stool culture

- ■ Differential Diagnosis
  - • Shigellosis
  - • Salmonellosis
  - • Viral gastroenteritis
  - • Amebic dysentery
  - • Food poisoning
  - • Ulcerative colitis

- ■ Treatment
  - • Erythromycin or ciprofloxacin will shorten the duration of illness by approximately 1 day, although quinolone resistance is increasing
  - • Disease is self-limited but can be severe

- ■ Pearl

The most commonly isolated pathogen in dysentery.

Reference

Bereswill S, Kist M: Recent developments in *Campylobacter* pathogenesis. Curr Opin Infect Dis 2003;16:487. [PMID: 14502003]

Cat-Scratch Disease (*Bartonella henselae*)

- **Essentials of Diagnosis**
  - History of cat scratch or contact with cats; may be forgotten by patient
  - Primary lesion (papule, pustule, conjunctivitis) at site of inoculation in one-third of cases
  - One to three weeks after scratch, fever, malaise, and headache accompanied by regional lymphadenopathy
  - Sterile pus from node aspirate
  - Biopsy consistent with cat-scratch disease showing necrotizing lymphadenitis; positive skin test; positive serology for bacteria
  - Bacillary angiomatosis and peliosis hepatis in immunosuppressed patients

- **Differential Diagnosis**
  - Lymphadenitis due to other bacterial infections
  - Lymphoma
  - Tuberculosis
  - Toxoplasmosis
  - Kikuchi's disease

- **Treatment**
  - Nonspecific; exclusion of similar diseases most important
  - Erythromycin in immunocompromised patients

- **Pearl**

The involved cat is usually a kitten adopted from an animal shelter; though asymptomatic, these animals have enormous organism burdens.

Reference

Lamps LW, Scott MA: Cat-scratch disease: historic, clinical, and pathologic perspectives. Am J Clin Pathol 2004;121(Suppl):S71. [PMID: 15298152]

Chancroid (*Haemophilus ducreyi*)

- ■ Essentials of Diagnosis
  - A sexually transmitted disease with an incubation period of 3–5 days
  - Painful, tender genital ulcer
  - Inguinal adenitis with erythema or fluctuance and multiple genital ulcers often develop
  - Balanitis, phimosis frequent complications
  - Women have no external signs of infection

- ■ Differential Diagnosis
  - Behçet's syndrome
  - Syphilis
  - Pyogenic infection of lower extremity with regional lymphadenitis
  - Genital ulcers of other cause

- ■ Treatment
  - Appropriate antibiotic (azithromycin, ceftriaxone, erythromycin, or ciprofloxacin)
  - Rapid plasma reagin (RPR) for all, HIV when appropriate

- ■ Pearl

Tender inguinal lymphadenopathy in overweight patients may not be nodes; an incarcerated femoral hernia may be the problem.

Reference

Sehgal VN, Srivastava G: Chancroid: contemporary appraisal. Int J Dermatol 2003;42:182. [PMID: 12653911]

Cholera (*Vibrio cholerae*)

- ■ Essentials of Diagnosis
  - • Acute diarrheal illness leading to profound hypovolemia and death if not addressed promptly
  - • History of travel to endemic area or contact with infected person
  - • Occurs in epidemics under conditions of crowding and famine; acquired via ingestion of contaminated food or water
  - • Sudden onset of frequent, high-volume diarrhea
  - • Liquid ("rice water") stool is gray, turbid
  - • Rapid development of hypotension, marked dehydration, acidosis, and hypokalemia
  - • Positive stool culture confirmatory; serologic testing useful in first and second weeks

- ■ Differential Diagnosis
  - • Other small intestinal diarrheal illness (eg, salmonellosis, enterotoxigenic *E coli*)
  - • Viral gastroenteritis
  - • Vasoactive intestinal peptide (VIP)-producing pancreatic tumor (pancreatic cholera)

- ■ Treatment
  - • Vaccination preventive for travelers to endemic areas but is rarely indicated (*see* www.cdc.gov/travel)
  - • Rapid replacement of fluid and electrolytes, especially potassium
  - • Cola beverages inhibit cyclic adenosine monophosphate (cAMP) reduce diarrhea, for use in areas where standard volume repletion is unavailable
  - • Tetracycline and many other antibiotics may shorten duration of *Vibrio* excretion

- ■ Pearl

In cholera, a markedly elevated hematocrit from severe dehydration may lead to hyperviscosity and secondary venous thrombosis.

Reference

Kaper JB, Morris JG Jr, Levine MM: Cholera. Clin Microbiol Rev 1995;8:48. [PMID: 7704895]

Clostridial Myonecrosis (Gas Gangrene)

- ■ Essentials of Diagnosis
    - • Sudden onset of pain, swelling in an area of wound contamination
    - • Severe systemic toxicity and rapid progression of involved tissue
    - • Brown or blood-tinged watery exudate with surrounding skin discoloration
    - • Gas in tissue by palpated or auscultated crepitus or x-ray
    - • *Clostridium perfringens* in anaerobic culture or smear of exudate is the classic—but not the only—cause

- ■ Differential Diagnosis
    - • Other gas-forming infections (mixed aerobic and anaerobic enteric organisms)
    - • Cellulitis due to staphylococcal or streptococcal infection

- ■ Treatment
    - • Immediate surgical débridement and exposure of infected areas
    - • Hyperbaric oxygen of uncertain benefit
    - • Intravenous penicillin with clindamycin
    - • Tetanus prophylaxis

- ■ Pearl

In a patient severely symptomatic and extremely toxic with the clinical picture noted, a relatively low-grade fever is virtually diagnostic of clostridial gas gangrene.

Reference

Headley AJ: Necrotizing soft tissue infections: a primary care review. Am Fam Physician 2003;68:323. [PMID: 12892352]

Diphtheria (*Corynebacterium diphtheriae*)

- ■ Essentials of Diagnosis
  - An acute infection spread by respiratory secretions
  - Sore throat, rhinorrhea, hoarseness, malaise, relatively unimpressive fever (usually < 37.8°C)
  - Some cases confined to the skin
  - Tenacious gray membrane at portal of entry
  - Toxin-induced myocarditis and neuropathy may complicate, due to an exotoxin; more common in pharyngeal than cutaneous diphtheria
  - Smear and culture confirm diagnosis

- ■ Differential Diagnosis
  - Other causes of pharyngitis (streptococcal, infectious mononucleosis, adenovirus)
  - Necrotizing gingivostomatitis
  - Candidiasis
  - Myocarditis from other causes
  - Myasthenia gravis
  - Botulism

- ■ Treatment
  - Active immunization (usually as diphtheria-tetanus-pertussis [DTP]) is preventive
  - Diphtheria antitoxin
  - Penicillin or erythromycin
  - Corticosteroids in selected patients with severe laryngeal involvement, myocarditis, or neuropathy
  - Exposures of susceptible individuals call for booster toxoid, active immunization, antibiotics, and daily throat inspections

- ■ Pearl

Hyperesthetic shallow skin ulcers in homeless patients suggest the diagnosis of cutaneous diphtheria.

Reference

Galazka A: The changing epidemiology of diphtheria in the vaccine era. J Infect Dis 2000;181(Suppl 1):S2. [PMID: 10657184]

Enteric Fever (Typhoid Fever)

■ **Essentials of Diagnosis**

- Caused by several *Salmonella* species; in "typhoid fever," serotype *Salmonella typhi* is causative and accompanied by bacteremia
- Transmitted by contaminated food or drink; incubation period is 5–14 days
- Gradual onset of malaise, headache, sore throat, and cough, followed by diarrhea, or with *S typhi,* constipation; stepladder rise of fever to a maximum of 40°C over 7–10 days, then slow return to normal with little diurnal variation
- Rose spots, relative bradycardia, splenomegaly, abdominal distention and tenderness
- Leukopenia; blood, stool, and urine cultures positive for *S typhi* (group D) or other salmonellae

■ **Differential Diagnosis**

- Brucellosis
- Tuberculosis
- Infectious endocarditis
- Q fever and other rickettsial infections
- Yersiniosis
- Hepatitis
- Lymphoma
- Adult Still's disease

■ **Treatment**

- Active immunization helpful during epidemics for travelers to endemic areas or for household contacts of persons with the disease
- Ciprofloxacin or second-generation cephalosporin pending susceptibility results
- Cholecystectomy may be necessary for relapsed cases
- Complications in one-third of untreated patients include intestinal hemorrhage or perforation, cholecystitis, nephritis, and meningitis

■ **Pearl**

The development of tachycardia and leukocytosis in a patient with typhoid fever is considered to be ileal perforation until proven otherwise.

Reference

Parry CM, Hien TT, Dougan G, et al: Typhoid fever. N Engl J Med 2002;347:1770. [PMID: 12456854]

Gonorrhea (*Neisseria gonorrhoeae*)

■ Essentials of Diagnosis

- A common communicable venereal disease; incubation period is 2–8 days
- Purulent profuse urethral discharge (men); vaginal discharge rare (women); may be asymptomatic in both sexes
- Disseminated disease causes intermittent fever, skin lesions (few in number and peripherally located), tenosynovitis in numerous joints, and usually monarticular arthritis involving the knee, ankle, or wrist
- Conjunctivitis, pharyngitis, proctitis, endocarditis, meningitis also occur
- Gram-negative intracellular diplococci on urethral smear or culture from cervix, rectum, or pharynx; molecular testing of first 10 mL of urine superior to cervical or urethral cultures
- Synovial fluid cultures seldom positive early, may become positive later in disease course

■ Differential Diagnosis

- Cervicitis, vaginitis, or urethritis due to other causes
- Other causes of pelvic inflammatory disease
- Reactive arthritis
- Meningococcemia

■ Treatment

- Rapid plasma reagin (RPR) obtained in all, HIV in selected cases
- Ceftriaxone intramuscularly for suspected cases; treat all sexual partners
- Oral antibiotics for concurrent chlamydial infection also recommended
- Intravenous antibiotics required for salpingitis, prostatitis, arthritis, or endocarditis

■ Pearl

It is wise to empirically treat for gonococcal arthritis in a young patient with a septic joint with negative Gram's stain and culture.

Reference

Donovan B: Sexually transmissible infections other than HIV. Lancet 2004;363:545. [PMID: 14975619]

Granuloma Inguinale
(*Calymmatobacterium granulomatis*)

- **Essentials of Diagnosis**
  - A chronic relapsing granulomatous anogenital infection; incubation period is 1–12 weeks
  - Ulcerative lesions on the skin or mucous membranes of the genitalia or perianal area
  - Donovan bodies revealed by Wright's or Giemsa's stain of ulcer scrapings

- **Differential Diagnosis**
  - Venereal ulcers of other cause
  - Syphilis
  - Herpes simplex
  - Reactive arthritis
  - Behçet's disease

- **Treatment**
  - Appropriate antibiotic (erythromycin or tetracycline) for at least 21 days
  - Surveillance and counseling for other sexually-transmitted diseases (STDs) (eg, syphilis, gonorrhea, HIV)

- **Pearl**

The most indolent of the major venereal diseases.

Reference

O'Farrell N: Donovanosis. Sex Transm Infect 2002;78:452. [PMID: 12473810]

Legionnaire's Disease

- **Essentials of Diagnosis**
  - Caused by *Legionella pneumophila* and a common cause of community-acquired pneumonia in some areas
  - Seen in patients who are immunocompromised or have chronic lung disease
  - Malaise, dry cough, fever, headache, pleuritic chest pain, toxic appearance, purulent sputum
  - Chest x-ray with patchy infiltrates often unimpressive early; subsequent development of effusion or multiple lobar involvement common
  - Purulent sputum without organisms seen by Gram's stain; diagnosis confirmed by culture or special silver stains or direct fluorescent antibodies, urinary antigen

- **Differential Diagnosis**
  - Other infectious pneumonias
  - Pulmonary embolism
  - Pleurodynia
  - Myocardial infarction

- **Treatment**
  - Azithromycin at high doses; quinolones are an effective alternative

- **Pearl**

The early assertion that hyponatremia and gastrointestinal symptoms are diagnostic is erroneous; many atypical pneumonias have the same problem.

Reference

Sabria M, Campins M: Legionnaires' disease: update on epidemiology and management options. Am J Respir Med 2003;2:235. [PMID: 14720005]

Leprosy (*Mycobacterium leprae*)

- ■ Essentials of Diagnosis
  - A chronic infection due to *M leprae*
  - Pale, anesthetic macular (tuberculoid) or infiltrative erythematous (lepromatous) skin lesions
  - Superficial nerve thickening with associated sensory changes; progression slow and symmetric (lepromatous) or sudden and asymmetric (tuberculoid)
  - Skin test negative (lepromatous) or positive (tuberculoid)
  - History of residence in endemic area during childhood; mode of transmission probably is respiratory
  - Acid-fast bacilli in skin lesions or nasal scrapings; characteristic histologic nerve biopsy
  - Lepromatous type occurs in patients with defective cellular immunity, organisms numerous in tissue specimens; bacilli sparse in tuberculoid disease

- ■ Differential Diagnosis
  - Lupus erythematosus
  - Sarcoidosis
  - Syphilis
  - Erythema nodosum
  - Erythema multiforme
  - Vitiligo
  - Neuropathy due to other causes, particularly amyloidosis
  - Cutaneous tuberculosis
  - Scleroderma
  - Syringomyelia

- ■ Treatment
  - Combination therapy for months or years, including dapsone, rifampin, and clofazimine

- ■ Pearl

Mycobacterium leprae *can be grown experimentally only in the armadillo foot pad.*

Reference

Britton WJ, Lockwood DN: Leprosy. Lancet 2004;363:1209. [PMID: 15081655]

Leptospirosis (*Leptospira* Species)

■ **Essentials of Diagnosis**

- An acute and often severe infection transmitted to humans by ingestion of food and drink contaminated by the urine of reservoir animals (rats, dogs, cattle, swine)
- Biphasic course of 2–3 weeks: initially high fever, headache, myalgias and conjunctival injection, followed by apparent recovery and then return of fever associated with meningitis
- Jaundice, conjunctival hemorrhages, meningeal signs, abdominal tenderness
- Renal insufficiency, acalculous cholecystitis may occur
- Variable renal function abnormalities, elevated creatinine phosphokinase level, abnormal cerebrospinal fluid in 10%
- Culture of organism from blood, cerebrospinal fluid, or from urine, or direct darkfield microscopy of urine or cerebrospinal fluid is diagnostic
- Serologic tests positive after first week; rapid enzyme-linked immunosorbent assay (ELISA) for IgM now available

■ **Differential Diagnosis**

- Aseptic meningitis due to other causes
- Hepatitis
- Lymphoma
- Cholecystitis due to other causes
- Hepatorenal syndrome
- Halogenated hydrocarbon ingestion

■ **Treatment**

- Early treatment with penicillin or tetracycline may shorten course
- Herxheimer reaction may appear after therapy
- Doxycycline effective as prophylaxis for exposures

■ **Pearl**

Jaundice and conjunctivitis in a toxic patient exposed to brackish water is leptospirosis until proved otherwise.

Reference

Bharti AR, Nally JE, Ricaldi JN, et al: Leptospirosis: a zoonotic disease of global importance. Lancet Infect Dis 2003;3:757. [PMID: 14652202]

Lyme Disease (*Borrelia burgdorferi*)

- ■ Essentials of Diagnosis
  - • History of exposure to *Ixodes* species of tick in endemic area; most U.S. cases occur in the Northeast, upper Midwest, and along the Pacific Coast
  - • Stage I: Early flulike syndrome, erythema chronicum migrans (flat macular rash and erythema with central clearing); usually occurs about 1 week after tick bite
  - • Stage II: Neurologic (Bell's palsy, meningoencephalitis, aseptic meningitis, peripheral neuropathy, transverse myelitis)
  - • Stage III: Musculoskeletal, usually arthritis, monarticular or oligoarticular
  - • Overlap between clinical stages often observed
  - • Mild carditis may occur
  - • Serologic diagnosis is possible after 2–4 weeks of illness; rarely, organism can be cultured from blood, cerebrospinal fluid, or rash aspirate

- ■ Differential Diagnosis
  - • Stage I: Other causes of viral exanthems; rheumatic fever
  - • Stage II: Other causes of peripheral neuropathy, transverse myelitis, encephalitis, aseptic meningitis, Bell's palsy
  - • Stage III: Autoimmune disease, particularly seronegative spondyloarthropathies, Still's disease
  - • Other causes of myocarditis, arrhythmias, and heart block
  - • Chronic fatigue syndrome

- ■ Treatment
  - • Antibiotic chosen depends on stage of disease
  - • Prophylaxis of tick bites not recommended

- ■ Pearl

A disease of which many patients complain and in whom few have it.

Reference

Stanek G, Strle F: Lyme borreliosis. Lancet 2003;362:1639. [PMID: 14630446]

Lymphogranuloma Venereum (*Chlamydia trachomatis* types L1–L3)

- ■ Essentials of Diagnosis
  - A sexually transmitted disease with an incubation period of 5–21 days
  - Evanescent primary genital lesion
  - Inguinal lymphadenopathy and suppuration with draining sinuses
  - Proctitis; rectal stricture; systemic joint, eye, or central nervous system involvement may occur
  - Serologic tests positive in second to third week of illness

- ■ Differential Diagnosis
  - Syphilis
  - Genital herpes
  - Chancroid
  - Bacterial lymphadenitis of other cause (eg, tuberculosis, tularemia)
  - Cancer of rectosigmoid
  - Rectal stricture due to other causes

- ■ Treatment
  - Obtain rapid plasma reagin (RPR) test, consider HIV testing
  - Tetracyclines; erythromycin in pregnancy; quinolones also effective but expensive
  - Dilation or surgical repair of rectal stricture

- ■ Pearl

Early anorectal manifestations in women and homosexual men may simulate inflammatory bowel disease.

Reference

Mabey D, Peeling RW: Lymphogranuloma venereum. Sex Transm Infect 2002;78:90. [PMID: 12081191]

Meningococcal Meningitis (*Neisseria meningitidis*)

- **Essentials of Diagnosis**
  - Fever, headache, vomiting, confusion, delirium, or seizures; typically epidemic in young adults; onset may be astonishingly abrupt
  - Petechial or ecchymotic rash of skin and mucous membranes
  - May have positive Kernig's and Brudzinski's signs
  - Purulent spinal fluid with gram-negative intracellular and extracellular cocci
  - Culture of cerebrospinal fluid, blood, or petechial aspirate confirms diagnosis
  - Disseminated intravascular coagulation and shock may complicate

- **Differential Diagnosis**
  - Meningitis due to other causes
  - Petechial rash due to rickettsial, viral, or other bacterial infection
  - Idiopathic thrombocytopenic purpura

- **Treatment**
  - Active immunization available for selected susceptible groups (military recruits, college dormitory residents)
  - Penicillin or ceftriaxone
  - Mannitol and corticosteroids for elevated intracranial pressure
  - Ciprofloxacin (single dose) or rifampin (2 days) therapy for intimate exposures

- **Pearl**

The most common bacterial meningitis in which organisms are not seen on cerebrospinal fluid Gram's stain (50% of cases).

Reference

Roos KL: Acute bacterial meningitis. Semin Neurol 2000;20:293. [PMID: 11051294]

Nocardiosis

- **Essentials of Diagnosis**
  - *Nocardia asteroides* and *Nocardia brasiliensis* are aerobic soil bacteria causing pulmonary and systemic disease
  - Malaise, weight loss, fever, night sweats, cough
  - Pulmonary consolidation or thin-walled abscess; invasion through chest wall possible
  - Lobar infiltrates, air-fluid level, effusion by chest x-ray
  - Delicate branching, gram-positive filaments by Gram's stain, weakly positive acid-fast staining; culture identifies specific organism
  - Disseminated form may occur with abscess in any organ; brain, subcutaneous nodules most frequent
  - Alveolar proteinosis, corticosteroid use, immunodeficiency predispose to infection
  - The above are all due to *N asteroides; N brasiliensis* causes lymphangitis after skin inoculation and is common among gardeners

- **Differential Diagnosis**
  - Actinomycosis
  - Tuberculosis or atypical mycobacterial infections
  - Other causes of pyogenic lung abscess
  - Lymphoma
  - Coccidioidomycosis
  - Histoplasmosis
  - Herpetic whitlow (*N brasiliensis*)
  - Bacterial lymphangitis (*N brasiliensis*)

- **Treatment**
  - Parenteral and then oral trimethoprim-sulfamethoxazole for many months; shorter, oral course acceptable for *N brasiliensis*
  - Surgical drainage and resection may be needed

- **Pearl**

Nocardia, *like some endemic fungal infections, is a mimic of lung cancer.*

Reference

Corti ME, Villafane-Fioti MF: Nocardiosis: a review. Int J Infect Dis 2003;7:243. [PMID: 14656414]

Pertussis (*Bordetella pertussis*)

■ Essentials of Diagnosis

- An acute infection of the respiratory tract spread by respiratory droplets
- History of declined diphtheria-pertussis-tetanus (DPT) vaccination
- Two-week prodromal catarrhal stage of malaise, cough, coryza, and anorexia; seen predominantly in infants under age 2
- Paroxysmal cough ending in high-pitched inspiratory "whoop" (whooping cough)
- Absolute lymphocytosis with extremely high white counts possible
- Culture confirms diagnosis

■ Differential Diagnosis

- Viral pneumonia
- Foreign body aspiration
- Acute bronchitis
- Acute leukemia (when leukocytosis is marked)

■ Treatment

- Active immunization preventive (as part of DTP)
- Erythromycin with immune globulin in selected patients
- Treat secondary pneumonia and other complications

■ Pearl

The cause of the highest benign white counts in clinical medicine.

Reference

von Konig CH, Halperin S, Riffelmann M, Guiso N: Pertussis of adults and infants. Lancet Infect Dis 2002;2:744. [PMID: 12467690]

Plague (*Yersinia pestis*)

- **Essentials of Diagnosis**
  - History of exposure to rodents in endemic area of southwestern United States; by bites of fleas or contact with infected rodents; human-to-human transmission with pneumonic plague only
  - Sudden onset of high fever, severe malaise, myalgias; stunning systemic toxicity
  - Regional lymphangitis and lymphadenitis with suppuration of nodes
  - Bacteremia, pneumonitis, or meningitis complicate
  - Positive smear and culture from aspirate or blood; striking leukopenia with marked left shift

- **Differential Diagnosis**
  - Tularemia
  - Lymphadenitis with bacterial disease of extremity
  - Lymphogranuloma venereum
  - Other bacterial pneumonia or meningitis
  - Typhoid fever
  - Various rickettsial diseases

- **Treatment**
  - Combination antibiotics required (eg, streptomycin plus tetracycline)
  - Tetracycline prophylaxis for persons exposed to patients with pneumonic plague
  - Strict isolation of pneumonic disease patients

- **Pearl**

Plague should be treated empirically in any case of meningitis encountered in the arid southwestern United States.

Reference

Lazarus AA, Decker CF: Plague. Respir Care Clin North Am 2004;10:83. [PMID: 15062229]

Pneumococcal Infections

- **Essentials of Diagnosis**
  - Pneumonia characterized by initial chill, severe pleuritis, fever without diurnal variation; signs of consolidation and lobar infiltrate on x-ray ensue rapidly
  - Leukocytosis, hyperbilirubinemia
  - Gram-positive diplococci in sputum; lancet-shaped only on stained culture colonies
  - Meningitis: rapid onset of fever, altered mental status, and headache; cerebrospinal fluid polymorphonuclear leukocytosis with elevated protein and decreased glucose; gram-stained smear of fluid obtained prior to receipt of antimicrobial therapy positive in 90% of cases
  - Endocarditis (50% cases with pneumonia and meningitis), empyema, pericarditis, and arthritis may also complicate, with empyema most common
  - Predisposition to bacteremia in children under 24 months of age or in asplenic or immunocompromised adults (eg, AIDS, elderly)

- **Differential Diagnosis**
  - Pneumonia, meningitis of other cause
  - Pulmonary embolism
  - Myocardial infarction
  - Acute exacerbation of chronic bronchitis
  - Acute bronchitis
  - Gram-negative septicemia

- **Treatment**
  - Blood culture prior to antibiotics
  - Third-generation cephalosporin for severe disease; add empiric vancomycin for meningitis pending culture results
  - Adults over 50 with any serious medical illness, patients with sickle cell disease, and asplenic patients should receive pneumococcal vaccine
  - Penicillin unreliable pending results of susceptibility testing

- **Pearl**

Rigors after the first day of infection in a patient with pneumococcal pneumonia suggest a different etiology or an extrapulmonary complication.

Reference

Jacobs MR: *Streptococcus pneumoniae*: epidemiology and patterns of resistance. Am J Med 2004;117(Suppl 3A):3S. [PMID: 15360092]

Psittacosis (*Chlamydia psittaci*)

- ■ Essentials of Diagnosis
  - Contact with infected bird 7–15 days before onset of symptoms
  - Rapid onset of fever, chills, malaise, headache, dry cough, epistaxis
  - Temperature-pulse dissociation, meningismus, erythematous macular rash (Horder's spots), dry crackles, splenomegaly
  - Slightly delayed appearance of signs of pneumonitis; culture-negative endocarditis may occur
  - Serologic diagnosis by second week of illness; organism rarely isolated by culture of respiratory secretions

- ■ Differential Diagnosis
  - Other atypical pneumonias (eg, viral, mycoplasmal, rickettsial)
  - Typhoid fever
  - Lymphoma
  - Tuberculosis
  - Other culture-negative endocarditis

- ■ Treatment
  - Tetracycline

- ■ Pearl

The history of bird contact may be difficult to obtain, as many cases are transmitted by illegally imported parrots valued by patients as loyal pets.

Reference

Elliott JH: Psittacosis. A flu like syndrome. Aust Fam Physician 2001;30:739. [PMID: 11681143]

Rat-Bite Fever (*Spirillum minus*)

- **Essentials of Diagnosis**
  - History of rodent bite; one to several weeks after bite, the site becomes swollen, indurated, and painful
  - Fever, chills, nausea, vomiting, rash, headache, myalgia, and arthralgia; symptoms relapse at 24- to 48-hour intervals
  - Regional lymphangitis or adenopathy, splenomegaly
  - False-positive rapid plasma reagin (RPR) test
  - Diagnosis confirmed by serologic testing or Giemsa-stained darkfield examination of blood or exudate

- **Differential Diagnosis**
  - Malaria
  - Tularemia
  - Leptospirosis
  - Borreliosis
  - Rickettsial infection
  - Brucellosis
  - Lymphangitis caused by *Nocardia brasiliensis*

- **Treatment**
  - Penicillin or tetracycline

- **Pearl**

One of medicine's few relapsing fevers.

Reference

Freels LK, Elliott SP: Rat bite fever: three case reports and a literature review. Clin Pediatr (Phila) 2004;43:291. [PMID: 15094956]

Relapsing Fever (*Borrelia recurrentis*)

- **Essentials of Diagnosis**
  - History of exposure to ticks in endemic area
  - Abrupt fever and chills, nausea, headache, arthralgia lasting 3–10 days with relapse at intervals of 1–2 weeks
  - Tachycardia, hepatosplenomegaly, rash
  - Spirochetes seen on blood smear during fever; serologic diagnosis positive at second week of illness

- **Differential Diagnosis**
  - Malaria
  - Leptospirosis
  - Meningococcemia
  - Yellow fever
  - Typhus
  - Rat-bite fever
  - Hodgkin's disease with Pel-Ebstein fever

- **Treatment**
  - Single dose of tetracycline, erythromycin, or penicillin
  - Herxheimer reaction may occur after treatment with bactericidal agents

- **Pearl**

One of the few diseases in medicine in which the fever curve is diagnostic.

Reference

Dworkin MS, Schwan TG, Anderson DE Jr: Tick-borne relapsing fever in North America. Med Clin North Am 2002;86:417, viii. [PMID: 11982310]

Salmonella Gastroenteritis
(Various *Salmonella* Species)

- ■ Essentials of Diagnosis
  - The most common form of salmonellosis
  - Nausea, headache, meningismus, fever, high-volume diarrhea, usually without blood, and abdominal pain 8–48 hours after ingestion of contaminated food or liquid
  - Positive fecal leukocytes
  - Culture of organism from stool; bacteremia less common

- ■ Differential Diagnosis
  - Viral gastroenteritis, especially enterovirus
  - Dysenteric illness (*Shigella, Campylobacter,* amebic)
  - Enterotoxigenic *E coli* infection
  - Inflammatory bowel disease

- ■ Treatment
  - Rehydration and potassium repletion
  - Antibiotics (ciprofloxacin or ceftriaxone) essential in those with sickle cell anemia, immunosuppression, or severe vascular disease
  - In others, antimicrobials reduce symptoms by 1–2 days

- ■ Pearl

All patients continuously bacteremic with Salmonella *should be suspected of having a mycotic aortic aneurysm.*

Reference

Edwards BH: *Salmonella* and *Shigella* species. Clin Lab Med 1999;19:469, v. [PMID: 10549421]

Staphylococcal Soft Tissue or Skin Infections

- **Essentials of Diagnosis**
  - More often encountered in diabetics
  - Painful, pruritic erythematous rash with golden crusts or discharge
  - Folliculitis, furunculosis, carbuncle, abscess, and cellulitis all seen
  - Culture of abscess is diagnostic; gram-stained smear positive for large gram-positive cocci (*Staphylococcus aureus*) in clusters

- **Differential Diagnosis**
  - Streptococcal skin infections

- **Treatment**
  - Penicillinase-resistant penicillin or first-generation cephalosporin; erythromycin may also be effective in some cases
  - Drainage of abscess
  - Persistence of blood culture positivity suggests endocarditis or osteomyelitis

- **Pearl**

Microbiologic etiology is seldom in doubt; treatment more complicated than for Streptococcus *infections.*

Reference

Fung HB, Chang JY, Kuczynski S: A practical guide to the treatment of complicated skin and soft tissue infections. Drugs 2003;63:1459. [PMID: 12834364]

Staphylococcus aureus-Associated Toxic Shock Syndrome

- **Essentials of Diagnosis**
  - Association with tampon use, often postsurgical
  - Abrupt onset of fever, vomiting, diarrhea, sore throat, headache, myalgia
  - Toxic appearance, with tachycardia and hypotension
  - Diffuse maculopapular erythematous rash with desquamation on the palms and soles; nonpurulent conjunctivitis
  - Culture of nasopharynx, vagina, rectum, and wounds may yield staphylococci, but blood cultures usually negative
  - Usually caused by toxic shock syndrome toxin-1 (TSST-1)

- **Differential Diagnosis**
  - Streptococcal infection, particularly scarlet fever
  - Gram-negative sepsis
  - Rickettsial disease, especially Rocky Mountain spotted fever

- **Treatment**
  - Aggressive supportive care (eg, fluids, vasopressor medication, monitoring)
  - Antistaphylococcal antibiotics to eliminate source

- **Pearl**

Unlike streptococcal toxic shock syndrome, most patients with staphylococcal toxic shock do not have a clinically apparent infection.

Reference

Alouf JE, Muller-Alouf H: Staphylococcal and streptococcal superantigens: molecular, biological and clinical aspects. Int J Med Microbiol 2003;292:429. [PMID: 12635926]

Streptococcal Pharyngitis

- **■ Essentials of Diagnosis**
  - Abrupt onset of sore throat, fever, malaise, nausea, headache
  - Pharynx erythematous and edematous with exudate; cervical adenopathy
  - Strawberry tongue
  - Throat culture or rapid antigen detection confirmatory
  - If erythrotoxin (scarlet fever) is produced, scarlatiniform rash that is red and papular with petechiae and fine desquamation will be present; prominent in axilla, groin, behind knees
  - Glomerulonephritis, rheumatic fever may complicate

- **■ Differential Diagnosis**
  - Viral pharyngitis
  - Mononucleosis
  - Diphtheria
  - With rash: meningococcemia, toxic shock syndrome, drug reaction, viral exanthem

- **■ Treatment**
  - For two or more clinical criteria (cervical adenopathy, fever, exudate, and absence of rhinorrhea): empiric penicillin
  - If equivocal, await culture or antigen confirmation
  - If history of rheumatic fever, continuous antibiotic prophylaxis for 5 years

- **■ Pearl**

Despite the clinical severity of pharyngeal diphtheria, fever is higher in strep throat.

Reference

Vincent MT, Celestin N, Hussain AN: Pharyngitis. Am Fam Physician 2004;69:1465. [PMID: 15053411]

Streptococcal Skin Infection

- **Essentials of Diagnosis**
    - Erysipelas: rapidly spreading cutaneous erythema and edema with sharp borders
    - Impetigo: rapidly spreading erythema with vesicular or denuded areas and salmon-colored crust
    - Culture of wound or blood grows group A beta-hemolytic streptococci
    - Complication: glomerulonephritis

- **Differential Diagnosis**
    - Other causes of infectious cellulitis (eg, staphylococcal)
    - Toxic shock syndrome
    - Beriberi (in setting of thiamin deficiency)

- **Treatment**
    - Penicillin for culture-proved streptococcal infection
    - Staphylococcal coverage (nafcillin, dicloxacillin) for empiric therapy or uncertain diagnosis

- **Pearl**

Group A cutaneous infections can result in glomerulonephritis but not rheumatic fever.

Reference

Bonnetblanc JM, Bedane C: Erysipelas: recognition and management. Am J Clin Dermatol 2003;4:157. [PMID: 12627991]

Syphilis, Primary (*Treponema pallidum*)

- **Essentials of Diagnosis**
  - History of sexual contact, often of uncertain reliability or identity
  - Painless ulcer (chancre) on genitalia, perianal region, oropharynx, or elsewhere 2–6 weeks following exposure
  - Nontender regional adenopathy
  - Fluid expressed from lesion positive, and infectious, by immunofluorescence or darkfield microscopy
  - Rapid plasma reagin (RPR) positive in 60%

- **Differential Diagnosis**
  - Chancroid
  - Lymphogranuloma venereum
  - Genital herpes
  - Lymphadenitis of other causes
  - Lymphoma
  - Drug eruption
  - Reactive arthritis
  - Behçet's syndrome

- **Treatment**
  - Benzathine penicillin, 2.4 million units intramuscularly
  - With penicillin allergy, erythromycin or doxycycline acceptable

- **Pearl**

Any painless genital ulcer should be considered syphilitic until an alternative diagnosis is established.

Reference

Golden MR, Marra CM, Holmes KK: Update on syphilis: resurgence of an old problem. JAMA 2003;290:1510. [PMID: 13129993]

Syphilis, Secondary

- **Essentials of Diagnosis**
  - Develops coincident with, or more typically, 2 weeks to 6 months after appearance—and usually spontaneous disappearance—of chancre
  - Fever, generalized maculopapular skin rash (including palms, soles, and mucous membranes, the latter highly contagious)
  - Weeping papules (condyloma lata) in moist skin areas
  - Generalized tender lymphadenopathy
  - Meningitis, hepatitis, osteitis, arthritis, or iritis may occur
  - Many treponemes in scrapings of mucous membranes or skin lesions by immunofluorescence or darkfield microscopy
  - Rapid plasma reagin (RPR) test is uniformly positive in high titer; should be repeated 1–2 weeks later because of prozone effect with false-negative

- **Differential Diagnosis**
  - Viral exanthems
  - Pityriasis rosea
  - Drug rash, especially erythema multiforme
  - Multiple organ involvement may mimic meningitis, hepatitis, arthritis, uveitis, nephrotic syndrome of other etiology

- **Treatment**
  - Same as for primary syphilis; skin lesions may be temporarily exaggerated
  - If central nervous system disease present, treat as neurosyphilis, with longer course of therapy
  - Herxheimer reaction most common after bactericidal treatment of secondary syphilis

- **Pearl**

Any dermatologic eruption involving the palms should be considered secondary syphilis, regardless of history or appearance, until proved otherwise.

Reference

Golden MR, Marra CM, Holmes KK: Update on syphilis: resurgence of an old problem. JAMA 2003;290:1510. [PMID: 13129993]

Syphilis, Tertiary (or Late)

- **Essentials of Diagnosis**
  - Many asymptomatic
  - May occur at any time after secondary syphilis (occurs in one-third of untreated patients)
  - Infiltrative tumors of skin, bone, liver (gummas); vascular disease with aortitis, ascending aortic aneurysms with aortic insufficiency
  - Neurosyphilis, early latent: meningovascular, with presenting symptoms of basilar meningitis or stroke
  - Neurosyphilis, late latent: tabes dorsalis; wide-based gait, fleeting abdominal or leg pain, bladder symptoms all due to dorsal column disease; general paresis; slowly progressive dementia; Argyll-Robertson pupils (miotic, nonreactive but accommodating)
  - Tabes may result in severe knee arthropathy (Charcot's joint)

- **Differential Diagnosis**
  - Primary or secondary malignancy in any organ in which a gumma is involved
  - Aortic insufficiency due to other causes
  - Pernicious anemia (tabes)
  - Surgical causes of acute abdomen (tabes)
  - Viral or fungal meningitis (meningovascular)
  - Other causes of neurogenic bladder (tabes)

- **Treatment**
  - Lumbar puncture for patients with syphilis longer than 1 year or with peripheral titers > 1:32 (unless asymptomatic), HIV-positive, or with neurologic signs
  - For asymptomatic patients, treat with three doses 1 week apart of intramuscular benzathine penicillin
  - For neurosyphilis with symptomatic or central nervous system abnormality: 10–14 days of parenteral penicillin
  - Repeat lumbar puncture to follow cerebrospinal fluid abnormality to resolution
  - Treatment in HIV neurosyphilis controversial

- **Pearl**

One third of patients with tertiary lues are rapid plasma reagin (RPR)-negative; antitreponemal studies are required for diagnosis.

Reference

Golden MR, Marra CM, Holmes KK: Update on syphilis: resurgence of an old problem. JAMA 2003;290:1510. [PMID: 13129993]

Tetanus (*Clostridium tetani*)

- **Essentials of Diagnosis**
  - History of non-debrided wound or contamination may or may not be obtained
  - Jaw stiffness followed by spasms (trismus)
  - Stiffness of neck or other muscles, dysphagia, irritability, hyperreflexia; late, painful convulsions precipitated by minimal stimuli; fever is low-grade

- **Differential Diagnosis**
  - Infectious meningitis
  - Rabies
  - Strychnine poisoning
  - Malignant neuroleptic syndrome
  - Hypocalcemia

- **Treatment**
  - Active immunization preventive
  - Passive immunization with tetanus immune globulin and concurrent active immunization for all suspected cases
  - Chlorpromazine or diazepam for spasms or convulsions, with additional sedation by barbiturates as necessary
  - Vigorous supportive care with particular attention to airway and laryngospasm
  - Penicillin or clindamycin

- **Pearl**

Tetanus should be high on the list in "skin-popping" illicit drug users with increased muscle tone.

Reference

Farrar JJ, Yen LM, Cook T, et al: Tetanus. J Neurol Neurosurg Psychiatry 2000;69:292. [PMID: 10945801]

Tuberculosis (*Mycobacterium tuberculosis*)

- ■ Essentials of Diagnosis
  - • Most infections subclinical, with positive skin test only
  - • Symptoms progressive, and include cough, dyspnea, fever, night sweats, weight loss, and hemoptysis
  - • In primary infection, mid-lung field infiltrates with regional lymphadenopathy; pleural effusion common
  - • Apical fibronodular pulmonary infiltrate on chest film, with or without cavitation, is most typical in reactivation diseases
  - • Posttussive rales noted on auscultation
  - • Most common extrapulmonary manifestations include meningitis, genitourinary infection, miliary disease, arthritis, with localized symptoms and signs

- ■ Differential Diagnosis
  - • Pneumonia of other cause; bacterial and fungal (histoplasmosis, coccidioidomycosis) most similar
  - • Other mycobacterosis
  - • HIV infection (may be associated)
  - • Prolonged fever of other cause
  - • Urinary tract infection, oligoarticular arthritis of other cause
  - • Carcinoma of the lung
  - • Lung abscess

- ■ Treatment
  - • Four-drug regimens to include isoniazid and rifampin
  - • Attention must be paid to sensitivity patterns due to increasing prevalence of drug-resistant strains

- ■ Pearl

In HIV-infected patients, concerning tuberculosis and the clinical scenario: if it looks like TB, it's not, and if it doesn't, it is.

Reference

Frieden TR, Sterling TR, Munsiff SS, et al: Tuberculosis. Lancet 2003;362:887. [PMID: 13678977]

Tuberculous Meningitis (*Mycobacterium tuberculosis*)

- ■ Essentials of Diagnosis
  - Insidious onset of listlessness, irritability, headaches
  - Meningeal signs, cranial nerve palsies
  - Tuberculous focus evident elsewhere in half of patients
  - Cerebrospinal fluid with lymphocytic pleocytosis, low glucose, and high protein; culture positive for acid-fast bacilli in many but not all; polymerase chain reaction (PCR) often helpful
  - Chest x-ray may reveal abnormalities compatible with pulmonary tuberculosis

- ■ Differential Diagnosis
  - Chronic lymphocytic meningitis due to fungi, brucellosis, leptospirosis, HIV infection, neurocysticercosis, sarcoidosis
  - Carcinomatous meningitis
  - Unsuspected head trauma with subdural hematoma
  - Drug overdose
  - Psychiatric disorder

- ■ Treatment
  - Empiric antituberculous therapy essential in proper clinical setting
  - Concomitant corticosteroids reduce long-term complications

- ■ Pearl

Striking hypoglycorrhachia in lymphocytic meningitis means tuberculous meningitis until disproved; acellular hypoglycorrhachia should be assumed to be hypoglycemia until proven otherwise by blood glucose.

Reference

Thwaites G, Chau TT, Mai NT, et al: Tuberculous meningitis. J Neurol Neurosurg Psychiatry 2000;68:289. [PMID: 10675209]

Tularemia (*Francisella tularensis*)

- **Essentials of Diagnosis**
  - History of contact with rabbits, other rodents, and biting arthropods (eg, ticks) in endemic areas; incubation period 2–10 days
  - Fever, headache, nausea begin suddenly
  - Papule progressing to ulcer at site of inoculation; the conjunctiva may be the site in occasional patients
  - Prominent, tender regional lymphadenopathy, splenomegaly
  - Diagnosis confirmed by culture of ulcerated lesion, lymph node aspirate, or blood; serologic confirmation positive after second week of illness
  - Though primarily cutaneous, ocular, glandular, or typhoidal, only the very rare pneumonic form is transmissible between humans

- **Differential Diagnosis**
  - Cat-scratch disease
  - Infectious mononucleosis
  - Plague
  - Typhoid fever
  - Lymphoma
  - Various rickettsial infections
  - Meningococcemia

- **Treatment**
  - Combination antibiotics required; streptomycin and tetracycline are usually used

- **Pearl**

Although named for the index case in Tulare County in California, the most prominent epidemic was on Martha's Vineyard in Massachusetts; it is rarely encountered in Tulare County.

Reference

Choi E: Tularemia and Q fever. Med Clin North Am 2002;86:393. [PMID: 11982309]

FUNGAL INFECTIONS

Candidiasis (*Candida albicans*)

- ■ Essentials of Diagnosis
  - Plaquelike or ulcerative lesions of oral mucosa (thrush)
  - Vulvovaginitis, skin fold infections, or paronychia
  - Esophageal, pulmonary, central nervous system, or disseminated disease in immunosuppressed patients
  - Endocarditis in patients with prosthetic valves
  - A compatible clinical picture, susceptible host, and finding *Candida* in specimens establishes diagnosis

- ■ Differential Diagnosis
  - Severe atopic dermatitis
  - Herpetic or cytomegalovirus esophagitis in immunosupressed patients
  - Other fungal or basilar meningitides
  - Prosthetic valve endocarditis of other cause

- ■ Treatment
  - Nystatin, clotrimazole, miconazole for local lesions
  - Fluconazole for systemic infections
  - Amphotericin B or caspofungin for severe infection
  - Valve replacement obligatory in prosthetic valve endocarditis

- ■ Pearl

Candida glabrata—*once known as* Torulopsis glabrata—*is increasingly common and often resistant to fluconazole; it may cause a refractory prostatitis.*

Reference

Eggimann P, Garbino J, Pittet D: Management of *Candida* species infections in critically ill patients. Lancet Infect Dis 2003;3:772. [PMID: 14652203]

Coccidioidomycosis (*Coccidioides immitis*)

- **Essentials of Diagnosis**
  - Arthrospores in deserts of central and southern California and Arizona; highly infectious
  - Pulmonary form: fever, pleuritis, dry cough, anorexia, weight loss, erythema nodosum, and erythema multiforme with arthralgias; "desert rheumatism or valley fever"
  - Incubation period 10–30 days; not contagious between humans
  - Disseminated lesions involve skin, bones, and meninges
  - Eosinophilia and leukocytosis
  - Sporangia in pus, sputum, or cerebrospinal fluid may be seen
  - Radiographic studies show nodular pulmonary infiltrates with thin-walled cavities and hilar adenopathy
  - Skin test of limited value, but serologic testing helpful both diagnostically and prognostically; persistence of IgG in higher titer indicates disseminated disease

- **Differential Diagnosis**
  - Tuberculosis
  - Histoplasmosis
  - Blastomycosis
  - Osteomyelitis from other causes
  - Aseptic meningitis from other causes
  - Sarcoidosis

- **Treatment**
  - Fluconazole in mild disease
  - Amphotericin B for disseminated disease

- **Pearl**

Coccidioidomycosis cultured from pathologic material undergoes morphologic change to highly infectious arthrospores; immunologic confirmation of diagnosis safe and accurate.

Reference

Feldman BS, Snyder LS: Primary pulmonary coccidioidomycosis. Semin Respir Infect 2001;16:231. [PMID: 11740823]

Cryptococcosis (*Cryptococcus neoformans*)

- **Essentials of Diagnosis**
  - Opportunistic disease seen most commonly in AIDS patients or those with Hodgkin's disease
  - Findings subtle with fever, headache, photophobia, and neuropathies
  - Meningeal signs with positive Kernig's and Brudzinski's signs unusual
  - Solitary, local skin lesions may be seen
  - Subacute respiratory infection with low-grade fever, pleuritic pain, and cough seen as well
  - Spinal fluid findings include increased pressure, variable pleocytosis, increased protein, and decreased glucose
  - Large encapsulated yeasts by India ink mount of spinal fluid or cryptococcal antigen serology positive on both serum and spinal fluid

- **Differential Diagnosis**
  - Other causes of meningitis
  - Lymphoma
  - Tuberculosis

- **Treatment**
  - Amphotericin B and flucytosine for severe disease
  - Fluconazole can be used in many patients to complete therapy
  - All patients with serum antigen-positive and HIV disease should undergo lumbar puncture

- **Pearl**

Ninety-five percent of patients with cryptococcal meningitis have positive serum cryptococcal antigen.

Reference

Perfect JR, Casadevall A: Cryptococcosis. Infect Dis Clin North Am 2002;16: 837, v. [PMID: 12512184]

Histoplasmosis (*Histoplasma capsulatum*)

- **Essentials of Diagnosis**
  - History of bird or bat exposure or of living near a river valley; house painters at risk
  - Often asymptomatic; variable cough, fever, malaise, chest pain in self-limited infections
  - Ulceration of naso- and oropharynx, hepatosplenomegaly, generalized lymphadenopathy in disseminated disease (1 in 250,000 cases) if not immunocompromised; this is the typical presentation in HIV disease
  - Acute pericarditis an uncommon presentation; adrenalitis also observed in systemic disease
  - Fibrosing mediastinitis a long-term complication; may cause superior vena cava syndrome
  - Skin test of limited value
  - Urinary *Histoplasma* antigen is diagnostic; small budding fungus cells found in reticuloendothelial cells; biopsy and culture of organism confirms diagnosis

- **Differential Diagnosis**
  - Tuberculosis
  - Blastomycosis
  - Coccidioidomycosis
  - Lymphoma
  - Sarcoidosis

- **Treatment**
  - Oral itraconazole for most infections
  - Amphotericin B in severe disease or in those who have failed itraconazole treatment

- **Pearl**

Pulmonary calcifications on chest x-ray in patients whose social security number begins with 2, 3, or 4 is histoplasmosis.

Reference

Wheat LJ, Kauffman CA: Histoplasmosis. Infect Dis Clin North Am 2003;17:1, vii. [PMID: 12751258]

Pneumocystosis
(*Pneumocystis carinii* Pneumonia [PCP])

■ Essentials of Diagnosis

- Seen primarily in immunocompromised patients (AIDS, post–tissue transplantation, lymphoreticular malignancy); CD4 level less than 200 is the rule
- Fever, dyspnea, dry cough, often insidious onset
- Dry crackles upon auscultation
- Diffuse alveolar disease by chest x-ray; occasionally, small cavities
- Large alveolar-arterial gradient; decreased single-breath diffusing capacity; elevated serum lactate dehydrogenase; abnormal gallium scan
- Organism identified by silver stain, antibody staining, or polymerase chain reaction (PCR) of secretions or biopsy
- Extrapulmonary disease may be seen if patient is undergoing routine prophylactic therapy with pentamidine

■ Differential Diagnosis

- Atypical pneumonia due to other causes
- Congestive heart failure
- Tuberculosis
- Disseminated fungal disease

■ Treatment

- Many drug regimens effective; trimethoprim-sulfamethoxazole is first-line therapy
- Corticosteroids are adjunctive if moderate or severe hypoxemia present
- Chemoprophylaxis recommended for immunocompromised patients at risk

■ Pearl

A negative PCR or antibody staining from bronchoalveolar lavage virtually excludes PCP.

Reference

Thomas CF Jr, Limper AH: *Pneumocystis* pneumonia. N Engl J Med 2004;350:2487. [PMID: 15190141]

Sporotrichosis (*Sporothrix schenckii*)

- Essentials of Diagnosis
  - Ulcer following trauma to extremity
  - Occupationally associated with exposure to plants or soil; thorn inoculation typical
  - Nodules found along lymphatic drainage, which may ulcerate with a black eschar
  - Culture is needed to establish diagnosis
  - Serology helpful in disseminated disease (rare)

- Differential Diagnosis
  - Tularemia
  - Anthrax
  - Other mycotic infections
  - Cutaneous tuberculosis

- Treatment
  - Itraconazole for several months is the treatment of choice for localized disease
  - Amphotericin B used in severe systemic infection
  - Potassium iodide solution orally in some cases

- Pearl

Lymphadenopathy in a rose fancier is sporotrichosis until proven otherwise.

Reference

De Araujo T, Marques AC, Kerdel F: Sporotrichosis. Int J Dermatol 2001;40:737. [PMID: 11903665]

HELMINTHIC INFECTIONS

Ascariasis (*Ascaris lumbricoides*)

- **Essentials of Diagnosis**
  - Pulmonary phase: fever, cough, hemoptysis, wheezing, urticaria, and eosinophilia; fleeting pulmonary infiltrates be seen (Löffler's pneumonia)
  - Intestinal phase: vague abdominal discomfort and colic, vomiting
  - Inflammatory reactions in any organs and tissues invaded by wandering adult worms
  - Pancreatitis, appendicitis, intestinal obstruction may all complicate infection
  - Characteristic ascaritic ova in stool with larvae in sputum

- **Differential Diagnosis**
  - Pneumonitis due to other parasitic infiltrations (especially hookworm and *Strongyloides*)
  - Bacterial or viral pneumonia
  - Allergic disorders such as Löffler's syndrome, asthma, urticaria, allergic bronchopulmonary aspergillosis, Churg-Strauss syndrome
  - Eosinophilic pneumonia
  - Pancreatitis, peptic ulcer disease, appendicitis, and diverticulitis due to other causes

- **Treatment**
  - Mebendazole or albendazole

- **Pearl**

Consider ascariasis in appendicitis or pancreatitis with eosinophilia.

Reference

Crompton DW: Ascaris and ascariasis. Adv Parasitol 2001;48:285. [PMID: 11013758]

Cysticercosis (*Taenia solium*)

- Essentials of Diagnosis
  - History of exposure in endemic area
  - Infection by the larval (cysticercus) stage of *T solium;* locations of cysts in order of frequency are central nervous system, subcutaneous tissue, striated muscle, globe of eye, and rarely, other tissues
  - Seizure, headache, vomiting, blurred vision, fever
  - Focal neurologic abnormalities, papilledema, pear-shaped subcutaneous or muscular nodules
  - Eosinophilia; lymphocytic and eosinophilic pleocytosis, elevated protein, and decreased glucose in cerebrospinal fluid
  - Parasite seen upon histologic examination of skin or subcutaneous nodule
  - Plain radiograph of soft tissue reveals oval or linear calcifications in nodules
  - CT or MRI of the head reveals calcification of cysts and signs of elevated intracerebral pressure
  - Serologic testing is helpful to differentiate cysticercosis from echinococcosis

- Differential Diagnosis
  - Echinococcosis
  - Lymphoma
  - Toxoplasmosis
  - Brain abscess
  - Brain tumor
  - Coccidioidomycosis

- Treatment
  - Controversial in CNS disease
  - Praziquantel or albendazole
  - Concomitant treatment with steroids and mannitol for cerebral edema may be beneficial
  - Surgery in selected cases (orbital, retinal, spinal cord, or cisternal disease)

- Pearl

The most common cause of seizures in young adults in Mexico.

Reference

Garcia HH, Gonzalez AE, Gilman RH; Cysticercosis Working Group in Peru: Diagnosis, treatment and control of *Taenia solium* cysticercosis. Curr Opin Infect Dis 2003;16:411. [PMID: 14501993]

Echinococcosis (Hydatid Disease)

- **Essentials of Diagnosis**
  - A zoonosis in which humans are an intermediate host of the larval stage of the parasite
  - History of close association with dogs in endemic area
  - Often asymptomatic; signs of local obstruction or cyst rupture and leakage (pain, fever, or anaphylaxis)
  - Avascular cystic tumor of liver, lung, bone, brain, or other organs
  - Eosinophilia; serologic tests positive after 2–4 weeks

- **Differential Diagnosis**
  - Bacterial or amebic liver abscess
  - Tuberculosis
  - Other lung, bone, or brain tumors
  - Obstructive jaundice due to other causes
  - Cirrhosis from other causes
  - Anaphylaxis or eosinophilia from other causes

- **Treatment**
  - Surgical removal of cysts if location permits
  - Albendazole (or mebendazole) may be effective if surgery not possible
  - Treat pet dogs prophylactically (with praziquantel) in endemic areas

- **Pearl**

A liver cyst with rim calcification suggests the diagnosis.

Reference

McManus DP, Zhang W, Li J, Bartley PB: Echinococcosis. Lancet 2003;362:1295. [PMID: 14575976]

Enterobiasis (Pinworm; *Enterobius vermicularis*)

- ■ Essentials of Diagnosis
  - • Nocturnal perianal and vulvar pruritus; insomnia, restlessness, and irritability
  - • Children infected commonly
  - • Vague gastrointestinal symptoms
  - • Eggs of pinworms on skin or perianal area by cellulose tape test

- ■ Differential Diagnosis
  - • Perianal pruritus from other causes (mycotic infections, allergies, hemorrhoids, proctitis, fissures, strongyloidiasis)
  - • Enuresis, insomnia, or restlessness in children due to other causes

- ■ Treatment
  - • Pyrantel pamoate drug of choice
  - • Mebendazole also effective; do not give during pregnancy
  - • Treat all household members

- ■ Pearl

The nightmare—no pun intended—of any mother of a child with the problem.

Reference

Kucik CJ, Martin GL, Sortor BV: Common intestinal parasites. Am Fam Physician 2004;69:1161. [PMID: 15023017]

Hookworm Disease

- ■ Essentials of Diagnosis
  - • Widespread in the moist tropics and subtropics; occurs sporadically in southern U.S.
  - • Weakness, fatigue, pallor, palpitations, dyspnea, diarrhea, abdominal discomfort, and weight loss
  - • Transient episodes of coughing or wheezing with sore throat or bloody sputum sometimes seen
  - • Pruritic, erythematous, maculopapular or vesicular dermatitis; spoon-shaped nails
  - • Hypochromic microcytic anemia, eosinophilia
  - • Guaiac-positive stool
  - • Characteristic hookworm eggs in stool

- ■ Differential Diagnosis
  - • Iron deficiency due to other causes
  - • Recurrent pulmonary embolism
  - • Maculopapular or vesicular dermatitis due to other causes

- ■ Treatment
  - • Pyrantel pamoate or albendazole
  - • Mebendazole if ascariasis is also present
  - • Iron supplementation for anemia

- ■ Pearl

Iron deficiency with eosinophilia in endemic areas suggests hookworm.

Reference

Hotez PJ, Brooker S, Bethony JM, et al: Hookworm infection. N Engl J Med 2004;351:799. [PMID: 15317893]

Schistosomiasis (Bilharziasis; *Schistosoma* Species)

- **Essentials of Diagnosis**
  - Acute: Katayama fever (fever, diarrhea, dry cough, urticaria; cercarial dermatitis, a transient erythematous pruritic skin rash in areas of contact with water)
  - Chronic: Depends on species, with *S mansoni* producing severe portal hypertension and chronic portosystemic collateralization; terminal hematuria, urinary frequency, urethral and bladder pain in *S haematobium*
  - Eggs in systemic circulation obstruct pulmonary resistance vessels, causing pulmonary hypertension and cor pulmonale, ischemia in other organs including spinal cord
  - Demonstration of schistosome ova in stools or urine or rectal biopsy diagnostic

- **Differential Diagnosis**
  - Other causes of diarrhea (acute)
  - Cirrhosis
  - Hepatoma
  - Gastrointestinal neoplasm
  - Cystitis due to other causes
  - Genitourinary tumor
  - Transverse myelitis
  - Pulmonary hypertension due to other causes, especially mitral stenosis, primary pulmonary hypertension

- **Treatment**
  - Chemotherapy dependent upon species and site of disease; generally doesn't help chronic disease

- **Pearl**

Right heart failure of unknown cause in Puerto Ricans and East Asians should always raise the question of schistosomiasis, even years after they have left the endemic area.

Reference

Ross AG, Bartley PB, Sleigh AC, et al: Schistosomiasis. N Engl J Med 2002;346:1212. [PMID: 11961151]

Strongyloidiasis (*Strongyloides stercoralis*)

- **Essentials of Diagnosis**
  - Endemic in southeastern U.S.
  - Pruritic dermatitis at sites of larval penetration
  - Diarrhea, epigastric pain, nausea, malaise, weight loss, cough, rales and wheezing with chronic infection
  - Transient or fleeting pulmonary infiltrates
  - Eosinophilia; characteristic larvae in stool, duodenal aspirate, or sputum
  - Parasite may live in intestine for years after patient leaves endemic area
  - Hyperinfection syndrome: severe diarrhea with malabsorption, bronchopneumonia, gram-negative sepsis, with meningitis, often after corticosteroids given for "asthma"

- **Differential Diagnosis**
  - Eosinophilia due to other causes
  - Recurrent diarrhea due to other causes
  - Duodenal ulcer
  - Asthma
  - Recurrent pulmonary emboli
  - Cholecystitis or pancreatitis due to other causes
  - Intestinal malabsorption due to other causes

- **Treatment**
  - Thiabendazole or ivermectin
  - Mebendazole, pyrantel pamoate, cambendazole, levamisole less effective

- **Pearl**

Duodenal ulcer with eosinophilia is strongyloidiasis until proven otherwise.

Reference

Siddiqui AA, Berk SL: Diagnosis of *Strongyloides stercoralis* infection. Clin Infect Dis 2001;33:1040. Epub 2001 Sep 05. [PMID: 11528578]

Tapeworm Infections
(See also Echinococcosis and Cysticercosis)

- **Essentials of Diagnosis**
  - Six infect humans: *Taenia saginata* (beef tapeworm), *Taenia solium* (pork tapeworm), *Diphyllobothrium latum* (fish tapeworm), *Hymenolepis nana* (dwarf tapeworm), *Hymenolepis diminuta* (rodent tapeworm), *Dipylidium caninum* (dog tapeworm)
  - Usually asymptomatic but may cause nausea, diarrhea, abdominal cramps, malaise, weight loss
  - Segments of worm found in clothing or on bedding
  - Megaloblastic anemia (*D latum*) due to competition for intestinal vitamin B_{12}
  - Characteristic eggs or proglottid segments of tapeworms in stool

- **Differential Diagnosis**
  - Diarrhea due to other causes
  - Malabsorption states due to other causes
  - Pernicious anemia and folic acid deficiency

- **Treatment**
  - Niclosamide for all infections except *H nana*
  - Praziquantel for *H nana* infections

- **Pearl**

Ingestion of sushi and gefilte fish are occasional sources of fish tapeworms in Americans.

Reference

Hoberg EP: *Taenia* tapeworms: their biology, evolution and socioeconomic significance. Microbes Infect 2002;4:859. [PMID: 12270733]

Trichinosis (*Trichinella spiralis*)

- **Essentials of Diagnosis**
  - Vomiting, diarrhea, abdominal pain within first week of ingestion of inadequately cooked pork, boar, or bear; often in homemade sausage, but lean meat is most common cause in U.S.
  - Second week characterized by muscle pain and tenderness, fever (often herpetic), periorbital and facial edema, conjunctivitis; multiple splinter hemorrhages; symptoms due to dissemination of larvae
  - Eosinophilia and variably elevated serum CK, LDH, and AST; erythrocyte sedimentation rate low
  - Positive skin and serologic tests
  - Diagnosis confirmed by finding larvae in muscle biopsy

- **Differential Diagnosis**
  - Dermatomyositis
  - Polyarteritis nodosa
  - Endocarditis
  - Diarrhea due to other infections

- **Treatment**
  - Thiabendazole or mebendazole for intestinal phase
  - Corticosteroids during larval invasion and for systemic sequelae; should not be used during the intestinal phase

- **Pearl**

Clinical vasculitis with a low sedimentation rate suggests the diagnosis.

Reference

Kociecka W: Trichinellosis: human disease, diagnosis and treatment. Vet Parasitol 2000;93:365. [PMID: 11099848]

PROTOZOAL INFECTIONS

Amebiasis (*Entamoeba histolytica*)

- ■ Essentials of Diagnosis
  - May occur sporadically or in epidemics
  - Infection of the large intestine; the parasite may be carried to the liver, lungs, brain, or other organs
  - Recurrent bouts of diarrhea and abdominal cramps, often alternating with constipation
  - In fulminant cases, frank bloody dysentery
  - Tenderness and enlargement of liver with or without abscess
  - Colonic ameboma or liver cyst may occur without dysentery
  - Leukocytosis in some, but eosinophilia uncommon; positive fecal leukocytes
  - Organism demonstrable in stools or aspirate of liver abscess, with hematophagous amebas diagnostic
  - Cysts in stools in quiescent infection
  - Serologic tests very sensitive (99%) in invasive disease (liver abscess, ameboma), less so in intestinal disease (60%)
  - Ultrasound and CT scan useful to image hepatic abscesses

- ■ Differential Diagnosis
  - Other causes of acute or chronic diarrhea
  - Ulcerative colitis
  - Pyogenic liver abscess
  - Hepatoma
  - Echinococcal hepatic cyst
  - Carcinoma of sigmoid colon or cecum (ameboma)

- ■ Treatment
  - Metronidazole plus diloxanide or iodoquinol for nondysenteric colitis
  - Diloxanide or iodoquinol for asymptomatic intestinal infection
  - Chloroquine after metronidazole, diloxanide, or iodoquinol for clearing trophozoites or residual amebas from liver

- ■ Pearl

Amebiasis must be excluded before steroids are given for "inflammatory bowel disease."

Reference

Haque R, Huston CD, Hughes M, et al: Amebiasis. N Engl J Med 2003;348:1565. [PMID: 12700377]

American Trypanosomiasis
(Chagas' Disease; *Trypanosoma cruzi*)

- **Essentials of Diagnosis**
  - Transmitted by reduviid insects in endemic areas (Latin America and increasingly in the southwestern U.S.); most patients asymptomatic; some cases laboratory-acquired
  - Intermittent fever, with signs and symptoms of myocarditis or meningoencephalitis later in course
  - Unilateral bipalpebral or facial edema, conjunctivitis, (Romana's sign)
  - Hard, edematous, erythematous, furunclelike lesion with local lymphadenopathy (chagoma)
  - Cardiac disease with arrhythmias and right-sided congestive heart failure; gastrointestinal disease characterized by megacolon or megaesophagus
  - Trypanosomes in blood; isolation by animal inoculation or serologic testing confirmatory
  - Disease may occur after 30-year latent period

- **Differential Diagnosis**
  - Trichinosis
  - Kala-azar
  - Malaria
  - Congestive heart failure due to other causes
  - Meningoencephalitis due to other causes

- **Treatment**
  - Nifurtimox effective acutely but less valuable in chronic stage
  - Benznidazole effective (not available in the U.S.)
  - Ketoconazole of uncertain benefit

- **Pearl**

  The most common cause of congestive heart failure in South America.

Reference

Barrett MP, Burchmore RJ, Stich A, et al: The trypanosomiases. Lancet 2003;362:1469. [PMID: 14602444]

Babesiosis

- ■ Essentials of Diagnosis
  - • Exposure to *Ixodes* ticks in endemic area
  - • *B microti:* Irregular fever, chills, headache, diaphoresis, malaise without periodicity; hemolytic anemia and hepatosplenomegaly characteristic
  - • *B divergens:* High fever, toxic appearance, severe hemolytic anemia, liver and renal failure, with splenectomized patients particularly at risk
  - • Intraerythrocytic parasite on blood smear diagnostic; serologic test is available

- ■ Differential Diagnosis
  - • Malaria
  - • Lyme disease (may coinfect)
  - • Idiopathic autoimmune hemolytic anemia

- ■ Treatment
  - • None specific
  - • *B microti* infection usually benign and self-limited
  - • *B divergens* infection more severe
  - • Quinine and clindamycin, exchange transfusion of uncertain benefit in splenectomized patients

- ■ Pearl

If you diagnose babesiosis, take a second look for Lyme disease.

Reference

Krause PJ: Babesiosis. Med Clin North Am 2002;86:361. [PMID: 11982307]

Coccidiosis (*Isospora belli; Cryptosporidium*)

- **Essentials of Diagnosis**
  - An intestinal infection caused by one of three genera: *Isospora, Cryptosporidium,* and *Sarcocystis* most common in HIV disease
  - Watery diarrhea, crampy abdominal pain, nausea, low-grade fever, malaise
  - Fecal leukocytes absent
  - Usually self-limited disease over weeks to months in immuno-competent, but may be catastrophic or life-threatening in AIDS patients
  - Diagnosis with identification of parasite in feces or duodenal aspirate or biopsy (antigen test available for *Cryptosporidium*)

- **Differential Diagnosis**
  - Infectious enteritis (eg, *Giardia*)
  - Cholera
  - Infectious colitis
  - Ulcerative colitis or Crohn's disease
  - Viral gastroenteritis

- **Treatment**
  - *Isospora:* Sulfadiazine or trimethoprim-sulfamethoxazole; in AIDS patients, indefinite course
  - *Cryptosporidium:* No consistently effective therapy available; paromomycin and azithromycin often tried

- **Pearl**

Large outbreaks involving hundreds of thousands of people have occurred when sewage systems were overwhelmed by floods.

Reference

Chappell CL, Okhuysen PC: Cryptosporidiosis. Curr Opin Infect Dis 2002;15:523. [PMID: 12686887]

Giardiasis (*Giardia lamblia*)

- **Essentials of Diagnosis**

  - Infection of the upper small intestine that occurs worldwide; most infections asymptomatic
  - Outbreaks common in day care centers, individual cases from contaminated water
  - Acute or chronic diarrhea with bulky, greasy stools
  - Upper abdominal discomfort, cramps, distention
  - No fecal leukocytes
  - Cysts and occasionally trophozoites in stools, especially in high-volume diarrhea; trophozoites in duodenal aspirate or biopsy; IgA deficiency predisposes, antigen test widely available
  - Malabsorption syndrome may be seen in chronic disease

- **Differential Diagnosis**

  - Gastroenteritis or diarrhea due to other causes
  - Mucosal small bowel disease such as sprue
  - Other causes of malabsorption, such as pancreatic insufficiency

- **Treatment**

  - Metronidazole
  - Tinidazole, quinacrine, or furazolidone also effective
  - Recheck stools to ensure success of therapy

- **Pearl**

Diarrhea in a returned mountain hiker is giardiasis unless proved otherwise.

Reference

Ali SA, Hill DR: *Giardia intestinalis.* Curr Opin Infect Dis 2003;16:453. [PMID: 14501998]

Malaria (*Plasmodium* Species)

- ■ Essentials of Diagnosis
  - • History of exposure to mosquitoes in endemic area
  - • Paroxysms of periodic chills, fever, headache, myalgias, and sweating with delirium; periodicity of fever determined by species
  - • Jaundice, hepatosplenomegaly
  - • Hemolytic anemia, leukopenia with relative monocytosis, thrombocytopenia, and nonspecific liver function test abnormalities
  - • Characteristic plasmodia seen in erythrocytes in thick (experienced observers only) or thin blood smear
  - • Serologic test not available for acute diagnosis
  - • Pulmonary edema, hepatic failure, hypoglycemia, acute tubular necrosis (blackwater fever) may complicate falciparum malaria
  - • Recurrent attacks over months or years indicate *P vivax* infection

- ■ Differential Diagnosis
  - • Influenza
  - • Typhoid fever
  - • Infectious hepatitis
  - • Dengue
  - • Kala-azar
  - • Leptospirosis
  - • Borreliosis
  - • Lymphoma

- ■ Treatment
  - • Chemotherapy determined by species and drug sensitivities of endemic area
  - • Chemoprophylaxis for travel to endemic area: oral chloroquine with addition of primaquine after leaving endemic area; mefloquine, doxycycline, or proguanil and atovaquone if exposure to resistant falciparum malaria anticipated

- ■ Pearl

Wright's stain of insufficiently dried blood smears shows a central ring artifact similar to plasmodia in red cells.

Reference

Maitland K, Bejon P, Newton CR: Malaria. Curr Opin Infect Dis 2003;16:389. [PMID: 14501990]

Primary Amebic Meningoencephalitis (*Naegleria* Species; *Acanthamoeba* Species)

- **■ Essentials of Diagnosis**

  Naegleria:
  - Upper respiratory syndrome followed by rapidly progressing, usually fatal meningoencephalitis
  - Generally young, healthy persons with history of swimming in soil-contaminated fresh water 3–7 days prior to onset of symptoms
  - Amebas with large, central karyosome in fresh wet mount of uncentrifuged cerebrospinal fluid; can be cultured

  Acanthamoeba:
  - Skin lesions and ulceration with multiple organ dissemination, uveitis, chronic keratitis, or more insidious onset of severe meningoencephalitis
  - History of preexisting specific or nonspecific immunosuppression; trauma to skin, mucous membranes, or eye usually present

8

- **■ Differential Diagnosis**
  - Other causes of meningitis or encephalitis
  - Other causes of keratitis

- **■ Treatment**
  - Amphotericin B, miconazole, and rifampin with marginal success for *Naegleria* infections
  - Systemic ketoconazole, topical antifungals of uncertain benefit for *Acanthamoeba* infections

- **■ Pearl**

  One of medicine's few infectious diseases caused by free-living organisms...and also its most deadly prognosis.

Reference

Marciano-Cabral F, Cabral G: *Acanthamoeba* spp. as agents of disease in humans. Clin Microbiol Rev 2003;16:273. [PMID: 12692099]

Toxoplasmosis (*Toxoplasma gondii*)

- **Essentials of Diagnosis**
    - Serious disease encountered extremely rarely in immunocompetent adults
    - Fever, malaise, headache, sore throat, myalgia, blurred vision
    - Rash, hepatosplenomegaly, cervical lymphadenopathy, retinochoroiditis, focal neurologic findings
    - In immunocompromised patients, brain abscess with focal neurologic abnormalities most common; pneumonitis, myocarditis also occur, likewise lesions elsewhere including testes
    - IgM diagnostic in nonimmunosuppressed population; negative IgG makes CNS disease unlikely in HIV patients
    - Polymerase chain reaction (PCR) from bronchoalveolar lavage, CSF, blood, or tissue biopsies diagnostic; resolution of brain abscess with empiric therapy highly suggestive

- **Differential Diagnosis**
    - Other causes of space-occupying brain lesions (primary or secondary malignancy, bacterial abscess, lymphoma)
    - Other causes of encephalitis (herpes simplex, CMV, viral encephalitis)
    - CMV infection (may exist in HIV disease)
    - Epstein-Barr virus
    - Other causes of myocarditis
    - Other atypical pneumonias; *Pneumocystis*
    - Other causes of lymphadenopathy (sarcoidosis, tuberculosis, lymphoma)

- **Treatment**
    - Pyrimethamine-sulfadiazine and clindamycin effective
    - Corticosteroids useful adjuvant in ocular or severe CNS disease
    - Therapy in AIDS patients may be stopped if they are successfully treated with highly active antiretroviral therapy

- **Pearl**

Seronegative heart transplant recipients of seropositive donors have a very high incidence of systemic toxoplasmosis; prophylaxis for toxoplasmosis is obligatory in these individuals.

Reference

Montoya JG, Liesenfeld O: Toxoplasmosis. Lancet 2004;363:1965. [PMID: 15194258]

Visceral Leishmaniasis
(Kala-Azar; *Leishmania donovani* Complex)

- ■ Essentials of Diagnosis
  - • A zoonotic disease transmitted by bites of sandflies; incubation period is 4–6 months
  - • Local, typically inapparent nonulcerating nodule at site of sand-fly bite
  - • Irregular fever (often biquotidian) with progressive darkening of skin (especially on forehead and hands), diarrhea
  - • Cachexia, progressive and marked splenomegaly and hepatomegaly, generalized lymphadenopathy, petechiae
  - • Pancytopenia with relative lymphocytosis and monocytosis
  - • Leishman-Donovan bodies demonstrable in splenic, bone marrow, or lymph node smears or buffy coat blood smear; serologic tests diagnostic after second week of illness

8

- ■ Differential Diagnosis
  - • Malaria
  - • Lymphoma
  - • Brucellosis
  - • Schistosomiasis
  - • Infectious mononucleosis
  - • Myeloproliferative syndromes, especially myelofibrosis
  - • Anemia due to other causes
  - • Tuberculosis
  - • Leprosy
  - • African trypanosomiasis
  - • Subacute infective endocarditis
  - • Adult Still's disease

- ■ Treatment
  - • Sodium stibogluconate
  - • Pentamidine, liposomal amphotericin for treatment failures
  - • High fatality rate if not treated

- ■ Pearl

A biquotidian fever pattern and massive splenomegaly suggests the diagnosis in endemic regions.

Reference

Rosenthal E, Marty P: Recent understanding in the treatment of visceral leishmaniasis. J Postgrad Med 2003;49:61. [PMID: 12865573]

RICKETTSIAL INFECTIONS

Epidemic Louse-Borne Typhus (*Rickettsia prowazekii*)

■ Essentials of Diagnosis
  - Transmission of *R prowazekii* favored by crowded living conditions, famine
  - Headache, chills, fever, often severe or intractable
  - Maculopapular rash appears on fourth to seventh days on trunk and axillae, then extremities; spares face, palms, and soles
  - Conjunctivitis, rales, splenomegaly, hypotension, and delirium in some patients; renal insufficiency
  - Serologic confirmation by second week of illness
  - Brill's disease: Recrudescence of disease after apparent recovery

■ Differential Diagnosis
  - Other viral syndromes
  - Pneumonia
  - Other exanthems
  - Meningococcemia
  - Sepsis
  - Toxic shock syndrome

■ Treatment
  - Prevention with louse control
  - Vaccine available in some parts of the world (not in the U.S.)
  - Tetracycline and chloramphenicol equally effective

■ Pearl

A more lethal enemy for armies than combat in endemic countries during World War II.

Reference

Andersson JO, Andersson SG: A century of typhus, lice and *Rickettsia*. Res Microbiol 2000;151:143. [PMID: 10865960]

Q Fever (*Coxiella burnetii*)

■ Essentials of Diagnosis

- Infection following exposure to sheep, goats, cattle, or fowl
- Acute or chronic febrile illness with severe headache, cough, and abdominal discomfort
- Granulomatous hepatitis and culture-negative endocarditis in occasional cases
- Pulmonary infiltrates by chest x-ray; leukopenia
- Serologic confirmation by third to fourth weeks of illness using phase I and II antibodies to determine chronicity

■ Differential Diagnosis

- Atypical pneumonia
- Granulomatous hepatitis due to other cause
- Brucellosis
- Other causes of culture-negative endocarditis

■ Treatment

- Tetracyclines suppressive but not always curative, especially with endocarditis; surgery typically necessary given large, destructive vegetations
- Vaccine being developed

■ Pearl

The only rickettsial disease without a rash.

Reference

Marrie TJ: Q fever pneumonia. Curr Opin Infect Dis 2004;17:137. [PMID: 15021054]

Rocky Mountain Spotted Fever (*Rickettsia rickettsii*)

- **Essentials of Diagnosis**
  - Exposure to ticks in endemic area
  - Influenzal prodrome followed by chills, fever, severe headache, myalgias, occasionally delirium and coma
  - Red macular rash with onset between second and sixth days of fever; first on extremities, then centrally, may become petechial or purpuric
  - Leukocytosis, proteinuria, hematuria
  - Serologic tests positive by second week of illness, but diagnosis best made earlier by skin biopsy with immunologic staining

- **Differential Diagnosis**
  - Meningococcemia
  - Endocarditis
  - Gonococcemia
  - Ehrlichiosis
  - Measles

- **Treatment**
  - Tetracyclines or chloramphenicol
  - Vaccine in development

- **Pearl**

Despite the name, there are more cases in North Carolina than in Colorado.

Reference

Masters EJ, Olson GS, Weiner SJ, Paddock CD: Rocky Mountain spotted fever: a clinician's dilemma. Arch Intern Med 2003;163:769. [PMID: 12695267]

Scrub Typhus (Tsutsugamushi Disease)

- **Essentials of Diagnosis**

  - Caused by *Rickettsia tsutsugamushi,* parasite of rodents transmitted by mites
  - Exposure to mites in endemic area of Southeast Asia, western Pacific, Australia
  - Black eschar at site of bite with regional or generalized lymphadenopathy, malaise, chills, headache, backache
  - Conjunctivitis and fleeting macular rash
  - Pneumonitis, encephalitis, and cardiac failure may complicate
  - Serologic confirmation by second week of illness

- **Differential Diagnosis**

  - Typhoid fever
  - Dengue
  - Malaria
  - Leptospirosis
  - Other rickettsial infections

- **Treatment**

  - Tetracyclines or chloramphenicol, though some resistance is being encountered
  - Rifampin may also be effective

- **Pearl**

A particularly common cause of unexplained fever in the tropics, especially in children.

Reference

Watt G, Parola P: Scrub typhus and tropical rickettsioses. Curr Opin Infect Dis 2003;16:429. [PMID: 14501995]

VIRAL INFECTIONS

Colorado Tick Fever

- **Essentials of Diagnosis**
  - A self-limited acute viral (coltivirus) infection transmitted by *Dermacentor andersoni* tick bites
  - Onset 3–6 days following bite
  - Abrupt onset of fever, chills, myalgia, headache, photophobia
  - Occasional faint rash
  - Second phase of fever after remission of 2–3 days common
  - Imbedded ticks, especially in children's scalps, may cause marked muscle weakness

- **Differential Diagnosis**
  - Borreliosis
  - Influenza
  - Adult Still's disease
  - Other viral exanthems
  - Guillain-Barré syndrome (if paralysis present)

- **Treatment**
  - Supportive for uncomplicated cases
  - With paresis, removal of tick results in prompt resolution of symptoms

- **Pearl**

In endemic areas, search the entire epidermis for ticks prior to plasmapheresis for Guillain-Barré syndrome.

Reference

Klasco R: Colorado tick fever. Med Clin North Am 2002;86:435, ix. [PMID: 11982311]

Cytomegalovirus Disease

■ Essentials of Diagnosis

- Neonatal infection: Hepatosplenomegaly, purpura, central nervous system abnormalities
- Immunocompetent adults: Mononucleosislike illness characterized by fever, myalgias, hepatosplenomegaly, leukopenia with lymphocytic predominance, often following transfusion; pharyngitis less common
- Immunocompromised adults: Pneumonia, meningoencephalitis, polyradiculopathy, chorioretinitis, chronic diarrhea
- Fever may be prolonged in the latter group
- In immunocompetent adults, IgM is diagnostic
- In AIDS patients, funduscopic examination establishes the diagnosis, culture positivity does not
- Contributes to organ rejection and other infections in transplant patients

8

■ Differential Diagnosis

- Infectious mononucleosis (Epstein-Barr virus)
- Acute HIV infection
- Other causes of prolonged fever (eg, lymphoma, endocarditis)
- In immunocompromised patients: Other causes of atypical pneumonia, meningoencephalitis, or chronic diarrhea
- In infants: Toxoplasmosis, rubella, herpes simplex, syphilis

■ Treatment

- Appropriate supportive care
- Ganciclovir, foscarnet, or cidofovir intravenously in immunocompromised patients

■ Pearl

Acute cytomegalovirus infection should always be considered in a patient with "mononucleosis" without pharyngitis.

Reference

Taylor GH: Cytomegalovirus. Am Fam Physician 2003;67:519. [PMID: 12588074]

Dengue (Breakbone Fever, Dandy Fever)

- **Essentials of Diagnosis**
  - A viral (togavirus, flavivirus) illness transmitted by the bite of the *Aedes* mosquito
  - Sudden onset of high fever, chills, severe myalgias, headache, sore throat; rare orchitis
  - Biphasic fever curve with initial phase of 3–4 days, short remission, and second phase of 1–2 days
  - Rash is biphasic—first evanescent, followed by maculopapular, scarlatiniform, morbilliform, or petechial changes during remission or second phase of fever; first in the extremities and spreads to torso
  - Dengue hemorrhagic fever is a severe form in which gastrointestinal hemorrhage is prominent and patients often present with shock; occurs with repeat viral challenge with similar serotype

- **Differential Diagnosis**
  - Malaria
  - Yellow fever
  - Influenza
  - Typhoid fever
  - Borreliosis
  - Other viral exanthems

- **Treatment**
  - Supportive care
  - Vaccine has been developed but not commercially available

- **Pearl**

Dengue should always be considered in the febrile returned traveler with presumed influenza.

Reference

Mairuhu AT, Wagenaar J, Brandjes DP, van Gorp EC: Dengue: an arthropod-borne disease of global importance. Eur J Clin Microbiol Infect Dis 2004;23:425. Epub 2004 May 18. [PMID: 15148655]

Herpes Simplex

- **Essentials of Diagnosis**
  - Recurrent grouped small vesicles on erythematous base, usually perioral or perigenital
  - Primary infection more severe and often associated with fever, regional lymphadenopathy, and aseptic meningitis
  - Recurrences precipitated by minor infections, trauma, stress, sun exposure
  - Oral and genital lesions highly infectious
  - Systemic infection may occur in immunosuppressed patients
  - Proctitis, esophagitis, meningitis/encephalitis, and keratitis may complicate
  - Direct fluorescent antibody or culture of ulcer can be diagnostic

- **Differential Diagnosis**
  - Herpangina, hand-foot-and-mouth disease
  - Aphthous ulcers
  - Stevens-Johnson syndrome
  - Bacterial infection of the skin
  - Syphilis and other sexually transmitted diseases
  - Other causes of encephalitis, proctitis, or keratitis

- **Treatment**
  - Acyclovir, famciclovir, and valacyclovir may attenuate recurrent course of genital or oral lesions and are obligatory for systemic or central nervous system disease

- **Pearl**

In unexplained heel pain in a young person, inquire about genital herpes; the virus lives in the sacral ganglia.

Reference

Kimberlin DW, Rouse DJ: Clinical practice. Genital herpes. N Engl J Med 2004;350:1970. [PMID: 15128897]

HIV Infection

- **Essentials of Diagnosis**
  - Caused by a retrovirus slowly destroying CD4 lymphocytes
  - At-risk populations include intravenous drug users and their partners, blood product recipients prior to 1984, health care workers injured with needles used for HIV-positive patients, homosexual men; heterosexual transmission most common in much of the world
  - Coinfection with hepatitis C common
  - Acute HIV infection characterized by nonspecific flulike syndrome and aseptic meningitis
  - Later, opportunistic infections, certain malignancies, and AIDS wasting dictate the clinical picture, 2–15 years after primary infection
  - Picture deteriorates as CD4 count falls below 200; certain opportunistic infections occur predictably at various levels (eg, PCP < 200)

- **Differential Diagnosis**
  - Depends upon which infection is complicating
  - Interstitial lung diseases of numerous types
  - Non-AIDS lymphoma
  - Tuberculosis
  - Sarcoidosis
  - Brain abscess
  - Fever of unknown origin of other cause
  - Posterior uveitis of other causes

- **Treatment**
  - Combination antiretroviral treatment can restore lost immunity and dramatically extend life expectancy
  - Prophylaxis for *P carinii* pneumonia when CD4 count reaches 200, and *Mycobacterium avium* complex when CD4 is less than 75
  - Otherwise, treatment for associated lymphoma, toxoplasmosis, mycobacteriosis, CMV, Kaposi's sarcoma as indicated

- **Pearl**

Consider HIV testing in patients with abnormal liver functions and unexplained cytopenias; risk history may be difficult to secure.

Reference

Paredes R, Clotet B: New antiretroviral drugs and approaches to HIV treatment. AIDS. 2003;17(Suppl 4):S85. [PMID: 15080184]

Infectious Mononucleosis (Epstein-Barr Virus Infection)

- ■ Essentials of Diagnosis
  - An acute illness due to Epstein-Barr virus, usually occurring up to age 35 but possible throughout life
  - Transmitted by saliva; incubation period is 5–15 days or longer
  - Fever, severe sore throat, striking malaise
  - Maculopapular rash, lymphadenopathy, splenomegaly common
  - Leukocytosis and lymphocytosis with atypical large lymphocytes by smear; positive heterophil agglutination test (Monospot) by fourth week of illness; false-positive rapid plasma reagin test (RPR) in 10%
  - Clinical picture much less typical in older patients
  - Complications include splenic rupture, hepatitis, myocarditis, any cytopenia in the blood, and encephalitis

- ■ Differential Diagnosis
  - Other causes of pharyngitis
  - Other causes of hepatitis
  - Toxoplasmosis
  - Rubella
  - Acute HIV, CMV, or rubella infections
  - Acute leukemia or lymphoma
  - Kawasaki's syndrome
  - Hypersensitivity reaction due to carbamazepine

- ■ Treatment
  - Supportive care only; fever usually disappears in 10 days, lymphadenopathy and splenomegaly in 4 weeks
  - Ampicillin apt to cause rash
  - Avoid vigorous abdominal activity or exercise

- ■ Pearl

Mononucleosis is the most common cause of the otherwise rare anti-i hemolytic anemia.

Reference

Cohen JI: Epstein-Barr virus infection. N Engl J Med 2000;343:481. [PMID: 10944566]

Influenza

- **Essentials of Diagnosis**
  - Caused by an orthomyxovirus transmitted via the respiratory route
  - Abrupt onset of fever, headache, chills, malaise, dry cough, coryza, and myalgias; constitutional signs out of proportion to catarrhal symptoms
  - Epidemic outbreaks in fall or winter, with short incubation period
  - Rapid tests on nasopharyngeal swabs widely available, confirmed by viral culture or serology
  - Complications include bacterial sinusitis, otitis media, encephalitis, pneumonia
  - Myalgias occur early in course, rhabdomyolysis late

- **Differential Diagnosis**
  - Other viral syndromes
  - Primary bacterial pneumonia
  - Meningitis
  - Dengue in returned travelers
  - Rhabdomyolysis of other cause

- **Treatment**
  - Yearly active immunization of persons at high risk (eg, chronic respiratory disease, pregnant women, cardiac disease, health care workers, immunosuppressed); also for all over 50
  - Chemoprophylaxis for epidemic influenza A effective with amantadine; zanamivir and oseltamivir effective against influenza A and B
  - Antivirals reduce duration of symptoms and infectivity if given within 48 hours
  - Avoid salicylates in children because of association with Reye's syndrome

- **Pearl**

The 1918 worldwide epidemic killed as many in 20 weeks as has AIDS in 20 years: the importance of immunization cannot be overemphasized.

Reference

Barry JM: The Great Influenza—The Epic Story of the Deadliest Plague in History. New York, Viking Press, 2004.

Lymphocytic Choriomeningitis

- **Essentials of Diagnosis**
  - History of exposure to mice or hamsters
  - Influenzalike prodrome with fever, chills, headache, malaise, and cough followed by headache, photophobia, or neck pain
  - Kernig's and Brudzinski's signs positive
  - Cerebrospinal fluid with lymphocytic pleocytosis and slight increase in protein
  - Serology for arenavirus positive 2 weeks after onset of symptoms; virus recovered from blood and cerebrospinal fluid
  - Illness usually lasts 1–2 weeks

- **Differential Diagnosis**
  - Other aseptic meningitides
  - Bacterial or granulomatous meningitis

- **Treatment**
  - Supportive care

- **Pearl**

One of the few causes of hypoglycorrhachia in a patient who appears to be well.

Reference

Zinkernagel RM: Lymphocytic choriomeningitis virus and immunology. Curr Top Microbiol Immunol 2002;263:1. [PMID: 11987811]

Measles (Rubeola)

- **Essentials of Diagnosis**
  - An acute systemic viral illness transmitted by inhalation of infective droplets; 800,000 deaths yearly worldwide
  - Incubation period 10–14 days
  - Prodrome of fever, coryza, cough, conjunctivitis, photophobia
  - Progression of brick-red, irregular maculopapular rash 3 days after prodrome from face to trunk to extremities
  - Koplik's spots (tiny "table salt crystals") on the buccal mucosa are pathognomonic but appear and disappear rapidly
  - Leukopenia
  - Encephalitis in 1–3%

- **Differential Diagnosis**
  - Other acute exanthems (eg, rubella, enterovirus, Epstein-Barr virus infection, varicella, roseola)
  - Drug allergy
  - Pneumonia or encephalitis due to other cause

- **Treatment**
  - Primary immunization preventive after age 15 months; revaccination of adults born after 1956 without documented immunity recommended
  - Isolation for 1 week following onset of rash
  - Specific treatment of secondary bacterial complications

- **Pearl**

Of all the viral exanthems, systemic toxicity is most marked with measles.

Reference

Duke T, Mgone CS: Measles: not just another viral exanthem. Lancet 2003;361:763. [PMID: 12620751]

Mumps (Epidemic Parotitis)

- ■ Essentials of Diagnosis
  - • Incubation period 12–24 days
  - • Painful, swollen salivary glands, usually parotid; may be unilateral; systemic symptoms of infection
  - • Orchitis or oophoritis, meningoencephalitis, or pancreatitis may occur
  - • Cerebrospinal fluid shows lymphocytic pleocytosis in meningoencephalitis with hypoglycorrhachia
  - • Diagnosis confirmed by isolation of virus in saliva or appearance of antibodies after second week

- ■ Differential Diagnosis
  - • Parotitis or enlarged parotids due to other causes (eg, bacteria, sialolithiasis with sialadenitis, cirrhosis, diabetes, starch ingestion, Sjögren's syndrome, sarcoidosis, tumor)
  - • Aseptic meningitis, pancreatitis, or orchitis due to other causes

- ■ Treatment
  - • Immunization is preventive
  - • Supportive care with surveillance for complications

- ■ Pearl

Mumps orchitis is a potentially treatable cause of sterility, associated with high blood FSH and low testosterone levels.

Reference

McQuone SJ: Acute viral and bacterial infections of the salivary glands. Otolaryngol Clin North Am 1999;32:793. [PMID: 10477787]

Poliomyelitis

- ■ Essentials of Diagnosis
  - Enterovirus acquired via fecal-oral route; many cases asymptomatic, majority of symptomatic cases are not neurologic
  - Muscle weakness, malaise, headache, fever, nausea, abdominal pain, sore throat
  - Signs of lower motor neuron lesions: Asymmetric, flaccid paralysis with decreased deep tendon reflexes, muscle atrophy; may include cranial nerve abnormalities (bulbar form)
  - Cerebrospinal fluid lymphocytic pleocytosis with slight elevation of protein
  - Virus recovered from throat washings or stool

- ■ Differential Diagnosis
  - Other aseptic meningitides
  - Postinfectious polyneuropathy (Guillain-Barré syndrome)
  - Amyotrophic lateral sclerosis
  - Myopathy

- ■ Treatment
  - Vaccination is preventive and has eliminated the disease in the United States
  - Supportive care with particular attention to respiratory function, skin care, and bowel and bladder function

- ■ Pearl

Stiff neck after an enteric illness is a potential precursor of neurologic polio.

Reference

Minor PD: Polio eradication, cessation of vaccination and re-emergence of disease. Nat Rev Microbiol 2004;2:473. [PMID: 15152203]

Rabies

- **Essentials of Diagnosis**
  - A rhabdovirus encephalitis transmitted by infected saliva
  - History of animal bite (bats, bears, skunks, foxes, raccoons; dogs and cats in developing countries)
  - Paresthesias, hydrophobia, rage alternating with calm
  - Convulsions, paralysis, thick tenacious saliva, and muscle spasms

- **Differential Diagnosis**
  - Tetanus
  - Encephalitis due to other causes

- **Treatment**
  - Active immunization of household pets and persons at risk (eg, veterinarians)
  - Thorough, repeated washing of bite and scratch wounds
  - Postexposure immunization, both passive and active
  - Observation of healthy biting animals, examination of brains of sick or dead biting animals
  - Treatment is supportive only; disease is almost uniformly fatal

- **Pearl**

Bats are the most common vector for rabies in the United States, and even absent history of a bite, children exposed to bats indoors should be immunized.

Reference

Warrell MJ, Warrell DA: Rabies and other lyssavirus diseases. Lancet 2004;363:959. [PMID: 15043965]

Rubella

- **Essentials of Diagnosis**
  - A systemic illness transmitted by inhalation of infected droplets, with incubation period of 14–21 days
  - No prodrome in children (mild in adults); fever, malaise, coryza coincide with eruption of fine maculopapular rash on face to trunk to extremities which rapidly fades
  - Arthralgias common, particularly in young women
  - Posterior cervical, suboccipital, and posterior auricular lymphadenopathy 5–10 days before rash
  - Leukopenia, thrombocytopenia
  - In one out of 6000 cases, postinfectious encephalopathy develops 1–6 days after the rash; mortality rate is 20%

- **Differential Diagnosis**
  - Other acute exanthems (eg, rubeola, enterovirus, Epstein-Barr virus infection, varicella)
  - Drug allergy

- **Treatment**
  - Active immunization after age 15 months; girls should be immunized before menarche though not during pregnancy
  - Symptomatic therapy only

- **Pearl**

Rubella-associated arthritis is more symptomatic after vaccination than with natural infection.

Reference

Banatvala JE, Brown DW: Rubella. Lancet 2004;363:1127. [PMID: 15064032]

Smallpox (Variola)

- Diagnosis
  - Generally requires prolonged close contact for transmission
  - Incubation period 1–2 weeks
  - Initial symptoms include fever, malaise, headache
  - Rash progresses rapidly from mouth sores to macules then papules and pustules
  - Central umbilication characteristic
  - Unlike most other viral vesicular diseases, lesions in any part of the body are all at the same stage at the same time
  - Suspected cases should be reported to public health authorities; confirmation requires polymerase chain reaction (PCR) or culture

- Differential Diagnosis
  - Varicella
  - Herpes simplex virus
  - Other viral exanthema
  - Drug reaction
  - Other pox viruses (eg, monkey pox)

- Treatment
  - Contact and airborne isolation critical
  - Supportive care as no specific treatment is available

- Pearl

As smallpox has been eradicated, any future case should raise suspicion of a bioterrorist attack or of severe varicella.

Reference

Dacko A, Hardick K, Yoshida T: Smallpox. Cutis 2003;71:319. [PMID: 12729099]

Varicella (Acute Chickenpox, Zoster [Shingles])

- **Essentials of Diagnosis**
  - Incubation period 14–21 days
  - Acute varicella: Fever, malaise with eruption of pruritic, centripetal, papular rash, becoming vesicular and pustular before crusting; lesions in all stages at any given time; "drop on rose petal" is the first lesion
  - Bacterial infection, pneumonia, and encephalitis may complicate
  - Reactivation varicella (herpes zoster): Dermatomal distribution, vesicular rash with pain often preceding eruption; thoracic and cranial nerve V most commonly involved

- **Differential Diagnosis**
  - Other viral infections
  - Drug allergy
  - Dermatitis herpetiformis
  - Pemphigus

- **Treatment**
  - Supportive measures with topical lotions and antihistamines; antivirals (acyclovir, valacyclovir, famciclovir) for all adults with varicella
  - Immune globulin or antivirals for exposed susceptible immunosuppressed or pregnant patients
  - Acyclovir early for immunocompromised or pregnant patients, severe disease (eg, pneumonitis, encephalitis), or ophthalmic division of trigeminal nerve involvement with zoster signaled by vesicle on tip of nose
  - Corticosteroids combined with antiviral agent with rapid taper may diminish postherpetic neuralgia in older patients with zoster

- **Pearl**

Varicella pneumonia in adults is the only cause in medicine of densely calcified, perfectly round, numerous, 2- to 3-mm nodules at both bases.

Reference

Gilden DH, Cohrs RJ, Mahalingam R: Clinical and molecular pathogenesis of varicella virus infection. Viral Immunol 2003;16:243. [PMID: 14583142]

Viral Encephalitis

- **Essentials of Diagnosis**
  - Most common agents include enterovirus, Epstein-Barr virus, herpes simplex, measles, rubella, rubeola, varicella, West Nile, St. Louis, Western and Eastern equine
  - Some sporadic, some epidemic
  - Fever, malaise, stiff neck, nausea, altered mentation
  - Signs of upper motor neuron lesion: exaggerated deep tendon reflexes, absent superficial reflexes, spastic paralysis
  - Increased cerebrospinal fluid protein with lymphocytic pleocytosis, occasional hypoglycorrhachia
  - Polymerase chain reaction (PCR) for HSV is sensitive and specific
  - Isolation of virus from blood or cerebrospinal fluid; serology positive in paired specimens 3–4 weeks apart
  - Brain imaging shows temporal lobe abnormalities in herpetic encephalitis

- **Differential Diagnosis**
  - Other noninfectious encephalitides (postvaccination, Reye's syndrome, toxins)
  - Lymphocytic choriomeningitis
  - Primary or secondary neoplasm
  - Brain abscess or partially treated bacterial meningitis
  - Fungal meningitis, especially coccidioidomycosis

- **Treatment**
  - Vigorous supportive measures with attention to elevated central nervous system pressures
  - Mannitol in selected patients
  - Acyclovir for suspected herpes simplex encephalitis; other specific antiviral therapy is under study

- **Pearl**

In patients with suspected encephalitis, acyclovir is given immediately and continued until herpes is excluded.

Reference

Whitley RJ, Gnann JW: Viral encephalitis: familiar infections and emerging pathogens. Lancet 2002;359:507. [PMID: 11853816]

Yellow Fever

- **Essentials of Diagnosis**
  - Arbovirus or togavirus transmitted by mosquito bites
  - Endemic only in Africa and South America
  - Sudden onset of severe headache, photophobia, myalgias, and palpitations
  - Early tachycardia with late bradycardia and hypotension, jaundice, hemorrhagic phenomena (gastrointestinal bleeding, mucosal lesions) in the severe form
  - Proteinuria, leukopenia, hyperbilirubinemia
  - Virus isolated from blood; serologic tests positive after second week of illness

- **Differential Diagnosis**
  - Leptospirosis
  - Viral hepatitis
  - Typhoid fever
  - Biliary tract disease
  - Malaria
  - Dengue

- **Treatment**
  - Active immunization of persons living in or traveling to endemic areas
  - Supportive care

- **Pearl**

A yearly epidemic occurrence treated by phlebotomy by the most distinguished physicians (eg, Benjamin Rush) in 18th-century urban America.

Reference

Gubler DJ: The global emergence/resurgence of arboviral diseases as public health problems. Arch Med Res 2002;33:330. [PMID: 12234522]

9

Oncologic Diseases

Adenocarcinoma of the Kidney (Renal Cell Carcinoma)

- **Essentials of Diagnosis**
  - Pleomorphic clinical manifestations: The internist's tumor
  - Gross or microscopic hematuria, back pain, fever, weight loss, night sweats
  - Flank or abdominal mass may be palpable
  - Anemia in 30%, erythrocytosis in 3%; hypercalcemia, liver function test abnormalities, hypoglycemia sometimes seen
  - Tumor invasion of renal vein and inferior vena cava on occasion causes superior vena cava syndrome
  - Renal ultrasound, CT, or MRI reveals characteristic lesion

- **Differential Diagnosis**
  - Polycystic kidney disease; simple cyst
  - Single complex renal cyst; 70% of these are malignant
  - Renal tuberculosis, calculi, or infarction
  - Endocarditis

- **Treatment**
  - Nephrectomy curative for patients with early-stage lesions
  - Poor response to chemotherapy or radiation in metastatic disease
  - Small response rate to combination bio-chemotherapy (interleukin 2 plus cytotoxic agents), though very toxic
  - Resection of primary lesion has been documented to result in regression of metastases on rare occasions and may improve response to subsequent immunotherapy
  - Nonmyeloablative allogeneic bone marrow transplantation has significant response rate in highly selected patients

- **Pearl**

A small proportion of patients have a nonmetastatic hepatopathy, with elevation of alkaline phosphatase; this abnormality does not imply inoperability and disappears with resection of the tumor.

Reference

Curti BD: Renal cell carcinoma. JAMA 2004;292:97. [PMID: 15238597]

Bronchogenic Carcinoma (Lung Cancer)

- **Essentials of Diagnosis**
  - Smoking most important cause, asbestos exposure synergistic
  - Chronic cough, dyspnea; chest pain, hoarseness, hemoptysis, weight loss; may be asymptomatic, however
  - Examination depends on disease stage; localized wheezing, clubbing, superior vena cava syndrome in some
  - Enlarging mass, infiltrate, atelectasis, pleural effusion, or cavitation by chest x-ray; peripheral coin lesions in a minority
  - Diagnostic: Presence of malignant cells by sputum or pleural fluid cytology or on histologic examination of tissue biopsy
  - Metastases or paraneoplastic effects may dominate
  - PET scanning before resection

- **Differential Diagnosis**
  - Tuberculosis
  - Pulmonary mycoses, lung abscess
  - Metastasis from extrapulmonary primary tumor
  - Benign lung tumor, eg, hamartoma
  - Noninfectious granulomatous disease

- **Treatment**
  - Resection for appropriate non-small-cell carcinomas and all coin lesions, assuming no evidence of spread or other primary
  - Concurrent chemotherapy and radiation for limited-stage small-cell carcinoma; may be curative
  - Prophylactic cranial radiation probably beneficial for those patients with small cell carcinoma
  - Palliative therapy for metastatic non-small-cell carcinoma
  - Advanced small cell carcinoma has excellent response rate to combination therapy, but responses seldom durable

- **Pearl**

Although digital clubbing is common in lung cancer generally, it is typically absent in small cell tumors.

Reference

Spira A, Ettinger DS: Multidisciplinary management of lung cancer. N Engl J Med 2004;350:379. [PMID: 14736930]

Cancer of the Cervix

- ■ Essentials of Diagnosis
  - • Abnormal uterine bleeding, vaginal discharge, pelvic or abdominal pain
  - • Cervical lesion may be visible on inspection as tumor or ulceration
  - • Vaginal cytology is usually positive; must be confirmed by biopsy
  - • CT or MRI of abdomen and pelvis, examination under anesthesia useful for staging disease

- ■ Differential Diagnosis
  - • Cervicitis
  - • Chronic vaginitis or infection (tuberculosis, actinomycosis)
  - • Sexually transmitted diseases (syphilis, lymphogranuloma venereum, chancroid, granuloma inguinale)
  - • Aborted cervical pregnancy

- ■ Treatment
  - • Stage-dependent and requires input of surgeons, medical oncologists, and radiation oncologists
  - • Radical or extended hysterectomy curative in patients with early-stage disease
  - • Combination of radiation therapy and radiosensitizing chemotherapy curative in majority of patients with localized disease not amenable to primary resection
  - • Role of surgery following chemotherapy and radiotherapy still being defined
  - • Combination chemotherapy for metastatic disease has significant response rate, but unclear magnitude of benefit on survival

- ■ Pearl

Adherence to screening guidelines prevents the invasive stage of this disease.

Reference

Waggoner SE: Cervical cancer. Lancet 2003;361:2217. [PMID: 12842378]

Carcinoma of the Bladder (Transitional Cell Carcinoma)

- **Essentials of Diagnosis**
  - More common in men over 40 years of age; predisposing factors include smoking and alcohol as well as chronic *Schistosoma haematobium* infection, exposure to certain industrial toxins, or previous cyclophosphamide therapy
  - Microscopic or gross hematuria with no other symptoms is the most common presentation
  - Suprapubic pain, urgency, and frequency when concurrent infection present
  - Occasional uremia if both ureterovesical orifices obstructed
  - Tumor visible by cystoscopy

- **Differential Diagnosis**
  - Other urinary tract tumor
  - Acute cystitis
  - Renal tuberculosis
  - Urinary calculi
  - Glomerulonephritis or interstitial nephritis

- **Treatment**
  - Endoscopic transurethral resection for superficial or submucosal tumors; intravesical chemotherapy reduces the likelihood of recurrence
  - Radical cystectomy standard with muscle-invasive tumors, though less morbid procedures with intensive follow-up may provide similar outcomes
  - Role of adjuvant chemotherapy or radiation for completely resected patients unclear, but generally offered to those at high risk of recurrence
  - Combination chemotherapy for metastatic disease has a high response rate and may be curative in a small percentage of patients

- **Pearl**

Remember Kaposi's sarcoma of the bladder in an AIDS patient with a urinary catheter and gross hematuria; cutaneous disease is not invariably present.

Reference

Borden LS Jr, Clark PE, Hall MC: Bladder cancer. Curr Opin Oncol 2003;15:227. [PMID: 12778017]

Carcinoma of the Female Breast

- ■ Essentials of Diagnosis
  - • Increased incidence in those with a family history of breast cancer and in nulliparous or late-childbearing women
  - • Painless lump, often found by the patient; nipple or skin changes over breast (peau d'orange, redness, ulceration) later findings; axillary mass, malaise, or weight loss even later findings
  - • Minority found by mammography
  - • Metastatic disease to lung, bone, or central nervous system may dominate clinical picture
  - • Staging based on size of tumor, involvement of lymph nodes, and presence of metastases
  - • Extent of involvement of axillary lymph nodes is most powerful prognostic indicator in localized disease

- ■ Differential Diagnosis
  - • Mammary dysplasia (fibrocystic disease)
  - • Benign tumor (fibroadenoma, ductal papilloma)
  - • Fat necrosis
  - • Mastitis
  - • Thrombophlebitis (Mondor's disease)

- ■ Treatment
  - • Treatment decisions require careful consideration of stage and other prognostic factors
  - • Resection (lumpectomy plus radiation therapy versus modified radical mastectomy) in early-stage disease
  - • Adjuvant chemotherapy or hormonal therapy recommended for many with completely resected disease except those at very low risk for recurrence
  - • Menopausal and tumor hormone receptor status dictate best adjuvant therapy
  - • Metastatic disease is incurable, but treatment with hormonal manipulation, chemotherapy, radiation, and monoclonal antibody therapy may provide long-term remission or disease stabilization

- ■ Pearl

Denial is common in this feared disease; it should be addressed by all primary care providers.

Reference

Mincey BA, Perez EA: Advances in screening, diagnosis, and treatment of breast cancer. Mayo Clin Proc 2004;79:810. [PMID: 15182098]

Carcinoma of the Head and Neck

- **Essentials of Diagnosis**
  - Most common between ages 50 and 70; occurs in heavy smokers, with alcohol as an apparent cocarcinogen
  - Early hoarseness in true cord lesions; sore throat, otalgia fairly common; odynophagia, hemoptysis indicate more advanced disease
  - Comorbid lung cancer in some patients; may appear clinically up to several years later
  - Lesions found by physical examination or direct or indirect laryngoscopy; regional lymphadenopathy common at presentation

- **Differential Diagnosis**
  - Chronic laryngitis, including reflux laryngitis
  - Laryngeal tuberculosis
  - Myxedema
  - Vocal cord paralysis due to laryngeal nerve palsy caused by left hilar lesion
  - Serous otitis media
  - Herpes simplex

- **Treatment**
  - Treatment varies by stage and tumor location and may include surgery, radiation, concurrent chemotherapy and radiation, or combinations of above
  - Chemotherapy may provide palliative benefit for metastatic or recurrent disease
  - Smoking cessation crucial for increasing treatment efficacy and preventing second malignancies

- **Pearl**

The typical head-neck squamous cancer remains undiagnosed for 9 months after patient or physician awareness of the first symptom or sign.

Reference

Mao L, Hong WK, Papadimitrakopoulou VA: Focus on head and neck cancer. Cancer Cell 2004;5:311. [PMID: 15093538]

Carcinoma of the Male Breast

- ■ Essentials of Diagnosis
    - Painless lump or skin changes of breast
    - Nipple discharge, retraction or ulceration, palpable mass, gynecomastia
    - Staging as in women

- ■ Differential Diagnosis
    - Gynecomastia due to other causes
    - Benign tumor

- ■ Treatment
    - Modified radical mastectomy with staging as in women
    - For metastatic disease, endocrine manipulation (physical or chemical castration) with tamoxifen or related compounds, aminoglutethimide, or corticosteroids often quite effective

- ■ Pearl

This constitutes only 1% of all breast cancer, but it is invariably diagnosed later in its course because men are neither suspected nor screened.

Reference

Giordano SH, Buzdar AU, Hortobagyi GN: Breast cancer in men. Ann Intern Med 2002;137:678. [PMID: 12379069]

Carcinoma of the Pancreas

- **Essentials of Diagnosis**
  - Peak incidence in seventh decade; more common in blacks, patients with chronic pancreatitis, and debatably, diabetes mellitus
  - Upper abdominal pain with radiation to back, weight loss, diarrhea, pruritus, thrombophlebitis; painless jaundice, with symptoms depending on where tumor is located, most being in the head of the pancreas
  - Palpable gallbladder or abdominal mass in some
  - Elevated amylase with liver function abnormalities; anemia, hyperglycemia, or frank diabetes in minority
  - Dilated common hepatic ducts by ultrasound or endoscopic retrograde cholangiogram
  - CT, MRI, and endoscopic ultrasound may delineate extent of disease and guide biopsy
  - Often, true extent of disease not appreciated before exploratory laparotomy

- **Differential Diagnosis**
  - Choledocholithiasis
  - Drug-induced cholestasis
  - Hepatitis
  - Cirrhosis
  - Carcinoma of ampulla of Vater

- **Treatment**
  - Surgical diversion for palliation in most cases
  - Radical pancreaticoduodenal resection for disease limited to head of pancreas or periampullary zone (Whipple resection) curative in rare cases, but more so in ampullary tumors
  - Chemotherapy, radiation, or combination in patients with advanced local disease may improve outcomes
  - Chemotherapy for metastatic disease may improve quality of life and prolong survival

- **Pearl**

A palpable periumbilical node—Sister Mary Joseph's node—was described by a scrub nurse at the Mayo Clinic, who noticed it while preoperatively sterilizing the abdominal walls of afflicted patients.

Reference

Li D, Xie K, Wolff R, Abbruzzese JL: Pancreatic cancer. Lancet 2004;363:1049. [PMID: 15051286]

Carcinoma of the Prostate

- **Essentials of Diagnosis**
  - Family history and African-American race are risk factors; African-Americans tend to have more aggressive disease
  - Routine screening with serum PSA remains controversial; likely to be of greatest benefit in men > age 50 (especially blacks) with life expectancy > 10 years
  - Symptoms of prostatism more often absent than present; bone pain (especially back) if metastases present; asymptomatic in many, however
  - Stony, hard, irregular prostate palpable, usually lateral part of gland
  - Osteoblastic osseous metastases visible by plain radiograph
  - Prostate-specific antigen (PSA) is age-dependent and is elevated in older patients with benign prostatic hyperplasia and also acute prostatitis; reliably predicts extent of neoplastic disease and recurrence after prostatectomy

- **Differential Diagnosis**
  - Benign prostatic hyperplasia (may be associated)
  - Scarring secondary due to tuberculosis or calculi
  - Urethral stricture
  - Neurogenic bladder

- **Treatment**
  - Radiation therapy (external beam, brachytherapy, or combination) or radical prostatectomy, ideally nerve-sparing for localized disease
  - Providers must apprise patients of the significant risk of erectile dysfunction and urinary incontinence complicating treatments for localized prostate cancer
  - Radiation or surgical therapy for local nodal metastases in selected patients after prostatectomy
  - Androgen ablation (chemical or surgical) for metastatic disease, though exact timing of initiation of therapy (at diagnosis or at onset of symptoms) is unclear
  - Combination chemotherapy may benefit selected patients with hormone-refractory metastatic disease

- **Pearl**

About 1% of prostate tumors—most of these are highly aggressive small-cell carcinomas—are not adenocarcinoma and thus do not express PSA.

Reference

Hernandez J, Thompson IM: Diagnosis and treatment of prostate cancer. Med Clin North Am 2004;88:267, ix. [PMID: 15049578]

Carcinoma of the Stomach

- **Essentials of Diagnosis**
  - Few early symptoms, but abdominal pain not unusual; late complaints include dyspepsia, anorexia, nausea, early satiety, weight loss
  - Palpable abdominal mass (late)
  - Iron deficiency anemia, fecal occult blood positive; achlorhydria present in minority of patients
  - Mass or ulcer visualized radiographically; endoscopic biopsy and cytologic examination diagnostic
  - Associated with atrophic gastritis, *Helicobacter pylori;* role of diet, previous partial gastrectomy controversial

- **Differential Diagnosis**
  - Benign gastric ulcer
  - Gastritis
  - Functional or irritable bowel syndrome
  - Other gastric tumors, eg, leiomyosarcoma, lymphoma

- **Treatment**
  - Resection for cure; palliative resection with gastroenterostomy in selected cases
  - Adjuvant chemotherapy or chemoradiotherapy improves long-term survival in high-risk patients postsurgery and may achieve remission in a minority of patients with metastatic disease
  - For patients with metastatic disease, combination chemotherapy has significant response rate and may prolong survival; endoscopic laser ablation, venting gastrostomy, and stenting may palliate symptoms

- **Pearl**

A gastric ulcer with histamine-fast achlorhydria is carcinoma in 100% of cases; no acid, no ulcer.

Reference

Hohenberger P, Gretschel S: Gastric cancer. Lancet 2003;362:305. [PMID: 12892963]

Carcinoma of the Vulva

- **Essentials of Diagnosis**
  - Prolonged vulvar irritation, pruritus, local discomfort, slight bloody discharge
  - History of genital warts common; association with human papillomavirus established
  - Early lesions may suggest chronic vulvitis
  - Late lesions may present as a mass, exophytic growth, or firm ulcerated area in vulva
  - Biopsy makes diagnosis

- **Differential Diagnosis**
  - Sexually transmitted diseases (syphilis, lymphogranuloma venereum, chancroid, granuloma inguinale)
  - Crohn's disease
  - Benign tumors (granular cell myoblastoma)
  - Reactive or eczematoid dermatitis
  - Vulvar dystrophy

- **Treatment**
  - Local resection for cases of in situ squamous cell carcinoma
  - Wide surgical excision with lymph node dissection for invasive carcinoma
  - Radiation or radiation plus radiosensitizing chemotherapy in addition to surgery may improve outcomes in patients with locally advanced disease

- **Pearl**

Diagnosis of this disorder is often delayed; it resembles many sexually transmitted diseases.

Reference

de Hullu JA, Oonk MH, van der Zee AG: Modern management of vulvar cancer. Curr Opin Obstet Gynecol 2004;16:65. [PMID: 15128010]

Cervical Intraepithelial Neoplasia
(CIN; Dysplasia or Carcinoma in Situ of the Cervix)

- ■ Essentials of Diagnosis
  - • Associated with human papillomavirus (HPV) infection in up to 90% of advanced CIN (almost 100% of invasive cervical cancers)
  - • Other risk factors include multiple sexual partners, HIV, cigarette smoking, other sexually transmitted diseases
  - • Asymptomatic in many
  - • Cervix appears grossly normal with dysplastic or carcinoma in situ cells by cytologic smear preparation
  - • Culdoscopic examination with coarse punctate or mosaic pattern of surface capillaries, atypical transformation zone, and thickened white epithelium
  - • Iodine-nonstaining (Schiller-positive) squamous epithelium is typical

- ■ Differential Diagnosis
  - • Cervicitis

- ■ Treatment
  - • Varies depending upon degree and extent of cervical or intraepithelial neoplasia; thus, staging crucial
  - • Observation for mild dysplasia
  - • Cryosurgery or CO_2 laser vaporization for moderate dysplasia
  - • Cone biopsy or hysterectomy for severe dysplasia or carcinoma in situ
  - • Repeat examinations to detect recurrence
  - • HPV vaccination may prevent CIN or recurrence in at-risk individuals

- ■ Pearl

One of the relatively few cancers or precancerous conditions for which screening has made an important difference.

Reference

Wright TC Jr, Cox JT, Massad LS, et al; American Society for Colposcopy and Cervical Pathology: 2001 Consensus guidelines for the management of women with cervical intraepithelial neoplasia. Am J Obstet Gynecol 2003;189:295. [PMID: 12861176]

Colorectal Carcinoma

■ Essentials of Diagnosis

- Risk factors include colonic polyposis, Lynch syndrome (hereditary nonpolyposis colon cancer), and ulcerative colitis
- Altered bowel habits, rectal bleeding from left-sided carcinoma; occult blood in bowel movements; iron deficiency anemia in right-sided lesions
- Palpable abdominal or rectal mass in minority
- Characteristic barium enema or colonoscopic appearance; tissue biopsy is diagnostic
- Elevated carcinoembryonic antigen (CEA) useful as marker of disease recurrence in patients with elevated CEA at diagnosis but is not useful as a diagnostic tool

■ Differential Diagnosis

- Hemorrhoids
- Diverticular disease
- Benign colonic polyps
- Peptic ulcer disease
- Ameboma
- Functional bowel disease
- Iron deficiency anemia due to other causes

■ Treatment

- Dukes staging predicts prognosis
- Surgical resection for cure, also for palliation
- Adjuvant chemotherapy recommended for those with significant risk of recurrence based on unfavorable Dukes stage after potentially curative surgery
- Combination chemotherapy palliative for distant metastatic disease; novel agents targeting angiogenesis and growth factor pathways now available
- Radiation with concurrent chemotherapy useful adjuvant to surgery for rectal cancer
- Chemotherapy and radiotherapy curative in majority of localized anal cancers without need for surgery
- Screening with colonoscopy will probably prove superior to flexible sigmoidoscopy

■ Pearl

Patients with Streptococcus bovis *endocarditis have colonic neoplasia until proved otherwise.*

Reference

Blumberg D, Ramanathan RK: Treatment of colon and rectal cancer. J Clin Gastroenterol 2002;34:15. [PMID: 11743241]

Endometrial Carcinoma

■ Essentials of Diagnosis
- Higher incidence in obesity, diabetes, nulliparity, polycystic ovaries, and women receiving tamoxifen as adjuvant therapy for breast cancer
- Abnormal uterine bleeding, pelvic or abdominal pain
- Uterus frequently not enlarged on palpation
- Endometrial biopsy or curettage is required to confirm diagnosis after negative pregnancy test; vaginal cytologic examination is negative in high percentage of cases
- Examination under anesthesia, chest x-ray, CT, or MRI required in staging

■ Differential Diagnosis
- Pregnancy, especially ectopic
- Atrophic vaginitis
- Exogenous estrogens
- Endometrial hyperplasia or polyps
- Other pelvic or abdominal neoplasms

■ Treatment
- Hysterectomy and salpingo-oophorectomy for well-differentiated or localized tumors
- Combined surgery and radiation for poorly differentiated tumors, cervical extension, deep myometrial penetration, and regional lymph node involvement
- Radiotherapy for unresectable localized malignancies
- Palliative chemotherapy may benefit those with metastatic disease, though role and optimal regimen still being defined
- Progestational agents may help some women with metastatic disease

■ Pearl

Unlike cervical cancers, screening is less helpful than having a high index of suspicion.

Reference

Levine DA, Hoskins WJ: Update in the management of endometrial cancer. Cancer J 2002;8(Suppl 1):S31. [PMID: 12075700]

Epithelial Ovarian Cancer

■ Essentials of Diagnosis

- Family history, BRCA1 or 2 mutations, nulliparity, long total duration of ovulation are risk factors; oral contraceptives, breast-feeding, multiparity
- Abdominal distention, pelvic pain, vaginal bleeding
- Ascites, abdominal or pelvic mass
- Ultrasonography, CT scan, or MRI delineates extent
- Laparoscopy or laparotomy to obtain tissue from mass or ascites for cytologic examination
- CA 125 useful for recurrence, not screening

■ Differential Diagnosis

- Uterine leiomyoma
- Endometriosis
- Tubal pregnancy
- Pelvic kidney
- Retroperitoneal tumor or fibrosis
- Colorectal carcinoma
- Chronic pelvic inflammatory disease (especially tuberculosis)
- Benign ovarian masses

■ Treatment

- Premenopausal women with small ovarian masses can be observed with a trial of ovulation suppression for two cycles followed by repeat examination to exclude physiologic cysts
- Simple excision with ovarian preservation for many benign cell types
- Unilateral salpingo-oophorectomy for certain cell types in younger women
- Hysterectomy with bilateral salpingo-oophorectomy in post-menopausal women, or premenopausal women with resectable disease not candidates for more conservative surgery
- Adjuvant chemotherapy for most patients with resected disease
- Cytoreductive surgery followed by combination chemotherapy for women with advanced disease without distant metastases
- Combination chemotherapy has high response rate and may provide durable remissions in women with metastatic disease

■ Pearl

A woman with a personal history of breast cancer, or a family history of breast or ovarian cancer, has a two- to sixfold increase in risk of ovarian cancer.

Reference

Schwartz PE: Diagnosis and treatment of epithelial ovarian cancer. Minerva Ginecol 2003;55:315. [PMID: 14581856]

Gestational Trophoblastic Neoplasia (Hydatidiform Mole & Choriocarcinoma)

- ■ Essentials of Diagnosis
  - Uterine bleeding in first trimester
  - Uterus larger than expected for duration of pregnancy
  - No fetus demonstrated by ultrasound with sometimes characteristic findings of mole; excessively elevated levels of serum β-hCG for gestational duration of pregnancy
  - Vesicles may be passed from vagina
  - Preeclampsia seen in first trimester

- ■ Differential Diagnosis
  - Multiple pregnancy
  - Threatened abortion
  - Ectopic pregnancy

- ■ Treatment
  - Suction curettage for hydatidiform mole
  - For nonmetastatic malignant disease, single-agent chemotherapy (eg, methotrexate or dactinomycin) very effective, but the role of hysterectomy is uncertain
  - For metastatic disease, single-agent or combination chemotherapy depending upon clinical setting
  - Follow quantitative β-hCG until negative and then frequently for surveillance of tumor recurrence

- ■ Pearl

Remember a mole in a young woman who has hyperthyroidism without a palpable thyroid gland.

Reference

Soper JT, Mutch DG, Schink JC; American College of Obstetricians and Gynecologists: Diagnosis and treatment of gestational trophoblastic disease: ACOG Practice Bulletin No. 53. Gynecol Oncol 2004;93:575. [PMID: 15196847]

Hepatocellular Carcinoma

■ Essentials of Diagnosis

- Most common visceral malignancy worldwide; usually asymptomatic until disease advanced
- Alcoholic cirrhosis, chronic hepatitis B or C, and hemochromatosis are risk factors
- Abdominal enlargement, pain, jaundice, weight loss
- Hepatomegaly, abdominal mass; rub or bruit heard over right upper quadrant in some
- Anemia or erythrocytosis; liver function test abnormalities
- Dramatic elevation in alpha-fetoprotein (AFP) helpful in diagnosis, though significant percentage have normal AFPs
- Tendency to ascend hepatic vein and inferior vena cava
- Angiography (though rarely performed) with characteristic abnormality; CT or MRI suggests diagnosis; tissue biopsy for confirmation

■ Differential Diagnosis

- Benign liver tumors: Hemangioma, adenoma, focal nodular hyperplasia
- Bacterial hepatic abscess
- Amebic liver cyst
- Metastatic tumor

■ Treatment

- Therapeutic options often limited by severe underlying liver disease; no surgical option if cirrhosis is present in remainder of liver
- Surgical resection thought best curative option if lesions are resectable and patient is operative candidate
- Liver transplant may be curative in small percentage of highly selected patients
- Many intralesional therapies being developed for unresectable disease, though indications and timing of these interventions are not well established
- Little benefit from chemotherapy in advanced disease

■ Pearl

In a patient with known cirrhosis and a normal hematocrit, think hepatocellular carcinoma; it pseudonormalizes the anemia typical of cirrhosis.

Reference

Llovet JM, Burroughs A, Bruix J: Hepatocellular carcinoma. Lancet 2003;362:1907. [PMID: 14667750]

Malignant Tumors of the Bile Ducts

- **Essentials of Diagnosis**
  - Predisposing factors include choledochal cysts, primary sclerosing cholangitis, ulcerative colitis with sclerosing cholangitis, *Clonorchis sinensis* infection
  - Jaundice, pruritus, anorexia, right upper quadrant pain
  - Hepatomegaly, ascites, right upper quadrant tenderness
  - Dilated intrahepatic bile ducts by ultrasound or CT scan
  - Retrograde endoscopic cholangiogram characteristic; tissue biopsy is diagnostic
  - Hyperbilirubinemia (conjugated), markedly elevated alkaline phosphatase and cholesterol

- **Differential Diagnosis**
  - Choledocholithiasis
  - Drug-induced cholestasis
  - Cirrhosis
  - Chronic hepatitis
  - Metastatic hepatic malignancy
  - Pancreatic or ampullary carcinoma
  - Biliary stricture

- **Treatment**
  - Palliative surgical bypass of biliary flow
  - Stent bypass of biliary flow in selected patients
  - Pancreaticoduodenectomy for resectable distal duct tumors curative in minority

- **Pearl**

Half of cholangiocarcinoma patients have had ulcerative colitis; a far smaller number of patients with ulcerative colitis have cholangiocarcinoma.

Reference

Anderson CD, Pinson CW, Berlin J, Chari RS: Diagnosis and treatment of cholangiocarcinoma. Oncologist 2004;9:43. [PMID: 14755014]

Malignant Tumors of the Esophagus

- ■ Essentials of Diagnosis
  - Progressive dysphagia—initially during ingestion of solid foods, later with liquids; progressive weight loss and inanition ominous
  - Smoking, alcoholism, chronic esophageal reflux with Barrett's esophagus, achalasia, caustic injury, and asbestos are risk factors
  - Noninvasive imaging (barium swallow, CT scan) suggestive, diagnosis confirmed by endoscopy and biopsy
  - Staging of disease aided by endoscopic ultrasound
  - Squamous histology more common, though incidence of adenocarcinoma increasing rapidly in Western countries for unclear reasons

- ■ Differential Diagnosis
  - Benign tumors of the esophagus
  - Benign esophageal stricture or achalasia
  - Esophageal diverticulum
  - Esophageal webs
  - Achalasia (may be associated)
  - Globus hystericus

- ■ Treatment
  - Combination chemotherapy and radiotherapy or surgery for localized disease, though long-term remission or cure is achieved in only 10–15%
  - Dilation or esophageal stenting may palliate advanced disease; little role for chemotherapy or radiation in advanced or metastatic disease

- ■ Pearl

Dysphagia is one of the few symptoms in medicine for which anatomic correlation always exists—too often it represents carcinoma.

Reference

Enzinger PC, Mayer RJ: Esophageal cancer. N Engl J Med 2003;349:2241. [PMID: 14657432]

Pleural Mesothelioma

- **Essentials of Diagnosis**
  - Insidious dyspnea, nonpleuritic chest pain, weight loss
  - Dullness to percussion, diminished breath sounds, pleural friction rub, clubbing
  - Nodular or irregular unilateral pleural thickening, often with effusion by chest radiograph; CT scan often helpful
  - Pleural biopsy usually necessary for diagnosis, though malignant nature of tumor only confirmed by natural history; pleural fluid exudative and usually hemorrhagic
  - Strong association with asbestos exposure, with usual latency from time of exposure 20 years or more

- **Differential Diagnosis**
  - Primary pulmonary parenchymal malignancy
  - Empyema
  - Benign pleural inflammatory conditions (posttraumatic, asbestosis)

- **Treatment**
  - Surgical approaches for localized disease range from palliative plurodesis to attempted curative resection of involved lung and pleura
  - Combination chemotherapy with pemetrexed and cisplatin has significant response rate, but response duration still short
  - Investigations with combination surgery, radiotherapy, and chemotherapy are under way
  - One-year mortality rate > 75%

- **Pearl**

Consider this when empyema develops in patients irradiated for malignancy years earlier—it's a rare complication.

References

Pass HI, Vogelzang N, Hahn S, Carbone M: Malignant pleural mesothelioma. Curr Probl Cancer 2004;28:93. [PMID: 15197388]; Singhal S, Kaiser LR. Malignant mesothelioma: options for management. Surg Clin North Am 2002;82:797. [PMID: 12472131]

Primary Intracranial Tumors

- ■ Essentials of Diagnosis
    - • Prognosis depends on histology; half are gliomas
    - • Most present with generalized or focal disturbances of cerebral function: Generalized symptoms include nocturnal headache, seizures, and projectile vomiting; focal deficits relate to location of the tumor
    - • CT or MRI with gadolinium enhancement defines the lesion; posterior fossa tumors are better visualized by MRI
    - • Biopsy is the definitive diagnostic procedure, distinguishes primary brain tumors from brain abscess or metastasis
    - • Glioblastoma multiforme: In strictest sense an astrocytoma, but rapidly progressive with a poor prognosis
    - • Astrocytoma: More chronic course than glioblastoma, with a variable prognosis
    - • Medulloblastoma: Seen primarily in children and arises from roof of fourth ventricle
    - • Cerebellar hemangioblastoma: Patients usually present with disequilibrium and ataxia, and occasional erythrocytosis
    - • Meningioma: Compresses rather than invades; benign
    - • CNS lymphoma: Usually in HIV-AIDS, though may occur rarely in immunocompetent individuals

9

- ■ Treatment
    - • Treatment depends upon the type and site of the tumor and the condition of the patient
    - • Maximal resection predicts outcome in most
    - • Radiation postsurgery is mainstay of therapy; newer conformal radiation techniques decrease toxicity to normal brain
    - • Combination chemotherapy or single-agent temozolomide active in some cases
    - • Herniation treated with intravenous corticosteroids, mannitol, and surgical decompression if possible
    - • Prophylactic anticonvulsants are also commonly given, but their role is uncertain in patients without history of seizure

- ■ Pearl

A headache that awakens a patient from sleep puts this diagnosis at the top of the list.

Reference

Behin A, Hoang-Xuan K, Carpentier AF, Delattre JY: Primary brain tumours in adults. Lancet 2003;361:323. [PMID: 12559880]

Thyroid Cancer

- **Essentials of Diagnosis**
  - History of irradiation to neck in some patients
  - Often hard, painless nodule; dysphagia or hoarseness occasionally
  - Cervical lymphadenopathy when local metastases present
  - Thyroid function tests normal; nodule is characteristically stippled with calcium on x-ray, cold by radioiodine scan, and solid by ultrasound; does not regress with thyroid hormone administration

- **Differential Diagnosis**
  - Thyroiditis
  - Other neck masses and other causes of lymphadenopathy
  - Thyroglossal duct cyst
  - Benign thyroid nodules

- **Treatment**
  - Fine-needle aspiration biopsy best differentiates benign from malignant nodules
  - Total thyroidectomy for carcinoma; radioactive iodine postoperatively for selected patients with iodine-avid metastases; combination chemotherapy in anaplastic tumors
  - Prognosis related to cell type and histology; papillary carcinoma offers excellent outlook, anaplastic the worst
  - Medullary thyroid cancer is typically refractory to chemotherapy and radiation; associated with MEN syndromes; diagnosable by calcitonin elevation

- **Pearl**

In patients who had thymus radiation during childhood—a common practice in past years—a thyroid nodule is malignant until proved otherwise.

Reference

Sherman SI: Thyroid carcinoma. Lancet 2003;361:501. [PMID: 12583960]

Tumors of the Testis

- ■ Essentials of Diagnosis
  - • Painless testicular nodule; peak incidence at age 20–35
  - • Testis does not transilluminate
  - • Gynecomastia, premature virilization in occasional patients
  - • Tumor markers (AFP, LDH, β-hCG) useful in diagnosis, prognosis/ treatment planning, monitoring response to therapy, and surveillance for relapse
  - • Pure seminoma produces β-hCG only, while nonseminomatous germ cell tumors may produce β-hCG and AFP

- ■ Differential Diagnosis
  - • Genitourinary tuberculosis
  - • Syphilitic orchitis
  - • Hydrocele
  - • Spermatocele
  - • Epididymitis

- ■ Treatment
  - • Orchiectomy, with lumbar and inguinal lymph nodes examined for staging
  - • Retroperitoneal lymph node dissection useful for accurate staging and prevention of relapse in early-stage disease but may be deferred in favor of close clinical follow-up
  - • Adjuvant retroperitoneal radiation or chemotherapy for early-stage disease based on histology and a variety of risk factors including tumor markers
  - • Combination platinum-based chemotherapy curative in appreciable majority of patients with advanced or metastatic disease
  - • Late relapses possible, especially with seminoma, requiring long-term surveillance posttherapy

- ■ Pearl

One of the great stories in oncology, with 5-year survival rate increasing from approximately 65% to > 90–95% with the advent of platinum-based combination chemotherapy.

Reference

Jones RH, Vasey PA: Part I: testicular cancer—management of early disease. Lancet Oncol 2003;4:730. [PMID: 14662429]

10

Fluid, Acid-Base, & Electrolyte Disorders

Dehydration (Simple & Uncomplicated)

- ### Essentials of Diagnosis
  - Thirst, oliguria
  - Decreased skin turgor, especially on anterior thigh; dry mucous membranes, postural hypotension, tachycardia; none sensitive or specific
  - Impaired renal function (BUN:creatinine ratio > 20), elevated urinary osmolality and specific gravity, decreased urinary sodium, fractional excretion of sodium < 1% (for most causes)

- ### Differential Diagnosis
  - Hemorrhage
  - Sepsis
  - Gastrointestinal fluid losses
  - Skin sodium losses associated with burns or sweating
  - Renal sodium loss
  - Adrenal insufficiency
  - Nonketotic hyperosmolar state in type 2 diabetics

- ### Treatment
  - Identify source of volume loss if present
  - Replete with normal saline, blood, or colloid as indicated
  - Half-normal saline may be substituted when blood pressure normalizes

- ### Pearl

Dry mucous membranes are more indicative of mouth breathing than of dehydration.

Reference

Kreimeier U: Pathophysiology of fluid imbalance. Crit Care 2000;4(Suppl 2):S3. Epub 2000 Oct 13. [PMID: 11255592]

Hypercalcemia

- **■ Essentials of Diagnosis**
  - Polyuria and constipation; bony and abdominal pain in some
  - Thirst and dehydration
  - Mild hypertension
  - Altered mentation, hyporeflexia, stupor, coma all possible
  - Serum calcium > 10.2 mg/dL (corrected with concurrent serum albumin)
  - Renal insufficiency or azotemia
  - Shortened QT interval due to short ST segment; ventricular extrasystoles

- **■ Differential Diagnosis**
  - Primary hyperparathyroidism
  - Adrenal insufficiency (rare)
  - Malignancy (multiple myeloma with osteoclast-activating factor; lymphoma secreting 1,25-vitamin D; other primary tumor or metastasis releasing parathyroid hormone–related peptide)
  - Vitamin D intoxication
  - Milk-alkali syndrome
  - Sarcoidosis
  - Tuberculosis
  - Paget's disease of bone, especially with immobilization
  - Familial hypocalciuric hypercalcemia
  - Hyperthyroidism
  - Thiazide diuretics

10

- **■ Treatment**
  - Identify and treat underlying disorder
  - Volume expansion, loop diuretics (once euvolemic)
  - Glucocorticoids, calcitonin, bisphosphonates, and dialysis all useful in certain instances
  - Resection of parathyroid adenoma, if present

- **■ Pearl**

Hypercalcemia begets hypercalcemia; polyuria causes hypovolemia and consequent increased tubular calcium reabsorption.

Reference

Inzucchi SE: Management of hypercalcemia. Diagnostic workup, therapeutic options for hyperparathyroidism and other common causes. Postgrad Med 2004;115:27. [PMID: 15171076]

Hyperkalemia

■ Essentials of Diagnosis
- Weakness or flaccid paralysis, abdominal distention, diarrhea
- Serum potassium > 5 mEq/L
- Electrocardiographic changes: Peaked T waves, loss of P wave with sinoventricular rhythm, QRS widening, ventricular asystole, cardiac arrest

■ Differential Diagnosis
- Renal failure with oliguria
- Hypoaldosteronism (hyporeninism, potassium-sparing diuretics, ACE inhibitors, adrenal insufficiency, interstitial renal disease)
- Acidemia; type IV RTA
- Burns, hemolysis
- Digitalis overdose, beta-blockers (rare), heparin
- Spurious in patients with thrombocytosis; clot releases potassium into serum prior to laboratory determination

10 ■ Treatment
- Emergency (cardiac toxicity, paralysis): Calcium gluconate, intravenous bicarbonate, glucose, and insulin
- Dietary potassium restriction and sodium polystyrene sulfonate or loop diuretic to lower potassium subacutely
- Dialysis if oliguric renal failure or severe acidosis complicates
- Anti-digitalis Tc antibodies in patients receiving digitalis

■ Pearl

Atria are more susceptible to hyperkalemia than ventricles; thus, a "junctional" rhythm in marked hyperkalemia may be sinus, with sinus impulse failing to depolarize atria.

Reference

Kim HJ, Han SW: Therapeutic approach to hyperkalemia. Nephron 2002; 92(Suppl 1):33. [PMID: 12401936]

Hypermagnesemia

- **Essentials of Diagnosis**
  - Weakness, hyporeflexia, respiratory muscle paralysis
  - Confusion, altered mentation
  - Serum magnesium > 3 mg/dL; renal insufficiency the rule; increased uric acid, phosphate, potassium, and decreased calcium may be seen
  - Increased PR interval → heart block → cardiac arrest when marked

- **Differential Diagnosis**
  - Renal insufficiency
  - Excessive magnesium intake (food, antacids, laxatives, intravenous administration)

- **Treatment**
  - Correct renal insufficiency, if possible (volume expansion)
  - Intravenous calcium chloride for severe manifestations (eg, electrocardiographic changes, respiratory embarrassment)
  - Dialysis

10

- **Pearl**

Be cautious about magnesium-containing antacids—available OTC— in patients with renal insufficiency; little is needed to elevate this cation.

Reference

Touyz RM: Magnesium in clinical medicine. Front Biosci 2004;9:1278. [PMID: 14977544]

Hypernatremia

■ Essentials of Diagnosis
  - Severe thirst unless mentation altered; oliguria
  - In severe cases altered mental status, delirium, seizures, coma
  - If hypovolemic, loose skin with poor turgor, tachycardia, hypotension
  - Serum sodium > 145 mEq/L, serum osmolality > 300 mEq/L caused by free water loss
  - Affected patients usually include the very old, very young, critically ill, or neurologically impaired

■ Differential Diagnosis
  - Diabetes insipidus, either idiopathic or drug-induced (eg, by lithium)
  - Loss of hypotonic fluid (insensible, diuretics, vomiting, diarrhea, nasogastric suctioning, osmotic diuresis due to hyperglycemia)
  - Salt intoxication
  - Volume resuscitation and continuation of normal saline (155 mEq/L) after euvolemia achieved
  - Mineralocorticoid excess

■ Treatment
  - Relatively rapid volume replacement (if hypovolemic) followed by free water replacement over 48–72 hours (beware of cerebral edema; correct sodium by no more than 0.5 mEq/L per hour)
  - Desmopressin acetate for central diabetes insipidus

■ Pearl
If a patient has received tetracyclines for teenage acne, diabetes insipidus with potential for hypernatremia is permanent.

Reference

Adrogue HJ, Madias NE: Hypernatremia. N Engl J Med 2000;342:1493. [PMID: 10816188]

10

Hyperphosphatemia

- **Essentials of Diagnosis**
  - Few distinct symptoms
  - Cataracts, basal ganglion calcifications in hypoparathyroidism
  - Serum phosphate > 5 mg/dL; renal failure, hypocalcemia occasionally seen

- **Differential Diagnosis**
  - Renal failure
  - Hypoparathyroidism
  - Excess phosphate intake, vitamin D toxicity
  - Phosphate-containing laxative use
  - Cell destruction (tumor lysis syndrome), rhabdomyolysis, respiratory or metabolic acidosis
  - Multiple myeloma

- **Treatment**
  - Treat underlying disease when possible
  - Oral calcium carbonate (use noncalcium binder in concomitant hypercalcemia) to reduce phosphate absorption
  - Hemodialysis if refractory

- **Pearl**

Overshoot hyperphosphatemia from therapy of hypophosphatemia may precipitate the acute onset of tetany.

Reference

Slatopolsky E: New developments in hyperphosphatemia management. J Am Soc Nephrol 2003;14(9 Suppl 4):S297. [PMID: 12939384]

Hypocalcemia

- **Essentials of Diagnosis**
  - Abdominal and muscle cramps, stridor; tetany and seizures
  - Diplopia, facial paresthesias, papilledema
  - Positive Chvostek's and Trousseau's signs
  - Cataracts if chronic, likewise basal ganglion calcifications
  - Serum calcium < 8.5 mg/dL (corrected with concurrent serum albumin); phosphate usually elevated; hypomagnesemia may cause or complicate
  - Electrocardiographic changes: Prolonged QT interval; ventricular arrhythmias, including ventricular tachycardia

- **Differential Diagnosis**
  - Vitamin D deficiency and osteomalacia
  - Malabsorption
  - Hypoparathyroidism
  - Hyperphosphatemia
  - Hypomagnesemia
  - Chronic renal failure
  - Hypoalbuminemia
  - Pancreatitis
  - Drugs (loop diuretics, aminoglycosides, foscarnet)
  - Citrate excess due to massive blood transfusions

- **Treatment**
  - Identify and treat underlying disorder
  - For tetany, seizures, or arrhythmias, give calcium gluconate intravenously
  - Magnesium replacement if renal function normal
  - Oral calcium and vitamin D supplements (calcitriol in renal failure)
  - Phosphate binders in chronic hypocalcemia with hyperphosphatemia

- **Pearl**

The prolonged QT of hypocalcemia results from a lengthened ST segment; T waves are normal.

Reference

Carmeliet G, Van Cromphaut S, Daci E, Maes C, Bouillon R: Disorders of calcium homeostasis. Best Pract Res Clin Endocrinol Metab 2003;17:529. [PMID: 14687587]

Hypokalemia

■ **Essentials of Diagnosis**

- Usually asymptomatic
- Muscle weakness, lethargy, paresthesias, polyuria, anorexia, constipation, nausea, vomiting
- Electrocardiographic changes: Ventricular ectopy; T-wave flattening and ST depression → development of prominent U waves → AV block → cardiac arrest
- Serum potassium < 3.5 mEq/L and metabolic alkalosis sometimes concurrent

■ **Differential Diagnosis/Causes**

- Diuretic use
- Alkalemia
- β-Agonists (eg, albuterol)
- Hyperaldosteronism (adrenal adenoma, primary hyperreninism, mineralocorticoid use, and European licorice ingestion)
- Magnesium depletion
- Hyperthyroidism
- Diarrhea
- Renal tubular acidosis (types I, II)
- Bartter's, Gitelman's, and Liddle's syndromes
- Familial hypokalemic periodic paralysis
- Severe dietary potassium restriction

■ **Treatment**

- Identify and treat underlying cause
- Oral or intravenous potassium supplementation
- Magnesium repletion if indicated

■ **Pearl**

Think of hypokalemia in unexplained orthostatic hypotension.

Reference

Cohn JN, Kowey PR, Whelton PK, Prisant LM: New guidelines for potassium replacement in clinical practice: a contemporary review by the National Council on Potassium in Clinical Practice. Arch Intern Med 2000;160:2429. [PMID: 10979053]

Hypomagnesemia

- **Essentials of Diagnosis**
  - Muscle restlessness or cramps, athetoid movements, twitching or tremor, delirium, seizures
  - Muscle wasting, hyperreflexia, Babinski's sign, nystagmus, hypertension
  - Serum magnesium < 1.5 mEq/L; decreased calcium, potassium often associated
  - Electrocardiographic changes: Tachycardia, premature atrial or ventricular beats, increased QT interval, ventricular tachycardia or fibrillation

- **Differential Diagnosis**
  - Inadequate dietary intake
  - Hypervolemia
  - Diuretics, cisplatin, aminoglycosides, amphotericin B
  - Malabsorption or diarrhea
  - Alcoholism
  - Hyperaldosteronism, hyperthyroidism, hyperparathyroidism
  - Respiratory alkalosis

- **Treatment**
  - Identify and treat underlying cause
  - Intravenous magnesium replacement followed by oral maintenance
  - Calcium and potassium supplements if needed

- **Pearl**

Many manifestations of hypomagnesemia relate to the hypocalcemia induced by concomitant resistance to parathyroid hormone.

Reference

Topf JM, Murray PT: Hypomagnesemia and hypermagnesemia. Rev Endocr Metab Disord 2003;4:195. [PMID: 12766548]

Hyponatremia

- **Essentials of Diagnosis**

  - Nausea, headache, weakness, irritability, mental confusion (especially with serum sodium < 120 mEq/L, developing rapidly)
  - Generalized seizures, lethargy, coma, respiratory arrest and death may result, yet slowly developing cases may be asymptomatic
  - Serum sodium < 135 mEq/L; osmolality < 280 mEq/L (hypotonic hyponatremia); hypouricemia if SIADH or primary polydipsia is the cause

- **Differential Diagnosis**

  - Hypovolemic causes (thiazides, osmotic diuresis, adrenal insufficiency, vomiting, diarrhea, fluid sequestration)
  - Hypervolemic causes (congestive heart failure, cirrhosis, nephrotic syndrome, advanced renal failure, pregnancy)
  - Euvolemic causes (hypothyroidism, SIADH, glucocorticoid insufficiency, reset osmostat, primary polydipsia)
  - Hypertonic or isotonic hyponatremia (hyperglycemia, intravenous mannitol)
  - Pseudohyponatremia (hypertriglyceridemia, paraproteinemia) caused by laboratory artifact

10

- **Treatment**

  - Treat underlying disorder
  - Corticosteroids empirically if adrenal insufficiency suspected
  - Gradual correction (serum sodium change of no more than 0.5 mEq/L per hour) unless severe central nervous system signs present; central pontine myelinolysis may result from rapid overcorrection
  - If hypovolemic, use normal saline
  - If hypervolemic, use water restriction, loop diuretics, and normal saline volume replacement of urine output
  - Demeclocycline in selected patients with SIADH

- **Pearl**

  A sodium level less than 130 mg/dL, BUN less than 10 mg/dL, and hypouricemia in a patient without liver, heart, or kidney disease is virtually diagnostic of SIADH.

Reference

Adrogue HJ, Madias NE: Hyponatremia. N Engl J Med 2000;342:1581. [PMID: 10824078]

Hypophosphatemia

- **Essentials of Diagnosis**
  - Seldom an isolated abnormality
  - Anorexia, myopathy, arthralgias
  - Irritability, confusion, seizures
  - Rhabdomyolysis if severe
  - Serum phosphate < 2.5 mg/dL, severe < 1 mg/dL; elevated creatine kinase if rhabdomyolysis-associated
  - Hemolysis in severe cases

- **Differential Diagnosis**
  - Hyperparathyroidism, hyperthyroidism
  - Alcoholism
  - Vitamin D–resistant osteomalacia
  - Malabsorption, starvation
  - Hypercalcemia, hypomagnesemia
  - Correction of hyperglycemia
  - Recovery from catabolic state

- **Treatment**
  - Intravenous phosphate replacement when severe
  - Oral phosphate supplements (unless hypercalcemic); be cautious about overshooting
  - Correct magnesium deficit, if present

- **Pearl**

Phosphate levels even as low as 0–0.1 mg/dL are possible without clinical manifestations.

Reference

Ritz E, Haxsen V, Zeier M: Disorders of phosphate metabolism—pathomechanisms and management of hypophosphataemic disorders. Best Pract Res Clin Endocrinol Metab 2003;17:547. [PMID: 14687588]

Metabolic Acidosis

- **Essentials of Diagnosis**
  - Dyspnea, hyperventilation, respiratory fatigue
  - Tachycardia, tachypnea, hypotension, shock (depending on cause)
  - Acetone on breath (in ketoacidosis)
  - Arterial pH < 7.35, serum bicarbonate decreased; anion gap may be normal or high; ketonuria

- **Differential Diagnosis**
  - Ketoacidosis (diabetic, alcoholic, starvation)
  - Lactic acidosis
  - Poisons (methyl alcohol, ethylene glycol, salicylates, isopropyl alcohol)
  - Uremia
  - With normal anion gap, diarrhea, renal tubular acidosis
  - Post-hyperventilation

- **Treatment**
  - Identify and treat underlying cause
  - Correct volume, electrolyte status
  - Bicarbonate therapy indicated in ethylene glycol or methanol toxicity, renal tubular acidosis, debated for other causes
  - Hemodialysis, mechanical ventilation if necessary

10

- **Pearl**

A low pH in diabetic ketoacidosis is not *the cause of an altered mental status—hyperosmolality is.*

Reference

Levraut J, Grimaud D: Treatment of metabolic acidosis. Curr Opin Crit Care 2003;9:260. [PMID: 12883279]

Metabolic Alkalosis

- **Essentials of Diagnosis**
  - Weakness, malaise, lethargy; other symptoms depend on cause
  - Hyporeflexia, tetany, ileus, muscle weakness
  - Arterial pH > 7.45, P_{CO_2} up to 45 mm Hg, serum bicarbonate > 30 mEq/L; potassium and chloride usually low; hypoventilation is seldom prominent regardless of pH

- **Differential Diagnosis**
  - Loss of acid (vomiting or nasogastric aspiration)
  - Diuretic overuse or other volume contraction
  - Exogenous bicarbonate load
  - Aldosterone excess: Hyperreninemia, ingestion of some types of licorice, adrenal tumor or hyperplasia, Bartter's or Gitelman's syndrome

- **Treatment**
  - Identify and correct underlying cause
  - Replenish volume and electrolytes (use 0.9% sodium chloride)
  - Hydrochloric acid rarely if ever needed
  - Supplemental KCl in most

- **Pearl**

Vomiting causes mild metabolic alkalosis from contraction; only if associated with gastric outlet obstruction are abnormalities marked, as vomitus is pure HCl.

Reference

Galla JH: Metabolic alkalosis. J Am Soc Nephrol 2000;11:369. [PMID: 10665945]

Respiratory Acidosis

- **Essentials of Diagnosis**
    - Central to all is alveolar hypoventilation
    - Confusion, altered mentation, somnolence in many
    - Cyanosis and asterixis may or may not be present
    - Arterial P_{CO_2} increased; arterial pH decreased
    - Lung disease may be acute (pneumonia, asthma) or chronic (COPD)
    - Lung disease not present in all

- **Differential Diagnosis**
    - Chronic obstructive lung disease
    - Central nervous system depressants
    - Structural disorders of the thorax
    - Myxedema
    - Neurologic disorders, eg, Guillain-Barré syndrome, amyotrophic lateral sclerosis, myasthenia gravis

- **Treatment**
    - Address underlying cause
    - Artificial ventilation if necessary to oxygenate, invasive or noninvasive

10

- **Pearl**

Hypoxemia must be corrected before ascribing mental status changes to an elevated P_{CO_2}; it's the case in most chronically hypercapnic patients.

Reference

Epstein SK, Singh N: Respiratory acidosis. Respir Care 2001;46:366. [PMID: 11262556]

Respiratory Alkalosis

■ Essentials of Diagnosis
  • Lightheadedness, numbness or tingling of extremities, perioral paresthesias
  • Tachypnea; positive Chvostek's and Trousseau's signs in acute hyperventilation; carpopedal spasm and tetany
  • Arterial pH > 7.45, P_{CO_2} < 30 mm Hg

■ Differential Diagnosis
  • Restrictive lung disease or hypoxia
  • Pulmonary embolism
  • Salicylate toxicity
  • Anxiety or pain
  • End-stage cirrhosis
  • Sepsis
  • Pregnancy
  • High-altitude residence

■ Treatment
  • Correct hypoxia or underlying ventilatory stimulant
  • Increase ventilatory dead space (eg, breathe into paper bag, but only in anxiety-induced hyperventilation)

■ Pearl
A lowered P_{CO_2} is a dependable early sign of sepsis syndrome.

Reference

Foster GT, Vaziri ND, Sassoon CS: Respiratory alkalosis. Respir Care 2001; 46:384. [PMID: 11262557]

Shock

- **Essentials of Diagnosis**
  - History of hemorrhage, myocardial infarction, sepsis, trauma, or anaphylaxis
  - Tachycardia, hypotension, hypothermia, tachypnea
  - Cool, sweaty skin with pallor; however, may be warm or flushed with early sepsis; altered level of consciousness
  - Oliguria, acute tubular necrosis (if perfusion prolonged), anemia, disseminated intravascular coagulation, metabolic acidosis may complicate
  - Hemodynamic measurements depend upon underlying cause

- **Differential Diagnosis**
  - Numerous causes of the syndrome, as noted above
  - Adrenal insufficiency

- **Treatment**
  - Correct cause of shock (ie, control hemorrhage, treat infection, correct metabolic disease)
  - Empiric broad-spectrum antibiotics (gram-positive and gram-negative coverage) if cause not apparent
  - Restore hemodynamics with fluids; vasopressor medications may be required; early hemodynamic correction associated with improved outcome
  - Maintain urine output
  - Treat contributing disease (eg, diabetes mellitus)

- **Pearl**

A hypertensive patient appearing to be in shock has aortic dissection until proved otherwise.

Reference

Moore FA, McKinley BA, Moore EE: The next generation in shock resuscitation. Lancet 2004;363:1988. [PMID: 15194260]

11

Genitourinary & Renal Disorders

GENITOURINARY DISORDERS

Acute Epididymitis

- **■ Essentials of Diagnosis**
  - Sudden unilateral testicular pain and palpable swelling of epididymis, with fever, dysuria, urinary urgency, and frequency of less than 6 weeks' duration
  - Marked epididymal, testicular, or spermatic cord tenderness with symptomatic relief upon elevation of scrotum (Prehn's sign)
  - Leukocytosis, pyuria, bacteriuria
  - Usually caused by *Neisseria gonorrhoeae* or *Chlamydia trachomatis* in heterosexual men under age 40 and by Enterobacteriaceae in homosexual men of all ages and heterosexual men over age 40
  - Doppler ultrasonography differentiates from testicular torsion

- **■ Differential Diagnosis**
  - Testicular torsion
  - Testicular tumor
  - Orchitis
  - Prostatitis
  - Testicular trauma

- **■ Treatment**
  - Empiric antibiotics after culture of urine obtained
  - In men under age 40, treat for *N gonorrhoeae* and *C trachomatis* infection for 10–21 days
  - Consider examination and treatment of sexual partners
  - In men over age 40, treat for Enterobacteriaceae for 21–28 days
  - Analgesics and bed rest with elevation and support of scrotum

- **■ Pearl**

Consider the pathogenesis; a VDRL and an HIV test for all patients.

Reference

Luzzi GA, O'Brien TS: Acute epididymitis. BJU Int 2001;87:747. [PMID: 11350430]

Bacterial Prostatitis

■ Essentials of Diagnosis

- Acute bacterial prostatitis: Fever, dysuria, urinary urgency and frequency, perineal or suprapubic pain; very tender prostate; leukocytosis, pyuria, bacteriuria, and hematuria
- Caused by *Escherichia coli* most commonly, also by *Neisseria gonorrhoeae, Chlamydia trachomatis,* other gram-negative rods (eg, *Proteus, Pseudomonas*) or gram-positive organisms (eg, enterococcus)
- Vigorous prostatic massage may produce septicemia
- Chronic prostatitis: Usually in older men, may be asymptomatic; in some, urgency and frequency, dysuria, perineal or suprapubic pain; prostate boggy, not tender; pathogenic organisms can persist despite treatment
- Expressed prostatic secretions demonstrate increased numbers of leukocytes; culture often sterile

■ Differential Diagnosis

- Urethritis
- Cystitis
- Epididymitis
- Prostatodynia
- Nonbacterial prostatitis
- Perirectal abscess

■ Treatment

- Symptomatic treatment with hot sitz baths, NSAIDs, and stool softeners
- For acute bacterial prostatitis in men under 35 years of age, treat for *N gonorrhoeae* and *C trachomatis* infection
- For acute bacterial prostatitis in men over age 35 years or homosexual men, treat for Enterobacteriaceae with oral or intravenous antibiotics (eg, trimethoprim-sulfamethoxazole or ciprofloxacin) for 21 days
- For chronic bacterial prostatitis, treat for Enterobacteriaceae with oral antibiotics (eg, trimethoprim-sulfamethoxazole or ciprofloxacin) for 6–12 weeks; cure rate is often less than 50%

■ Pearl

Trimethoprim-sulfamethoxazole achieves one of the highest intraprostatic levels of all antibiotics; an ideal drug for this process.

Reference

Gurunadha Rao Tunuguntla HS, Evans CP: Management of prostatitis. Prostate Cancer Prostatic Dis 2002;5:172. [PMID: 12496977]

Benign Prostatic Hyperplasia

- **Essentials of Diagnosis**
  - Urinary hesitancy, intermittent stream, straining to initiate micturition, reduced force and caliber of the urinary stream, nocturia, frequency, urgency
  - Palpably enlarged prostate
  - Hematuria, pyuria when infection complicates
  - High postvoid residual volume as determined by ultrasonography or excretory urography; not always prognostic of outcome
  - May be complicated by acute urinary retention or azotemia following prolonged obstruction

- **Differential Diagnosis**
  - Urethral stricture
  - Vesicular stone
  - Neurogenic bladder
  - Prostate cancer
  - Bladder tumor
  - Urinary tract infection
  - Prostatitis

- **Treatment**
  - Treat associated infection if present; trimethoprim-sulfamethoxazole is usually best
  - Minimize evening fluid intake
  - Alpha$_1$-blockers for symptom relief; 5-α-reductase inhibitors (eg, finasteride) in patients with marked prostatic enlargement
  - Utilization of symptom scoring instruments to follow success of treatment
  - Transurethral resection for intolerable symptoms, refractory urinary retention, recurrent gross hematuria, and progressive renal insufficiency with demonstrated obstruction

- **Pearl**

In acute urinary retention in older men, ask about recent upper respiratory infections; anticholinergic medications in over-the-counter remedies may be the answer.

Reference

Thorpe A, Neal D: Benign prostatic hyperplasia. Lancet 2003;361:1359. Erratum in: Lancet 2003;362:496. [PMID: 12711484]

Testicular Torsion

- ■ Essentials of Diagnosis
  - Usually occurs in males under 25 years of age; may present as an acute abdomen
  - Sudden onset of severe, unilateral scrotal or inguinal pain
  - Exquisitely tender and swollen testicle and spermatic cord; pain worsened with elevation
  - Leukocytosis and pyuria
  - Technetium Tc99m sodium pertechnetate scan shows decreased uptake on the affected side (versus increased uptake with epididymitis)
  - Doppler ultrasonography confirms diagnosis

- ■ Differential Diagnosis
  - Epididymitis
  - Orchitis
  - Testicular trauma
  - Testicular tumor
  - Torsion of the appendix testis

- ■ Treatment
  - Inability to rule out testicular torsion requires surgical consult
  - Diagnostic confirmation requires immediate surgery

11

- ■ Pearl

Probably the diagnosis least easily forgotten by the affected patient in all of medicine.

Reference

Cuckow PM, Frank JD: Torsion of the testis. BJU Int 2000;86:349. [PMID: 10930945]

Tuberculosis of the Genitourinary Tract

- **Essentials of Diagnosis**
  - Fever, malaise, night sweats, weight loss; evidence of pulmonary tuberculosis in 50%
  - Symptoms or signs of urinary tract infection may be present
  - Nodular, indurated epididymis, testes, or prostate
  - Sterile pyuria or hematuria without bacteriuria; white blood cell casts can be seen with renal parenchymal involvement
  - Positive culture of morning urine on one of three consecutive samples
  - Proteinuria may indicate development of secondary amyloidosis
  - Plain radiographs may show renal and lower tract calcifications
  - Excretory urogram reveals "moth-eaten" calices, papillary necrosis, and beading of ureters
  - Occasionally, ulcers or granulomas of bladder wall at cystoscopy

- **Differential Diagnosis**
  - Other causes of chronic urinary tract infections
  - Interstitial nephritis, especially drug-induced
  - Nonspecific urethritis
  - Urinary calculi
  - Epididymitis
  - Bladder cancer

- **Treatment**
  - Standard combination antituberculosis therapy
  - Surgical procedures for obstruction and severe hemorrhage
  - Nephrectomy for extensive destruction of the kidney

- **Pearl**

Tuberculosis of the genitourinary tract is the only descending urinary tract infection; all others ascend.

Reference

Wise GJ, Marella VK: Genitourinary manifestations of tuberculosis. Urol Clin North Am 2003;30:111. [PMID: 12580563]

Urinary Calculi

- **Essentials of Diagnosis**
  - Most common in the stone belt, extending from central Ohio through mid-Florida
  - Sudden, severe colicky pain localized to the flank, commonly associated with nausea, vomiting, and fever; marked urinary urgency and frequency if stone lodged at ureterovesical junction
  - Occasionally asymptomatic
  - Hematuria in 90%, pyuria with concurrent infection; presence of crystals in urine may be diagnostically helpful
  - Plain films of the abdomen (stone seen in 90%), spiral CT, or sonography may be used to visualize location of stone
  - Depending on the metabolic abnormality (ie, hypercalcemia, hypercalciuria, hyperuricosuria, hypocitraturia, hyperoxaluria), stones can be composed of calcium oxalate or phosphate, struvite, uric acid, or cystine; over 50% of patients develop recurrent stones

- **Differential Diagnosis**
  - Acute pyelonephritis
  - Chronic prostatism
  - Tumor of genitourinary system
  - Renal tuberculosis
  - Renal infarction
  - Ectopic pregnancy

11

- **Treatment**
  - Stones usually pass spontaneously with analgesia and hydration
  - Antibiotics if concurrent infection present
  - Patient should filter urine and save stone for analysis
  - Hydration to produce at least 2 liters per day of urine output is a mainstay to prevent recurrence; also dietary change, thiazides, allopurinol, citrate, or a combination of these may be used to prevent recurrence, depending on composition of the stone
  - Refer to specialist for recurrent stones
  - Lithotripsy or surgical lithotomy may be necessary in refractory cases

- **Pearl**

Analyze all stones; it is a noninvasive metabolic biopsy of the disease process.

Reference

Parmar MS: Kidney stones. BMJ 2004;328:1420. [PMID: 15191979]

RENAL DISORDERS

Acute & Chronic Tubulointerstitial Nephritis

- **Essentials of Diagnosis**
  - Responsible for 10–15% of cases of acute renal failure
  - Most drug-related (acutely beta-lactam antibiotics or NSAIDs; chronically lead or lithium), but may be idiopathic, or rarely associated with sarcoidosis or certain infections (eg, legionellosis, leptospirosis, viral)
  - Sudden decrease in renal function, associated with fever, maculopapular rash, and eosinophilia; flank pain may be present
  - Hematuria, pyuria, proteinuria, white blood cell casts, and occasionally eosinophils in urine (Wright's stain necessary)
  - Chronic tubulointerstitial nephritis characterized by polyuria and nocturia, salt wasting, mild proteinuria, small kidneys, isosthenuria, hyperchloremic metabolic acidosis
  - Chronic form may result from prolonged obstruction, analgesic abuse, sickle cell trait, chronic hypercalcemia, uric acid nephropathy, or exposure to heavy metals
  - Signs of tubulointerstitial injury include Fanconi's syndrome and renal tubular acidosis
  - Clinical diagnosis which can only be confirmed by renal biopsy

- **Differential Diagnosis**
  - Acute or chronic glomerulonephritis
  - Prerenal azotemia
  - Primary obstructive uropathy

- **Treatment**
  - Discontinue all possible offending drugs or treat associated infection in patients with acute tubulointerstitial nephritis
  - Corticosteroids of debatable benefit but often used if renal function does not improve shortly after discontinuation of drug
  - Temporary dialysis may be necessary in up to one-third of patients with drug-induced acute interstitial nephritis

- **Pearl**

In ill-defined pain syndromes (headache, low back pain) with moderate renal insufficiency, over-the-counter analgesics used to great excess by the patient may be the culprit.

Reference

Harris DC: Tubulointerstitial renal disease. Curr Opin Nephrol Hypertens 2001;10:303. [PMID: 11342791]

Acute Cystitis & Pyelonephritis

- **Essentials of Diagnosis**
  - Dysuria with urinary frequency and urgency, hematuria, abdominal or flank pain
  - Fever, flank or suprapubic tenderness, and vomiting with pyelonephritis
  - Pyuria, bacteriuria, hematuria, positive urine culture, white cell casts on urinalysis (latter in pyelonephritis)
  - Usually caused by gram-negative bacteria (eg, *E coli, Proteus, Klebsiella,* Enterobacteriaceae) but may be due to gram-positive organisms (eg, *Enterococcus faecalis, Staphylococcus saprophyticus*)

- **Differential Diagnosis**
  - Urethritis
  - Nephrolithiasis
  - Prostatitis
  - Pelvic inflammatory disease or vaginosis
  - Lower lobe pneumonia
  - Surgical abdomen due to any cause, eg, appendicitis

- **Treatment**
  - Urine culture in complicated infections (pregnancy, male, elderly, hospital-acquired, recent antibiotics, immunocompromised, obstruction or instrumentation)
  - Empiric oral antibiotics (eg, trimethoprim-sulfamethoxazole, cephalexin, or ciprofloxacin) for 3 days for uncomplicated cystitis
  - Oral or intravenous antibiotics (eg, fluoroquinolone or cephalosporin) for 7–14 days for pyelonephritis
  - Intravenous antibiotics and fluids if dehydration or vomiting present
  - Pyridium for early symptomatic relief
  - Consider hospitalization for patients with single kidney, immunosuppression, or elderly
  - Pursue evaluation for anatomic abnormalities in men who develop cystitis or pyelonephritis
  - Recurrent episodes of cystitis (more than two per year) often treated with low-dose prophylactic antibiotics

- **Pearl**

Pyelonephritis is one of the reasons no one should have an exploratory laparotomy without a urinalysis.

Reference

Hooton TM: The current management strategies for community-acquired urinary tract infection. Infect Dis Clin North Am 2003;17:303. [PMID: 12848472]

Acute Glomerulonephritis

- ■ Essentials of Diagnosis
  - • History of preceding streptococcal or other infection, evidence of systemic vasculitis, or presence of occult malignancy
  - • Malaise, headache, fever, dark urine, hypertension, edema
  - • Renal insufficiency, low fractional excretion of sodium, or oligo/anuria with azotemia in severe cases
  - • Urinary abnormalities include: Hematuria (with or without dysmorphic red cells and red cell casts), proteinuria (usually not nephritic range), lipiduria
  - • Depending on the patient's age and history, further tests may include complement levels (CH50, C3, C4), antistreptolysin O (ASO) titer, antideoxyribonuclease B (anti-DNA B) titer, antinuclear antibody (ANA) titers, anti-GBM antibody levels, antineutrophil cytoplasmic antibodies, hepatitis B and C antibodies, cryoglobulins, and renal biopsy to establish cause

- ■ Differential Diagnosis
  - • IgA nephropathy
  - • Goodpasture's syndrome (anti-GBM antibody syndrome)
  - • Other vasculitides (eg, polyarteritis nodosa, SLE)
  - • Membranoproliferative glomerulonephritis
  - • Hepatitis B– or C–associated glomerulonephritis, other postinfectious glomerulonephritides
  - • Infective endocarditis
  - • Wegener's granulomatosis
  - • Henoch-Schönlein purpura
  - • Tubulointerstitial disease

- ■ Treatment
  - • Steroids and cytotoxic agents are used for rapidly progressive glomerulonephritis, more effective at higher GFRs
  - • Plasmapheresis occasionally of value in anti-GBM disease
  - • Lower blood pressure slowly to prevent sudden decreases in renal perfusion
  - • Supportive therapy with fluid and sodium restriction
  - • Monitor for malignant hypertension, congestive heart failure

- ■ Pearl

A red cell cast indicates glomerulonephritis; a urine specimen after 1000 mL of water and an hour of lordosis increases the yield.

Reference

Vinen CS, Oliveira DB: Acute glomerulonephritis. Postgrad Med J 2003;79:206; quiz 212. [PMID: 12743337]

Acute Renal Failure

- ## Essentials of Diagnosis
  - Usually caused by acute tubular necrosis
  - Nausea, vomiting, mental status changes, edema, hypertension
  - History can include exposure to nephrotoxic agents, sepsis, trauma, surgery, shock, or hemorrhage
  - Oliguria or discolored urine in many patients
  - Pericardial friction rub, asterixis may be present
  - Hyperkalemia, hyperphosphatemia, decreased serum bicarbonate
  - Kidneys of normal size or enlarged on imaging studies; small kidneys or renal osteodystrophy suggests chronic renal failure
  - Hematuria, proteinuria, and isosthenuria with tubular casts
  - Urinalysis with manual microscopy to guide diagnostic approach

- ## Differential Diagnosis
  - Prerenal azotemia (eg, cirrhosis, nephrosis, heart failure, hypovolemia)
  - Intrinsic causes (eg, vascular, glomerular, tubulointerstitial)
  - Postrenal azotemia (eg, obstructive uropathy)

- ## Treatment
  - Volume resuscitation with isotonic fluid for hypovolemia
  - Ultrasonography to rule out obstructive process
  - Renal biopsy (when glomerulonephritis suspected)
  - Supportive care for uncomplicated cases: Minimize fluid intake, follow potassium, phosphorus and bicarbonate levels
  - Oliguric renal failure with worse prognosis than a nonoliguric process; role of diuretics to convert to latter process recommended but unproved
  - Dialysis for fluid overload, hyperkalemia, pericarditis, symptoms of uremia
  - Adjust dosage of renally-metabolized medications
  - Avoid contrast exposure; N-acetylcysteine prophylaxis in high-risk patients prior to unavoidable contrast studies

- ## Pearl

If a contrast study is performed (however inappropriately), capture the first specimen thereafter for analysis; it has the highest yield for diagnostic casts.

Reference

Schrier RW, Wang W, Poole B, Mitra A: Acute renal failure: Definitions, diagnosis, pathogenesis, and therapy. J Clin Invest 2004;114:5. Erratum in: J Clin Invest 2004;114:598. [PMID: 15232604]

Anti–Glomerular Basement Membrane Nephritis (Goodpasture's Syndrome)

- ■ Essentials of Diagnosis
  - • Triad of pulmonary hemorrhage with hemoptysis, circulating anti-GBM antibody, and glomerulonephritis due to anti-GBM
  - • Most common in young (18–30) and middle-aged (50–60s) white men; smokers also have a predilection
  - • Extrarenal manifestations may be absent
  - • On immunofluorescence, renal biopsy reveals linear deposition of IgG with or without C3 deposition along the glomerular basement membrane
  - • Serum anti-GBM antibody is pathognomonic

- ■ Differential Diagnosis
  - • Wegener's granulomatosis
  - • Polyarteritis nodosa
  - • SLE
  - • Endocarditis
  - • Postinfectious glomerulonephritis
  - • Primary pulmonary hemorrhage

11

- ■ Treatment
  - • Plasmapheresis to remove circulating anti-GBM antibody
  - • Prednisone and cyclophosphamide for at least 3 months
  - • Recovery of renal function more likely if treatment is begun prior to a serum creatinine of 6–7 mg/dL; hemodialysis as necessary
  - • Renal transplant delayed for 12 months after disappearance of antibody from the serum

- ■ Pearl

One of the few causes in medicine of a dramatically elevated D$_{LCO}$.

Reference

Hudson BG, Tryggvason K, Sundaramoorthy M, Neilson EG: Alport's syndrome, Goodpasture's syndrome, and type IV collagen. N Engl J Med 2003;348:2543. [PMID: 12815141]

Asymptomatic Bacteriuria

- **Essentials of Diagnosis**
  - History of recurring urinary tract infections may be present
  - Bacteriuria with absence of symptoms or signs referable to the urinary tract
  - May be associated with obstruction, anatomic or neurologic abnormalities, pregnancy, indwelling catheter, urologic procedures, diverted urinary stream (eg, ileal loop conduit), diabetes, or old age
  - Usually caused by Enterobacteriaceae, *Pseudomonas,* or enterococci

- **Differential Diagnosis**
  - Drug-induced nephropathy, especially analgesics
  - Contaminated urine specimen

- **Treatment**
  - Indications for treatment include pregnancy, persistent bacteriuria in certain patients and prior to urologic procedures
  - Urine culture to guide antimicrobial therapy
  - Surgical relief of obstruction if present
  - In selected cases, chronic antibiotic suppression

11

- **Pearl**

Most patients with asymptomatic bacteriuria should not *be given antibiotics; prognosis is excellent.*

Reference

Raz R: Asymptomatic bacteriuria. Clinical significance and management. Int J Antimicrob Agents 2003;22(Suppl 2):45. [PMID: 14527770]

Chronic Kidney Disease

- ■ Essentials of Diagnosis
  - • Early usually asymptomatic
  - • Advanced dysfunction with volume overload, hypertension, metabolic acidosis, hyperkalemia, hyperphosphatemia, hypocalcemia, anemia, renal osteodystrophy
  - • Uremic symptoms over weeks to years include anorexia, nausea, vomiting, hiccups, CNS abnormalities
  - • Pericarditis, neuropathy
  - • Oliguria or polyuria; isosthenuria; benign sediment with broad waxy casts
  - • Bilateral shrunken kidneys on imaging studies; exceptions include polycystic kidney disease, diabetic nephropathy, myeloma kidney, HIV-associated nephropathy, amyloidosis

- ■ Differential Diagnosis
  - • Obstructive uropathy or prerenal azotemia
  - • Acute renal failure

- ■ Treatment
  - • Preventing or slowing progression by controlling underlying disease and hypertension, preferably with ACE inhibitor or ARB therapy
  - • Regular estimation of GFR, and urinary proteinuria with spot urine protein or albumin:creatinine ratio
  - • Attention to comorbid factors, especially cardiovascular disease, as well as hyperlipidemia and anemia
  - • Low-protein diet, salt and water restriction for patients with hypertension and edema
  - • Potassium, phosphorus, and magnesium restriction once GFR is below 30–60 mL/min
  - • Phosphorus binders for associated hyperphosphatemia with avoidance of chronic aluminum hydroxide if possible; calcium and vitamin D supplements to prevent osteodystrophy; aim for intact parathyroid hormone of two to three times normal values
  - • Bicarbonate therapy for chronic metabolic acidosis
  - • Erythropoietin for anemia after replacing iron stores
  - • In progressive disease, referral for dialysis or renal transplantation

- ■ Pearl

Patients with chronic kidney disease are far more likely to die of cardiovascular causes than of end-stage kidney disease.

Reference

Yu HT: Progression of chronic renal failure. Arch Intern Med 2003;163:1417. [PMID: 12824091]

11

Diabetic Nephropathy

- **Essentials of Diagnosis**
  - Seen in diabetes mellitus of 15–20 years' duration
  - Diabetic retinopathy often present
  - GFR increases initially, returns to normal as further renal damage occurs, then continues to fall
  - Proteinuria > 1 g/d, often nephrotic range
  - Normal to enlarged kidneys on ultrasound
  - Biopsy can show mesangial matrix expansion, diffuse glomerulosclerosis and nodular intercapillary glomerulosclerosis, the latter pathognomonic

- **Differential Diagnosis**
  - Nephrotic syndrome due to other cause, especially amyloidosis
  - Glomerulonephritis with nephrotic features such as that seen in systemic lupus erythematosus, membranous glomerulonephritis, or IgA nephropathy

- **Treatment**
  - ACE inhibition, or probably, angiotensin II receptor blockade early may reduce hyperfiltration, proteinuria, and progression
  - Strict glycemic and blood pressure control
  - Supportive care for progression of chronic renal insufficiency— includes treatment of anemia, acidosis and elevated phosphorus
  - Protein restriction has been advocated but not proved in clinical trials
  - Transplantation an alternative to dialysis at end stage, but comorbid vasculopathy can be daunting; may have significant survival benefit with pre-emptive (before ESRD) transplantation

11

- **Pearl**

One of medicine's few causes of massive albuminuria sustained in the end stages of renal function.

Reference

Jawa A, Kcomt J, Fonseca VA: Diabetic nephropathy and retinopathy. Med Clin North Am 2004;88:1001, xi. [PMID: 15308388]

Focal Segmental Glomerulosclerosis

- **Essentials of Diagnosis**
  - May be primary (idiopathic) or secondary (physiologic response to hyperfiltration or glomerular hypertrophy as in disorders with decreased renal mass such as unilateral renal agenesis, after nephrectomy, massive obesity, reflux nephropathy; or nonspecific healing from prior inflammatory injury)
  - Other causes include familial forms, toxin related (heroin), infections (HIV)
  - Along with membranous nephropathy, most common cause of nephrotic syndrome in nondiabetic adults
  - Primary form often presents with acute nephrotic syndrome: Proteinuria, hypoalbuminemia, edema, hyperlipidemia
  - Secondary forms often asymptomatic, presenting with non-nephrotic proteinuria and slowly progressive renal insufficiency
  - Depending on the history, further tests may include serologies (HIV), renal ultrasound, and renal biopsy (treatment implications present)

- **Differential Diagnosis**
  - Membranous nephropathy
  - Diabetic nephropathy
  - Minimal change disease
  - Pre-eclampsia
  - Amyloid, primary or secondary
  - Postinfectious glomerulonephritis (later stages)
  - IgA nephropathy
  - Membranoproliferative glomerulonephritis

- **Treatment**
  - General measures similar to those for nephrotic syndrome, especially use of ACE inhibitor for proteinuria and lipid-lowering agents for hyperlipidemia
  - Steroid treatment initially for symptomatic idiopathic FSGS; favorable prognosis for complete or partial responders
  - Steroid resistance associated with poor renal prognosis; additional therapy with cyclosporine, tacrolimus, mycophenolate mofetil, cytotoxic agents (cyclophosphamide, chlorambucil), or plasmapheresis

- **Pearl**

Among African-Americans, FSGS is the most common form of idiopathic nephrotic syndrome; untreated, it rapidly progresses to end-stage renal disease.

Reference

Cameron JS: Focal segmental glomerulosclerosis in adults. Nephrol Dial Transplant 2003;18(Suppl 6):vi, 45. [PMID: 12953042]

Hypertensive Nephrosclerosis

- **Essentials of Diagnosis**
  - Poorly controlled hypertension for over 15 years; alternatively, severe, aggressive hypertension, especially in young blacks
  - With extreme blood pressure elevation, papilledema and encephalopathy may occur
  - Ultrasound reveals bilateral small, echogenic kidneys in advanced disease
  - Proteinuria is usual
  - Biopsy can show thickened vessels and sclerotic glomeruli; malignant nephrosclerosis reveals characteristic onion-skinning

- **Differential Diagnosis**
  - Atheroembolic or atherosclerotic renal disease
  - Renal artery stenosis, especially bilateral
  - End-stage renal disease due to any other cause

- **Treatment**
  - Strict sodium restriction
  - Aggressive control of hypertension, including ACE inhibitor if possible
  - If patient presents with hypertensive urgency or emergency, decrease blood pressure slowly over several days to prevent decreased renal perfusion
  - May take up to 6 months of adequate blood pressure control to achieve improved baseline of renal function

- **Pearl**

In benign nephrosclerosis, the rule is for serum creatinine to rise after beginning antihypertensive therapy; stay the course with blood pressure control and improved renal function will follow.

Reference

Luft FC: Hypertensive nephrosclerosis: update. Curr Opin Nephrol Hypertens 2004;13:147. [PMID: 15202608]

IgA Nephropathy (Berger's Disease)

■ Essentials of Diagnosis

- Most common form of acute and chronic glomerulonephritis in Caucasians and Asians
- Focal proliferative glomerulonephritis of unknown cause
- Secondary causes include hepatic cirrhosis, celiac disease, inflammatory bowel disease, dermatitis herpetiformis, psoriasis, minimal change disease
- First episode: Macroscopic hematuria, often associated with a viral infection, with or without upper respiratory ("synpharyngitic") and gastrointestinal symptoms
- Malaise, fatigue, myalgias, hypertension, edema may be present
- Recurrent hematuria and mild proteinuria over decades, with same precipitants
- Often detected incidentally with microscopic hematuria
- Serum IgA increased in 30–50%; renal biopsy reveals inflammation and deposition of IgA with or without C3 and IgM in the mesangium of all glomeruli
- Usually indolent; 20–30% of patients progress to end-stage renal disease over 2–3 decades

11

■ Differential Diagnosis

- Hereditary nephritis (Alport's syndrome)
- Thin basement membrane disease
- Henoch-Schönlein purpura
- Poststreptococcal acute glomerulonephritis
- Infective endocarditis
- Goodpasture's syndrome
- Other vasculitides (eg, polyarteritis nodosa, SLE)
- Wegener's granulomatosis

■ Treatment

- Supportive therapy for patients with < 1 g/d of proteinuria with yearly monitoring of renal function
- In patients with proteinuria > 1 g/d or hypertension, treat with ACE inhibitors
- Fish oil of questionable benefit but not harmful
- Steroids, cytotoxic agents, and immunosuppressants in selected cases

■ Pearl

Berger's disease is not Buerger's disease—the latter is thromboangiitis obliterans.

Reference

Donadio JV, Grande JP: IgA nephropathy. N Engl J Med 2002;347:738. [PMID: 12213946]

Lupus Nephritis

- **Essentials of Diagnosis**
  - Can be the initial presentation of systemic lupus erythematosus
  - WHO classification of renal biopsy: Normal renal biopsy (class I); mesangial proliferation (class II); focal proliferation (class III); diffuse proliferation (class IV); membranous (class V)
  - Proteinuria or hematuria of glomerular origin; hypocomplementemia common
  - Glomerular filtration rate need not be depressed
  - Chronic tubulointerstitial changes on biopsy portend a worse prognosis

- **Differential Diagnosis**
  - Glomerulonephritis due to other diseases, including anti-GBM disease, microscopic polyarteritis, Wegener's membranous nephropathy, IgA nephropathy, thrombotic thrombocytopenic purpura
  - Nephrotic syndrome due to other causes
  - Vascular thrombi secondary to antiphospholipid antibodies

- **Treatment**
  - Follow serial measures of renal function and urinalysis
  - Strict control of hypertension
  - ACE inhibitor to reduce proteinuria
  - Steroids and cytotoxic agents for severe class III or any class IV
  - Early treatment of renal relapses may prevent severe flare
  - Repeat biopsy for flare of renal disease; lupus nephritis can change forms
  - Upon reaching end-stage renal disease, renal transplantation is an excellent alternative to dialysis

- **Pearl**

Kidney involvement is not encountered when SLE is drug-induced.

Reference

Flanc RS, Roberts MA, Strippoli GF, et al: Treatment for lupus nephritis. Cochrane Database Syst Rev 2004;1:CD002922. [PMID: 14973998]

Membranous Nephropathy

- ■ Essentials of Diagnosis
  - • Common; may be primary (idiopathic) or secondary (malignancy, usually solid organ; autoimmune diseases such as lupus or rheumatoid arthritis; systemic infections such as hepatitis B or C)
  - • Anorexia, dyspnea, foamy urine; anasarca
  - • Proteinuria, hypoalbuminemia, hyperlipidemia
  - • Hypercoagulability due to anticoagulant urinary loss; hematuria in half
  - • Renal ultrasound; renal biopsy to establish diagnosis
  - • Limit malignancy evaluation to age-appropriate screening or evaluation of abnormalities from history and physical

- ■ Differential Diagnosis
  - • Focal segmental glomerulosclerosis
  - • Diabetic nephropathy
  - • Minimal change disease
  - • Amyloidosis
  - • Membranoproliferative glomerulonephritis

11

- ■ Treatment
  - • General measures similar to those for nephrotic syndrome
  - • Spontaneous or partial ($\leq$ 2 g/d proteinuria) remission in 70%; thus if non-nephrotic proteinuria and asymptomatic, or symptoms of edema easily controlled, observe without treatment
  - • Risk factors for progressive disease: Men > age 50, proteinuria > 6 g/d, abnormal renal function at presentation, and tubulointerstitial disease on biopsy; active therapy with steroids and cytotoxic agent (cyclophosphamide or chlorambucil)
  - • Alternative agents in selected cases: Cyclosporine, mycophenolate mofetil, azathioprine, intravenous immunoglobulin
  - • Good long-term prognosis after spontaneous or drug-induced remission, although relapses may occur in one-quarter of cases

- ■ Pearl

Membranous nephropathy is one of three renal manifestations of hepatitis C virus; the others are mixed cryoglobulinemia and membranoproliferative glomerulonephritis.

Reference

Glassock RJ: Diagnosis and natural course of membranous nephropathy. Semin Nephrol 2003;23:324. [PMID: 12923720]

Myeloma Kidney

- **Essentials of Diagnosis**
  - May be initial presentation of multiple myeloma
  - The systemic disease with easily the most renal and metabolic complications
  - Classic definition: Light chain of immunoglobulins (Bence Jones proteins) directly toxic to tubules, or causing intratubular obstruction by precipitation
  - Myeloma may also be associated with glomerular amyloidosis, hypercalcemia, nephrocalcinosis, nephrolithiasis, plasma cell infiltration of the renal parenchyma, hyperviscosity syndrome compromising renal blood flow, proximal (Fanconi-like syndrome) or distal renal tubular acidosis, type IV renal tubular acidosis, and progressive renal insufficiency
  - Serum anion gap is low in the majority due to positively charged paraprotein
  - Serum and urinary electrophoresis reveals monoclonal spike in over 90% of patients; some cases are nonsecretory and are very aggressive clinically

- **Differential Diagnosis**
  - Interstitial nephritis
  - Prerenal azotemia
  - Obstructive nephropathy
  - Nephrotic syndrome of other cause
  - Drug-induced nephropathy

11

- **Treatment**
  - Therapy for myeloma; prognosis for renal survival is better if serum creatinine is < 2 mg/dL prior to treatment
  - Treat hypertension and hypercalcemia if present
  - Avoid contrast agents and other nephrotoxins
  - Avoid dehydration and maintain adequate intravascular volume; remember that hypercalcemia causes nephrogenic diabetes insipidus, and this worsens dehydration

- **Pearl**

The urine dipstick detects only albumin and intact globulin, as light chains are missed even when present in large amounts; suspect if negative dipstick with positive spot urine protein:creatinine ratio.

Reference

Pandit SR, Vesole DH: Management of renal dysfunction in multiple myeloma. Curr Treat Options Oncol 2003;4:239. [PMID: 12718801]

Nephrotic Syndrome

- **Essentials of Diagnosis**
  - May be primary or secondary to systemic infections (eg, secondary syphilis, endocarditis), diabetes, multiple myeloma with or without amyloidosis, heavy metals, and autoimmune diseases
  - Anorexia, dyspnea, anasarca, foamy urine
  - Proteinuria (> 3 g/d), hypoalbuminemia (< 3 g/dL), edema, hyperlipidemia in < 50% upon presentation
  - Hypercoagulability with peripheral renal vein thrombosis
  - Lipiduria with oval fat bodies, maltese crosses, and fatty and waxy casts in urinary sediment
  - Further tests may include complement levels (CH50, C3, C4), serum and urine electrophoresis, antinuclear antibody (ANA), serologies (hepatitis B and C, syphilis), renal ultrasound, and renal biopsy if treatment implications present

- **Differential Diagnosis/Causes**
  - CHF, cirrhosis, constriction
  - Minimal change disease
  - Focal segmental glomerulosclerosis and membranous GNPP
  - Diabetic nephropathy
  - Amyloidosis (primary or secondary)
  - Membranoproliferative glomerulonephritis

- **Treatment**
  - Supportive therapy with fluid and sodium restriction, diuretics to control edema, control of hypertension (with ACE inhibitor when possible), lipid-lowering agents, chronic anticoagulation for severe hypoalbuminemia or thrombotic events
  - Maintenance of adequate nutrition
  - Corticosteroids for minimal change disease (lipoid nephrosis); in focal and segmental glomerular sclerosis, longer courses of steroid therapy often necessary; membranous nephropathy may be treated with corticosteroids and cytotoxic agents; in membranoproliferative glomerulonephropathy, steroid use less well established

- **Pearl**

Membranous glomerulonephritis in patients over 50 obligates consideration of a visceral malignancy; it may be a paraneoplastic phenomenon.

Reference

Eddy AA, Symons JM: Nephrotic syndrome in childhood. Lancet 2003;362:629. [PMID: 12944064]

Obstructive Nephropathy

- ■ Essentials of Diagnosis
  - • Most cases are postvesical and usually of prostatic origin
  - • A few cases result from bilateral ureteral obstruction, usually from stones, which can present with sudden pain
  - • Obstruction may be acute or chronic, partial or complete
  - • Postvesical obstruction presents with nocturia, incontinence, malaise, nausea, with normal 24-hour urine output, but in swings
  - • Palpable bladder, suprapubic pain
  - • Renal insufficiency, hypertension may be present
  - • Renal ultrasound localizes site of obstruction with proximal tract dilation and hydronephrosis
  - • Spectrum of causes includes anatomic abnormalities, stricture, retroperitoneal or pelvic tumor, prostatic hypertrophy, bilateral renal stones, drug effect (methysergide), and neuromuscular disorders

- ■ Differential Diagnosis
  - • Prerenal azotemia
  - • Interstitial nephritis
  - • Acute or chronic renal failure due to any cause

- ■ Treatment
  - • Urinary catheter or ultrasonography to rule out obstruction secondary to enlarged prostate
  - • Nephrostomy tubes if significant bilateral hydronephrosis present with bilateral ureteral obstruction
  - • Treatment of concurrent infection if present
  - • Observe for postobstructive diuresis; can be brisk

- ■ Pearl

One stone can cause obstructive nephropathy in the one in 500 patients born with a single kidney.

Reference

Klahr S: Obstructive nephropathy. Intern Med 2000;39:355. [PMID: 10830173]

Polycystic Kidney Disease

- ■ Essentials of Diagnosis
  - Autosomal dominant inheritance and nearly complete penetrance, thus strikingly positive family history (autosomal recessive form rare, usually discovered in childhood)
  - Abdominal or flank pain associated with hematuria, frequent urinary tract infections, nephrolithiasis
  - Hypertension, large palpable kidneys, positive family history
  - Renal insufficiency in 50% of patients by age 70; unlikely to develop renal disease if no cystic renal lesions by age 30
  - Normal or elevated hematocrit common: Interstitial cells near cysts may elaborate erythropoietin
  - Diagnosis confirmed by multiple renal cysts on ultrasonography or CT scan
  - Increased incidence of cerebral aneurysms (10% of affected patients), aortic aneurysms, and abnormalities of the mitral valve; 40–50% have concomitant hepatic cysts; colonic diverticula; abdominal wall hernias

- ■ Differential Diagnosis
  - Renal cell carcinoma
  - Simple renal cysts
  - Other causes of chronic renal failure

- ■ Treatment
  - Treat hypertension and nephrolithiasis
  - Observe for urinary tract infection; if present, may require prolonged treatment
  - Avoid high-protein diet
  - Patients with family history of cerebral aneurysm should have screening cerebral CT or MR angiography
  - Occasional nephrectomy required for repeated episodes of pain and infection, or prior to transplant for very large kidneys
  - Excellent outcome with transplant

- ■ Pearl

Hypertension, an abdominal mass, and azotemia is polycystic disease until proven otherwise.

Reference

Wilson PD: Polycystic kidney disease. N Engl J Med 2004;350:151. [PMID: 14711914]

Renal Tubular Acidosis

- ■ Essentials of Diagnosis
  - • Unexplained metabolic acidosis with a normal anion gap
  - • Type I (distal): Impaired urinary acidification, plasma bicarbonate may be < 10 mEq/L, hypokalemia, abnormal (positive) urinary anion gap; may be familial or secondary to autoimmune disease, obstructive uropathy, drugs (eg, amphotericin B), hyperglobulinemia, hypercalciuria, renal transplantation, or sickle cell anemia
  - • Type II (proximal): Bicarbonaturia with serum bicarbonate usually 12–20 mEq/L, hypokalemia, often with Fanconi's syndrome (glycosuria, aminoaciduria, phosphaturia, uricosuria, and tubular proteinuria); may be secondary to myeloma, drugs, or renal transplant
  - • Type IV: Low renin and aldosterone; impaired ammoniagenesis with serum bicarbonate usually > 17 mEq/L; hyperkalemia, abnormal (positive) urinary anion gap; typical of renal insufficiency; others due to diabetes mellitus, drugs (eg, ACE inhibitors, NSAIDs, cyclosporine), tubulointerstitial disease, or nephrosclerosis

- ■ Differential Diagnosis
  - • Diarrhea
  - • Ileal loop constriction after surgery for bladder cancer
  - • Hypokalemia or hyperkalemia from other causes

11

- ■ Treatment
  - • Discontinue offending drug or treat underlying disease if present
  - • Bicarbonate or citrate and potassium replacement for types I and II
  - • Vitamin D and phosphate supplementation for type I to prevent osteomalacia, not type II because of possible hypercalcemia and further damage to the distal tubule
  - • Thiazides may increase bicarbonate reabsorption for type II
  - • Fludrocortisone for type IV only if volume repletion is difficult

- ■ Pearl

Along with SIADH, type II renal tubular acidosis is one of the few causes of hypouricemia in all of medicine.

Reference

Rodriguez Soriano J: Renal tubular acidosis: the clinical entity. J Am Soc Nephrol 2002;13:2160. [PMID: 12138150]

Uric Acid Nephropathy

■ Essentials of Diagnosis
  • Three distinct syndromes; terminology confusing
  • Uric acid nephrolithiasis: Radiolucent urate stones in 3% of patients with gout
  • Gouty kidney (chronic urate nephropathy): Interstitial sodium urate crystals of uncertain significance in patients with gout and interstitial nephropathy; no correlation with degree of elevation of serum uric acid
  • Uric acid nephropathy: Uric acid sludge within nephron due to cellular necrosis, typically after chemotherapy or radiation has induced rapid cell lysis

■ Differential Diagnosis
  • Renal failure due to other cause
  • Hypertensive nephrosclerosis
  • Nephrolithiasis due to other cause
  • Myeloma kidney

■ Treatment
  • Depends upon syndrome
  • Intravenous hydration and alkalinization of urine for uric acid stones
  • Pretreatment with allopurinol and intravenous hydration for selected patients at risk for tumor lysis syndrome; maintain urine pH > 6.5 and urine output > 2 L/d
  • In patients with gout, allopurinol and colchicine adjusted for renal function; NSAID use minimized in patients with renal dysfunction
  • Uricase prophylaxis in high-risk patients or treatment of acute uric acid nephropathy

■ Pearl
Remember aspirin and uric acid; at low dose (<3 g/d), aspirin causes hyperuricemia because of blockage of secretion; at higher doses, reabsorption is blocked more than secretion and hypouricemia ensues.

Reference
Steele TH: Hyperuricemic nephropathies. Nephron 1999;81(Suppl 1):45. [PMID: 9873214]

11

12

Neurologic Diseases

Arteriovenous Malformations

- **Essentials of Diagnosis**
  - Congenital vascular malformations that consist of arteriovenous communications without intervening capillaries
  - Patients typically under age 30 and normotensive
  - Initial symptoms include acute headache, seizures, abrupt onset of coma—the latter with rupture
  - May also present as transverse myelitis (spinal cord arteriovenous malformation)
  - Up to 70% of arteriovenous malformations bleed during their natural history, most commonly before age 40
  - CT of the brain suggests diagnosis; angiography characteristically diagnostic, but some types (eg, cavernous malformations) may not be visualized; MRI often helpful

- **Differential Diagnosis**
  - Dural arteriovenous fistulas
  - Seizures due to other causes
  - Hypertensive intracerebral hemorrhage
  - Ruptured intracranial aneurysm
  - Intracranial tumor
  - Meningitis or brain abscess
  - Transverse myelopathy due to other causes

- **Treatment**
  - Excision if malformation accessible and neurologic risk not great
  - Endovascular embolization in selected malformations
  - Radiosurgery for small malformations

- **Pearl**

The most common cause of intracranial hemorrhage between ages 15 and 30.

Reference

Fleetwood IG, Steinberg GK: Arteriovenous malformations. Lancet 2002; 359:863.

Bell's Palsy (Idiopathic Facial Paresis)

- **Essentials of Diagnosis**
  - An idiopathic facial paresis
  - Abrupt onset of hemifacial (including the forehead) weakness, difficulty closing eye; ipsilateral ear pain may precede or accompany weakness
  - Unilateral peripheral seventh nerve palsy on examination; taste lost on the anterior two-thirds of the tongue, and hyperacusis may occur

- **Differential Diagnosis**
  - Carotid distribution stroke
  - Intracranial mass lesion
  - Basilar meningitis, especially that associated with sarcoidosis
  - Lyme disease
  - First of multiple cranial neuropathies
  - Guillain-Barré syndrome

- **Treatment**
  - Treatment with corticosteroids and acyclovir may be beneficial when initiated early (48–72 hours)
  - Supportive measures with frequent eye lubrication and nocturnal eye patching
  - Only 10% of patients are dissatisfied with the final outcome of their disability or disfigurement

- **Pearl**

The Bell phenomenon: the eye on the affected side moves superiorly and laterally when the patient attempts to close his eyes.

Reference

Salinas R: Bell's palsy. Clin Evid 2002;8:1301. [PMID: 12603941]

Brain Abscess

- **Essentials of Diagnosis**
  - History of sinusitis, otitis, endocarditis, chronic pulmonary infection, or congenital heart defect common
  - Headache, focal neurologic symptoms, seizures may occur
  - Examination may confirm focal findings
  - The most common organisms are streptococci, staphylococci, and anaerobes; *Toxoplasma* in AIDS patients; commonly polymicrobial
  - Ring-enhancing lesion on CT scan or MRI; lumbar puncture potentially dangerous because of mass effect and not usually helpful diagnostically

- **Differential Diagnosis**
  - Primary or metastatic tumor
  - Cerebral infarction
  - Encephalitis
  - Subdural empyema
  - Neurosyphilis
  - Demyelination (eg, multiple sclerosis)

- **Treatment**
  - Intravenous broad-spectrum antibiotics (with coverage to include anaerobic organisms) may be curative if abscess smaller than 2 cm in diameter
  - Surgical aspiration through burr hole if no response to antibiotic drugs, either clinically or by CT scan

12

- **Pearl**

Frank brain abscess is the least common neurologic manifestation of endocarditis.

Reference

Calfee DP, Wispelwey B: Brain abscess. Semin Neurol 2000;20:353. [PMID: 11051299]

Combined System Disease (Posterolateral Sclerosis)

- ■ Essentials of Diagnosis
    - Numbness (pins and needles), tenderness, weakness; feeling of heaviness in toes, feet, fingers, and hands
    - Stocking and glove distribution of sensory loss in some patients
    - Extensor plantar response and hyperreflexia typical, as is loss of position and vibratory senses
    - May develop myelopathy in severe cases
    - Serum vitamin B_{12} level low; methylmalonic acid and homocysteine levels high
    - Megaloblastic anemia may be present but does not parallel neurologic dysfunction

- ■ Differential Diagnosis
    - Tabes dorsalis
    - Multiple sclerosis
    - Transverse myelitis of viral or other origin
    - Epidural tumor or abscess
    - Cervical spondylosis
    - Polyneuropathy due to toxin or metabolic abnormality
    - Nitric oxide abuse

- ■ Treatment
    - Vitamin B_{12} replacement, usually intramuscular

- ■ Pearl

When vitamin B_{12} deficiency is the cause, pharmacologic amounts of folic acid may worsen the neurologic picture.

Reference

Swain R: An update of vitamin B_{12} metabolism and deficiency states. J Fam Pract 1995;41:595. [PMID: 7500070]

Guillain-Barré Syndrome
(Acute Inflammatory Polyneuropathy)

■ Essentials of Diagnosis

- Associated with viral infections, stress, and preceding *Campylobacter jejuni* enteritis, but most cases do not have any definite link to pathogens
- Progressive, usually ascending, symmetric weakness with variable paresthesia or dysesthesia; autonomic involvement (eg, cardiac irregularities, hypertension, or hypotension) may be prominent
- Electromyography consistent with demyelinating injury; also a less common axonal form
- Lumbar puncture, normal in early or mild disease, shows high protein, normal cell count later in course

■ Differential Diagnosis

- Diphtheria, poliomyelitis (where endemic)
- Porphyria
- Heavy metal poisoning
- Botulism
- Transverse myelitis of any origin
- Familial periodic paralysis
- Tick paralysis
- Brainstem encephalitis

12

■ Treatment

- Plasmapheresis or intravenous immunoglobulin
- Pulmonary functions closely monitored, with intubation for impending respiratory failure
- Respiratory toilet with physical therapy
- Up to 20% of patients are left with persisting disability

■ Pearl

The occasional Guillain-Barré may start in the brainstem and descend— the C. Miller Fisher variant.

Reference

Newswanger DL, Warren CR: Guillain-Barré syndrome. Am Fam Physician 2004;69:2405. [PMID: 15168961]

Huntington's Disease

■ Essentials of Diagnosis

- Family history usually present (autosomal dominant)
- Onset at age 30–50, with gradual progressive chorea and dementia; death usually occurs within 20 years after onset
- Caused by a trinucleotide-repeat expansion in a gene located on the short arm of chromosome 4
- The earliest mental changes are often behavioral, including hypersexuality
- CT/MRI scan shows cerebral atrophy, particularly in the caudate

■ Differential Diagnosis

- Sydenham's chorea
- Tardive dyskinesia
- Lacunar infarcts of subthalamic nuclei
- Other causes of dementia

■ Treatment

- Primarily supportive
- Antidopaminergic agents (eg, haloperidol) or reserpine may reduce severity of movement abnormality
- Genetic counseling for offspring

12

■ Pearl

All movement abnormalities in Huntington's disease disappear when the patient is asleep.

Reference

Bonelli RM, Wenning GK, Kapfhammer HP: Huntington's disease: present treatments and future therapeutic modalities. Int Clin Psychopharmacol 2004; 19:51. [PMID: 15076012]

Idiopathic Epilepsy

- ■ Essentials of Diagnosis
  - Abrupt onset of paroxysmal, transitory, recurrent alterations of central nervous system function, often accompanied by alteration in consciousness
  - Family history common
  - Generalized tonic-clonic (grand mal): Loss of consciousness, generalized motor convulsions; altered mentation or focal abnormalities may persist for up to 48 hours postictally
  - Partial seizures: Focal motor convulsions or altered consciousness (complex); may become generalized
  - Absence seizures manifested typically as episodic inattention, usually in children
  - Characteristic EEG during seizures; often abnormal during interictal periods

- ■ Differential Diagnosis
  - Seizures due to metabolic disorders (hyponatremia, hypocalcemia most common), toxins (alcohol, cocaine), or vascular, infectious, neoplastic, or immunologic disease
  - Syncope
  - Narcolepsy
  - Psychiatric abnormalities (hysteria, panic attack)
  - Stroke (when patient first seen postictally)
  - Hypoglycemia

- ■ Treatment
  - Phenytoin, carbamazepine, and valproic acid for most types of epilepsy
  - Newer-generation anticonvulsants and phenobarbital may be helpful in patients unresponsive to other medications
  - For absence seizures, ethosuximide, valproic acid, and clonazepam are useful
  - Status epilepticus is treated as a medical emergency with intravenous diazepam or lorazepam and fosphenytoin; general anesthesia with barbiturates or halothane may be necessary in refractory cases

- ■ Pearl

Remember subclinical epilepsy in critically ill and unconscious patients; EEG may reveal status epilepticus.

Reference

Mattson RH: Overview: idiopathic generalized epilepsies. Epilepsia 2003; 44(Suppl 2):2. [PMID: 12752455]

12

Intracranial Aneurysms & Subarachnoid Hemorrhage

- **Essentials of Diagnosis**
  - Synonymous with berry aneurysm
  - Asymptomatic until expansion or rupture; sometimes preceded by abrupt onset of headaches that resolve (sentinel leaks)
  - Rupture characterized by sudden, severe headache, altered mental status, photophobia, nuchal rigidity, and vomiting
  - Focal neurologic signs unusual except for third nerve palsy with posterior communicating artery aneurysm
  - Multiple in 20% of cases; associated with polycystic renal disease, coarctation of aorta, fibromuscular dysplasia
  - CT scan or bloody cerebrospinal fluid confirmatory; MRI or MRA may reveal aneurysm; cerebral angiography indicates size, location, and number

- **Differential Diagnosis**
  - Primary or metastatic intracranial tumor
  - Hypertensive intraparenchymal hemorrhage
  - Ruptured arteriovenous malformation
  - Tension headache
  - Migraine headache
  - Meningitis

- **Treatment**
  - Nimodipine (calcium channel blocker) may reduce neurologic deficits
  - Induced hypertension and intracranial angioplasty may be useful for treating vasospasm, which often accompanies subarachnoid hemorrhage
  - Definitive therapy with surgical clipping or endovascular coil embolization of aneurysm if anatomy suitable and if patient's functional status is otherwise acceptable
  - Monitor electrolytes, especially sodium, closely
  - Small unruptured aneurysms may not require treatment

- **Pearl**

When a patient complains of "the worst headache of my life," it's a ruptured berry aneurysm until proven otherwise.

Reference

van Gijn J, Rinkel GJ: Subarachnoid haemorrhage: diagnosis, causes and management. Brain 2001;124(Pt 2):249. [PMID: 11157554]

Ischemic & Hemorrhagic Stroke

- **Essentials of Diagnosis**
  - May have history of atherosclerotic heart disease, hypertension, diabetes, valvular heart disease, or atrial fibrillation
  - Sudden onset of neurologic complaint, variably including focal weakness, sensory abnormalities, visual change, language defect, or altered mentation
  - Neurologic signs dependent on vessels involved: hemiplegia, hemianopia, and aphasia in anterior circulatory involvement; cranial nerve abnormalities, quadriplegia, cerebellar findings in posterior circulatory disease; hyperreflexia in both, but may be delayed
  - Deficits persist > 24 hours; if resolution in < 24 hours, transient ischemic attack or other process is present
  - CT of the head may be normal in the first 24 hours, depending on cause; hemorrhage visible immediately; MRI a superior imaging modality, especially in posterior fossa

- **Differential Diagnosis**
  - Primary or metastatic brain tumor
  - Subdural or epidural hematoma
  - Brain abscess
  - Multiple sclerosis
  - Any metabolic abnormality, especially hypoglycemia
  - Neurosyphilis
  - Seizure (and postictal state)
  - Migraine
  - Subarachnoid hemorrhage

- **Treatment**
  - Control of contributing factors, especially hypertension and hypercholesterolemia
  - Tissue plasminogen activator (t-PA) for selected patients with ischemic stroke who can be treated within 3 hours after onset
  - Anticoagulation for stroke due to known cardiac embolus
  - Aspirin, clopidogrel, or the combination dipyridamole and aspirin for thrombotic stroke
  - Carotid endarterectomy may be considered later in selected patients

- **Pearl**

A stroke is never a stroke until it's had 50 of D50.

Reference

Warlow C, Sudlow C, Dennis M, Wardlaw J, Sandercock P: Stroke. Lancet 2003;362:1211. [PMID: 14568745]

Migraine Headache

- **Essentials of Diagnosis**
  - Onset in adolescence or early adulthood
  - May be triggered by stress, foods (chocolate, red wine), birth control pills
  - Classic pattern: Unilateral throbbing pain, with prodrome including nausea, photophobia, scotomas
  - Basilar artery variant: Brainstem and cerebellar findings followed by occipital headache
  - Ophthalmic variant: Painless loss of vision, scotomas, usually unilateral

- **Differential Diagnosis**
  - Tension headache
  - Cluster headache
  - Giant cell arteritis
  - Subarachnoid hemorrhage
  - Mass lesion, eg, tumor or abscess
  - Meningitis
  - Increased intracranial pressure of other cause

- **Treatment**
  - Avoidance of precipitating factors
  - Acute treatment: Triptans, ergotamine with caffeine; analgesics (preferably at onset of prodrome)
  - Maintenance therapy includes NSAIDs, propranolol, amitriptyline, ergotamine, valproic acid

- **Pearl**

Interesting etymology: hemi *(mi)* cranium *(graine), a linguistic corruption here indicating the unilaterality of the process.*

Reference

Silberstein SD: Migraine. Lancet 2004;363:381. [PMID: 15070571]

Multiple Sclerosis

- ■ Essentials of Diagnosis
  - • Patient usually under 50 years of age at onset
  - • Episodic symptoms that may include sensory abnormalities, blurred vision due to optic neuritis, urinary sphincter disturbances, and weakness with or without spasticity
  - • Neurologic progression to fixed abnormalities occurs variably
  - • Classically, two clinical deficits separated by time and space with supportive imaging and laboratory data; however, one clinical event with characteristic brain MRI highly suggestive
  - • Multiple foci in white matter best demonstrated radiographically by MRI
  - • Finding of oligoclonal bands or elevated Ig index on lumbar puncture is nonspecific

- ■ Differential Diagnosis
  - • Vasculitis or systemic lupus erythematosus
  - • Small-vessel infarctions
  - • Neurosyphilis, Lyme disease, HIV-related illness, HTLV
  - • Optic neuritis due to other causes
  - • Primary or metastatic central nervous system neoplasm
  - • Cerebellar ataxia due to other causes
  - • Pernicious anemia
  - • Spinal cord compression or radiculopathy due to mechanical compression
  - • Syringomyelia

- ■ Treatment
  - • Beta-interferon reduces exacerbation rate; copolymer 1 (a random polymer-simulating myelin basic protein) may also be beneficial
  - • Steroids may hasten recovery from relapse, though do not change long-term disability
  - • Treatment with other immunosuppressants may be effective, but role is controversial
  - • Symptomatic treatment of spasticity and bladder dysfunction

- ■ Pearl

If you first diagnose multiple sclerosis in a patient over age 50, diagnose something else.

Reference

Hawker K, Frohman E: Multiple sclerosis. Prim Care 2004;31:201. [PMID: 15110166]

Myasthenia Gravis

- ■ Essentials of Diagnosis
  - • Symptoms due to a variable degree of block of neuromuscular transmission
  - • Fluctuating weakness of most-commonly used muscles; diplopia, dysphagia, ptosis, facial weakness with chewing and speaking
  - • Short-acting anticholinesterases transiently increase strength
  - • Electromyography and nerve conduction studies demonstrate decremental muscle response to repeated stimuli
  - • Associations include thymic tumors, thyrotoxicosis, rheumatoid arthritis, and SLE
  - • Elevated acetylcholine receptor antibody assay confirmatory but not completely sensitive

- ■ Differential Diagnosis
  - • Botulism
  - • Lambert-Eaton syndrome
  - • Polyneuropathy due to other causes
  - • Amyotrophic lateral sclerosis
  - • Bulbar poliomyelitis
  - • Neuromuscular blocking drug toxicity (aminoglycosides)
  - • Primary myopathy, eg, polymyositis

12

- ■ Treatment
  - • Anticholinesterase drugs—particularly pyridostigmine—may be effective
  - • Consider thymectomy in an otherwise healthy patient under age 60 if weakness not restricted to extraocular muscles
  - • Corticosteroids and immunosuppressants if response to above measures not ideal
  - • Plasmapheresis or intravenous immunoglobulin therapy provides short-term benefit in selected patients
  - • Avoid aminoglycosides
  - • Many other medications may lead to exacerbations

- ■ Pearl

Given the day-to-day variability of symptoms, many patients are labeled with a psychiatric diagnosis before myasthenia gravis is considered, let alone diagnosed.

Reference

Keesey JC: Clinical evaluation and management of myasthenia gravis. Muscle Nerve 2004;29:484. [PMID: 15052614]

Normal Pressure Hydrocephalus

- **Essentials of Diagnosis**
  - Subacute loss of higher cognitive function
  - Urinary incontinence
  - Gait apraxia
  - In some, history of head trauma or meningitis
  - Normal opening pressure on lumbar puncture
  - Enlarged ventricles without atrophy by CT or MRI

- **Differential Diagnosis**
  - Dementia or incontinence due to other cause
  - Parkinson's disease
  - Alcoholic cerebellar degeneration
  - Wernicke-Korsakoff syndrome
  - Encephalitis

- **Treatment**
  - Lumbar puncture provides temporary amelioration of symptoms
  - Ventriculoperitoneal shunting, most effective when precipitating event is identified and recent; gait is most likely symptom to improve

- **Pearl**

12

An apraxic gait differs from an ataxic gait—the former is magnetic, as though the floor were a magnet and the patient had shoes with metal soles.

Reference

Vanneste JA: Diagnosis and management of normal-pressure hydrocephalus. J Neurol 2000;247:5. [PMID: 10701891]

Parkinson's Disease

- **Essentials of Diagnosis**
  - Insidious onset in older patient of pill-rolling tremor (3–5/s), rigidity, bradykinesia, and progressive postural instability; tremor is the least disabling feature
  - Masklike facies, cogwheeling of extremities on passive motion; cutaneous seborrhea characteristic
  - Absence of tremor—not uncommon—may delay diagnosis
  - Reflexes normal
  - Mild intellectual deterioration often noted, but concurrent Alzheimer's disease may account for this in many

- **Differential Diagnosis**
  - Essential tremor
  - Phenothiazine, metoclopramide toxicity; also carbon monoxide, manganese poisoning
  - Hypothyroidism
  - Wilson's disease
  - Multiple system atrophy, progressive supranuclear palsy
  - Diffuse Lewy body disease
  - Depression
  - Normal pressure hydrocephalus

12

- **Treatment**
  - Carbidopa-levodopa is most effective medical regimen in patients with definite disability; dose should be reduced if dystonias occur
  - Dopamine agonists and bromocriptine may be of value as first-line therapy or in permitting reduction of carbidopa-levodopa dose
  - Anticholinergic drugs and amantadine are useful adjuncts
  - Inhibition of monoamine oxidase B with selegiline (L-deprenyl) offers theoretical advantage of preventing progression, but not yet established for this indication
  - Selected patients refractory to medications with good cognitive function, deep brain stimulators (in globus pallidus or subthalamic nucleus) useful

- **Pearl**

Autonomic abnormalities early in the course of a parkinsonian syndrome mean the diagnosis is not Parkinson's disease.

Reference

Samii A, Nutt JG, Ransom BR: Parkinson's disease. Lancet 2004;363:1783. [PMID: 15172778]

Periodic Paralysis Syndromes

- **Essentials of Diagnosis**

  - Episodes of flaccid weakness or paralysis with strength normal between attacks
  - Hypokalemic variety: Infrequent, prolonged, severe attacks; usually upon awakening, after exercise or after carbohydrate meals; familial and metabolic etiologies including hyperthyroidism especially in Asian men, chronic potassium wasting from medications, gastrointestinal or renal causes
  - Hyperkalemic or normokalemic variety: Frequent, short-duration, less severe attacks often after exercise; familial forms recognized; cause of nonfamilial forms less well known

- **Differential Diagnosis**

  - Myasthenia gravis
  - Polyneuropathies due to other causes, especially Guillain-Barré syndrome
  - Seizure
  - Myopathy

- **Treatment**

  - Hypokalemic variant: Potassium replacement for acute episode; low-carbohydrate, low-salt diet chronically, acetazolamide prophylactically; treatment of hyperthyroidism, when associated, reduces attacks, as does therapy with beta-blockers
  - Hyperkalemic-normokalemic variant: Intravenous calcium, intravenous diuretics useful for acute therapy; prophylactic acetazolamide or thiazides also beneficial

12

- **Pearl**

Despite dramatically lowered serum potassium during attacks of the hypokalemic variant, the level normalizes easily and often before therapy is begun.

Reference

Gutmann L: Periodic paralyses. Neurol Clin 2000;18:195. [PMID: 10658175]

Peripheral Neuropathy

- **Essentials of Diagnosis**
  - Polyneuropathies: Distal, symmetric (often subacute, slowly progressive) abnormalities of sensation, strength, or both usually secondary to metabolic, toxic, or inherited disorders
  - Mononeuropathies: Dysfunction of a single nerve (eg, carpal tunnel syndrome) usually secondary to focal nerve compression or stretch
  - Mononeuritis multiplex: Multiple individual nerves affected asymmetrically either at the same time or stepwise, usually secondary to inflammatory disorders
  - Causes of polyneuropathies: Diabetes mellitus (30%), alcohol (30%), idiopathic (30%), medication-related (especially chemotherapy agents), thyroid disease, syphilis, HIV-related, heavy metals and other toxins, vitamin B_{12} deficiency, amyloidosis, liver disease, renal disease, vasculitis and other rheumatologic disorders, sarcoidosis, inherited disorders such as Charcot-Marie-Tooth disease and chronic inflammatory demyelinating polyneuropathy

- **Differential Diagnosis**
  - Central nervous system process such as stroke or multiple sclerosis
  - Polyradiculopathy
  - Vascular insufficiency
  - Musculoskeletal disorder

- **Treatment**
  - Treat underlying cause if known, eg, stop alcohol or replace vitamin B_{12}
  - Treat pain with tricyclic antidepressants or gabapentin
  - Other anticonvulsants or topical capsaicin also may be tried
  - Consider bracing/padding and surgery for mononeuropathies (eg, carpal tunnel syndrome)

- **Pearl**

Typical distal symmetric polyneuropathies progress slowly; with rapid progression, think vasculitis, toxins, or a diagnosis other than peripheral neuropathy.

Reference

England JD, Asbury AK: Peripheral neuropathy. Lancet 2004;363:2151. [PMID: 15220040]

Pseudotumor Cerebri
(Benign Intracranial Hypertension)

- ■ Essentials of Diagnosis
  - • Headache, diplopia, nausea
  - • Papilledema, sixth nerve palsy
  - • Brain MRI brain and MR venogram normal except for small ventricles
  - • Lumbar puncture with elevated pressure but normal cerebrospinal fluid
  - • Associations include endocrinopathy (hypoparathyroidism, Addison's disease), hypervitaminosis A, drugs (tetracyclines, oral contraceptives), chronic pulmonary disease, obesity; often idiopathic
  - • Untreated pseudotumor cerebri may lead to secondary optic atrophy and permanent visual loss

- ■ Differential Diagnosis
  - • Venous sinus thrombosis
  - • Primary or metastatic tumor
  - • Optic neuritis
  - • Neurosyphilis
  - • Brain abscess or basilar meningitis
  - • Chronic meningitis (eg, coccidioidomycosis or cryptococcosis)
  - • Vascular headache, migraine headache

12

- ■ Treatment
  - • Treat underlying cause if present
  - • Acetazolamide or furosemide to reduce cerebrospinal fluid formation
  - • Repeat lumbar puncture with removal of cerebrospinal fluid
  - • Oral corticosteroids may be helpful; weight loss in obese patients
  - • Monitor visual fields and visual acuity closely
  - • Surgical therapy with placement of ventriculoperitoneal shunt or optic nerve sheath fenestration in refractory cases

- ■ Pearl

Pseudotumor may not be "pseudo" in women—mammography may indicate a primary breast cancer.

Reference

Brazis PW: Pseudotumor cerebri. Curr Neurol Neurosci Rep 2004;4:111. [PMID: 14984682]

Spinal Cord Compression

- ### Essential of Diagnosis
  - Weakness in legs or both arms and legs, sensory level, saddle anesthesia, hyperreflexia
  - Often early bowel/bladder dysfunction
  - Common causes: Trauma, vertebra or disc fragment, tumor, epidural abscess, epidural hematoma
  - Risk factors for cord compression in patient presenting with back pain: pain worse at rest, history of malignancy or trauma, presence of chronic infection, age > 50, pain for more than 1 month, current corticosteroid use, history of intravenous drug use, unexplained fever/weight loss, rapidly progressive neurologic deficit
  - Emergent MRI of spine diagnostic
  - Delayed diagnosis results in more severe neurologic impairment

- ### Differential Diagnosis
  - Cord contusion
  - Stroke of cord
  - Vascular malformation
  - Transverse myelitis
  - Intracranial midline anterior mass
  - Vitamin B_{12} deficiency
  - Infectious: HIV, HTLV-1 or -2, Lyme disease
  - Polyradiculopathy

- ### Treatment
  - Acute surgical decompression in cases of rapid neurologic deterioration
  - Intravenous corticosteroids; specialized protocol for acute traumatic cases
  - Chemotherapy/irradiation if tumor-associated
  - Bowel and bladder regimen

- ### Pearls

If the patient is able to walk at the time cord compression is recognized, that patient will likely walk after treatment; unfortunately, the converse is also true.

Reference

Schiff D: Spinal cord compression. Neurol Clin 2003;21:67, viii. [PMID: 12690645]

Syringomyelia

- ■ **Essentials of Diagnosis**
  - Characterized by destruction or degeneration of the gray and white matter adjacent to the central canal of the cervical spinal cord
  - Initial loss of pain and temperature sense with preservation of other sensory function; unrecognized burning or injury of hands a characteristic presentation
  - Weakness, hyporeflexia or areflexia, atrophy of muscles at level of spinal cord involvement (usually upper limbs and hands); hyperreflexia and spasticity at lower levels
  - Thoracic kyphoscoliosis common; associated with Arnold-Chiari malformation
  - Secondary to trauma in some cases, especially neck hyperextension/hyperflexion injuries
  - MRI of cervical cord confirms diagnosis

- ■ **Differential Diagnosis**
  - Spinal cord tumor or arteriovenous malformation
  - Transverse myelitis
  - Multiple sclerosis
  - Neurosyphilis
  - Degenerative arthritis of the cervical spine
  - Polyradiculopathy

- ■ **Treatment**
  - Surgical decompression of the foramen magnum
  - Syringostomy in selected cases

- ■ **Pearl**

One of the few causes of disassociation of pain and temperature from other sensory function on neurologic examination.

Reference

Levine DN: The pathogenesis of syringomyelia associated with lesions at the foramen magnum: a critical review of existing theories and proposal of a new hypothesis. J Neurol Sci 2004;220(1-2):3. [PMID: 15140600]

Tourette's Syndrome

■ **Essentials of Diagnosis**

- Motor and phonic tics; onset in childhood or adolescence
- Compulsive utterances are typical
- Hyperactivity, nonspecific electroencephalographic abnormalities in 50%
- Obsessive-compulsive disorder common

■ **Differential Diagnosis**

- Simple tic disorder
- Wilson's disease
- Focal seizures

■ **Treatment**

- Neuroleptics (eg, haloperidol) and α_2-adrenergic agonists (eg, clonidine)
- Clonazepam, phenothiazine, pimozide may also be tried
- Selective serotonin reuptake inhibitors for obsessive-compulsive symptoms

■ **Pearl**

When a child has no neurologic signs other than tics and Wilson's disease has been excluded, think Tourette's syndrome.

12

Reference

Leckman JF: Tourette's syndrome. Lancet 2002;360:1577. [PMID: 12443611]

Trigeminal Neuralgia (Tic Douloureux)

- ■ **Essentials of Diagnosis**
  - Characterized by momentary episodes of lancinating facial pain that arises from one side of the mouth and shoots toward the ipsilateral eye, ear, or nostril
  - Commonly affects women more than men in middle and later life
  - Triggered by touch, movement, and eating
  - Symptoms are confined to the distribution of the ipsilateral trigeminal nerve (almost always the second or third division)
  - Occasionally caused by multiple sclerosis or a brainstem tumor

- ■ **Differential Diagnosis**
  - Atypical facial pain syndrome
  - Glossopharyngeal neuralgia
  - Postherpetic neuralgia
  - Temporomandibular joint dysfunction
  - Angina pectoris
  - Giant cell arteritis
  - Brainstem gliosis

- ■ **Treatment**
  - Either carbamazepine or gabapentin is the drug of choice; if this is ineffective or poorly tolerated, phenytoin, valproic acid, or baclofen can be tried
  - Surgical exploration of posterior fossa successful in selected patients
  - Radiofrequency ablation useful in some

- ■ **Pearl**

The diagnosis can sometimes be made before the patient says a word: a man unshaven unilaterally in the V_2 distribution has tic douloureux until proven otherwise.

Reference

Rozen TD: Trigeminal neuralgia and glossopharyngeal neuralgia. Neurol Clin 2004;22:185. [PMID: 15062534]

13

Geriatric Disorders

Constipation

- **Essentials of Diagnosis**
  - Infrequent stools (less than three times a week)
  - Straining with defecation more than 25% of the time

- **Differential Diagnosis**
  - Normal bowel function that does not match patient expectations of bowel function
  - Anorectal dysfunction
  - Slow bowel transit
  - Dietary factors, including low-calorie diet
  - Obstructing cancer
  - Metabolic disorder, such as hypercalcemia
  - Medications (opioids, iron, calcium channel blockers)

- **Treatment**
  - In absence of pathology, increase fiber and liquid intake
  - In presence of slow transit constipation, stool softeners such as docusate, osmotically active agents such as sorbitol and lactulose
  - In refractory cases or with opioid use, stimulant laxatives (eg, senna) may be necessary
  - In presence of anorectal dysfunction, suppositories often necessary

- **Pearl**

One patient's constipation is another's diarrhea.

Reference

Lembo A, Camilleri M: Chronic constipation. N Engl J Med 2003;349:1360. [PMID: 14523145]

Decubitus Ulcers (Pressure Sores)

- ■ Essentials of Diagnosis
  - Ulcers over bony or cartilaginous prominences (sacrum, hips, heels)
  - Stage I (nonblanchable erythema of intact skin); stage II (partial thickness skin loss involving the epidermis or dermis); stage III (full-thickness skin loss extending to the deep fascia); stage IV (full-thickness skin loss involving muscle or bone)
  - Risk factors: immobility, incontinence, malnutrition, cognitive impairment, older age, impaired sensory perception

- ■ Differential Diagnosis
  - Herpes simplex virus ulcers
  - Venous insufficiency ulcers
  - Underlying osteomyelitis
  - Ulcerated skin cancer
  - Pyoderma gangrenosum

- ■ Treatment
  - Reduce pressure (reposition patient every 2 hours, use specialized mattress)
  - Treat underlying conditions that may prevent wound healing (infection, malnutrition, poor functional status, incontinence, comorbid illnesses)
  - Control pain
  - Select dressing to keep the wound moist and the surrounding tissue intact (hydrocolloids, silver sulfadiazine, or, if heavy exudate, calcium alginate or foams)
  - Perform debridement if necrotic tissue present (wet-to-dry dressings, sharp debridement with scalpel, collagenase, or moisture-retentive dressings)
  - Surgical procedures may be necessary to treat extensive pressure ulcers

13

- ■ Pearl

There is no "early" decubitus; pathogenesis begins from within, and skin loss is the last part of the process.

Reference

Thomas DR: Issues and dilemmas in the prevention and treatment of pressure ulcers: a review. J Gerontol A Biol Sci Med Sci 2001;56:M328.

Delirium

- **Essentials of Diagnosis**
  - Rapid onset of acute confusional state, usually lasting less than 1 week
  - Fluctuating mental status with marked deficit of short-term memory
  - Inability to concentrate, maintain attention, or sustain purposeful behavior
  - Increased anxiety and irritability or withdrawal
  - Risk factors include dementia, organic brain lesion, alcohol dependence, medications, and various medical problems
  - Mild to moderate delirium at night, often precipitated by hospitalization, drugs, or sensory deprivation ("sundowning")

- **Differential Diagnosis**
  - Depression or other psychiatric disorder
  - Alcohol or benzodiazepine withdrawal
  - Medication side effect
  - Subclinical status epilepticus
  - Pain

- **Treatment**
  - Identify and treat underlying cause
  - Manage pain; undertreatment or overtreatment of pain may contribute to delirium
  - Promote restful sleep; keep patient up and interactive during day
  - Frequent reorientation by staff, family, clocks, calendars
  - When medication needed, low-dose haloperidol or atypical antipsychotic; avoid benzodiazepines except in alcohol and benzodiazepine withdrawal
  - Avoid potentially offending medications, particularly anticholinergic and psychoactive medications
  - Avoid restraints, lines, and tubes

- **Pearl**

Delirium tremens is the most flagrant example of delirium, but the least common clinical expression.

Reference

Gleason OC: Delirium Am Fam Physician 2003;67:1027. Review. [PMID: 12643363]

13

Dementia

- **Essentials of Diagnosis**
  - Persistent and progressive impairment in intellectual function, including loss of short-term memory, word-finding difficulties, apraxia (inability to perform previously learned tasks), agnosia (inability to recognize objects), and visuospatial problems (becoming lost in familiar surroundings)
  - Impaired function
  - Behavioral disturbances, psychiatric symptoms common
  - Alzheimer's disease accounts for roughly two-thirds of cases; vascular dementia second most common; other causes include Lewy body and frontotemporal dementia

- **Differential Diagnosis**
  - Normal age-related cognitive changes or drug effects
  - Depression or other psychiatric disorder
  - Delirium
  - Metabolic disorder (eg, hypercalcemia, hyper- and hypothyroidism, or vitamin B_{12} deficiency)
  - Sensory impairment
  - Parkinson's disease

- **Treatment**
  - Correct sensory deficits, treat underlying disease, remove offending medications, and treat depression, when present
  - Caregiver education, referral to Alzheimer's Association, advanced care planning early
  - Consider anticholinesterase inhibitors (eg, donepezil) in Alzheimer's type dementia, vascular dementia, or dementia with Lewy bodies
  - Consider memantine in more advanced Alzheimer's type dementia
  - Treat behavioral problems (eg, agitation) with behavioral interventions or medications directed against target symptom
  - Late dementia can benefit from a hospice-type approach

13

- **Pearl**

In the demented patient, the real differential should be: reversible, reversible, reversible.

Reference

Casselli RJ: Current issues in the diagnosis and management of dementia. Semin Neurol 2003;23:231. Review. [PMID: 14722819]

Falls

- ■ **Essentials of Diagnosis**
  - • Frequently not mentioned to physicians
  - • Evidence of trauma or fractures, but this may be subtle, especially in the hip
  - • Decreased activity, social isolation
  - • Fear of falling
  - • Functional decline

- ■ **Differential Diagnosis**
  - • Visual impairment
  - • Gait impairment due to muscular weakness, podiatric disorder, or neurologic dysfunction
  - • Environmental hazards such as poor lighting, stairways, rugs, warped floors
  - • Polypharmacy (especially with use of sedative-hypnotics)
  - • Postural hypotension, particularly postprandial hypotension
  - • Presyncope, vertigo, dysequilibrium, and syncope

- ■ **Treatment**
  - • Review need for and encourage proper use of assistive devices (eg, cane, walker)
  - • Evaluate and treat for osteoporosis
  - • Evaluate vision
  - • Review medications
  - • Assess home and environmental safety and prescribe modifications as indicated

- ■ **Pearl**

The occasional older person crawls into bed after a fall causing a hip fracture and stays there, and presents with altered mental status only; look for shortening and external rotation of the hips in all older patients with new-onset dementia.

Reference

Tinetti M: Clinical practice. Preventing falls in elderly persons. N Engl J Med 2003;348:42. [PMID: 12510042]

Hearing Impairment

- **Essentials of Diagnosis**
  - Difficulty understanding speech, difficulty listening to television or talking on the telephone, tinnitus, hearing loss limiting personal or social life
  - "Whisper test": patient is unable to repeat numbers whispered in each ear
  - Hearing loss on formal audiologic evaluation (pure tone audiometry, speech reception threshold, bone conduction testing, acoustic reflexes, and tympanometry); hearing loss of > 40 dB will cause difficulty understanding normal speech

- **Differential Diagnosis**
  - Sensorineural hearing loss (presbyacusis, ototoxicity due to medications, tumors or infections of cranial nerve VIII, injury by vascular events)
  - Conductive hearing loss (cerumen impaction, otosclerosis, chronic otitis media, Meniere's disease, trauma, tumors)

- **Treatment**
  - Cerumen removal if impaction present (carbamide peroxide drops, gentle irrigation with warm water)
  - Consider assistive listening devices (telephone amplifiers, low-frequency doorbells, closed-captioned television decoders) and hearing aids
  - Patients with sudden or asymmetric hearing loss should be referred to a specialist for further evaluation
  - Educate family to speak slowly and to face the patient directly when speaking

- **Pearl**

Impaired hearing and vision is devastating to the older patient, leading to the misdiagnosis of dementia.

Reference

Bogardus ST et al: Screening and management of adult hearing loss in primary care: clinical applications. JAMA 2003;15:1986.

Insomnia

- **Essentials of Diagnosis**
  - Difficulty in initiating or maintaining sleep, or nonrestorative sleep that causes impairment of social or occupational functioning
  - For acute insomnia (< 3 weeks), presence of recent life stress or new medications
  - May be related to a psychiatric disorder, such as major depression or posttraumatic stress disorder

- **Differential Diagnosis**
  - Psychiatric illness (depression, anxiety, mania, psychoses, stress, panic attacks)
  - Drug effect (caffeine, theophylline, selective serotonin reuptake inhibitors, diuretics, others); withdrawal from sedative-hypnotic medications or alcohol
  - Comorbid disease causing chronic pain, dyspnea, urinary frequency, reflux esophagitis, or delirium
  - Akathisia or restless legs
  - Noisy environment, excessive daytime napping
  - Disordered circadian rhythms (jet lag, shift work, dementia)

- **Treatment**
  - Treat underlying cause of insomnia by removing or modifying mitigating factors
  - Maintain good sleep hygiene (avoid stimulants, minimize noise, keep regular sleep schedule, avoid daytime naps, exercise regularly)
  - Refer for polysomnography if a primary sleep disorder, such as sleep apnea, is suspected
  - Consider short-term (< 4 weeks) intermittent use of trazodone or a sedative-hypnotic (eg, zolpidem or a benzodiazepine with a short half-life)
  - Diphenhydramine best avoided because of its anticholinergic side effects

- **Pearl**

Many over-the-counter medications, sodas, and foods contain caffeine, a common contributor to sleep problems in older adults.

Reference

Ancoli-Israel S: Sleep disorders in older adults: a primary care guide to assessing 4 common sleep problems in geriatric patients. Geriatrics 2004;59:37.

Polypharmacy

■ Essentials of Diagnosis

- Risk factors: Older age, cognitive impairment, taking five or more medications, multiple prescribing physicians, and recent discharge from a hospital
- A medical regimen that includes unnecessary or inappropriate medications, such that the likelihood of adverse effects (from the number or type of medications) exceeds the likelihood of benefit
- Medications used to prevent illness without improving symptoms have increasingly marginal risk-benefit profiles in patients with limited life expectancies
- Over-the-counter drugs and vitamin supplements often added on by patient without physician's awareness

■ Differential Diagnosis

- Appropriate use of multiple medications to treat older adults for multiple comorbid conditions

■ Treatment

- Regularly review all medications, instructions, and indications
- Keep dosing regimens as simple as possible
- Avoid managing an adverse drug reaction with another drug
- Select medications that can treat more than one problem
- Consider if benefit of adding a medication justifies the increase in complexity of the regimen and risk of side effects

13

■ Pearl

For any new symptom in an older patient, a medication side effect or drug-drug interaction is the simplest—and most overlooked—cause.

Reference

Beyth RJ, Shorr RI: Principles of drug therapy in older patients: rational drug prescribing. Clin Geriatr Med 2002;18:577.

Weight Loss (Involuntary)

- **Essentials of Diagnosis**
    - Weight loss exceeding 5% in 1 month or 10% in 6 months
    - Weight should be measured regularly and compared with previous measures and normative data for age and gender
    - The cause of weight loss is usually diagnosed by history and physical examination
    - Most useful tests for further evaluation: Chest x-ray, complete blood count, serum chemistries (including glucose, thyroid-stimulating hormone, creatinine, calcium, liver function tests, albumin), urinalysis, and fecal occult blood testing

- **Differential Diagnosis**
    - Medical disorders (congestive heart failure, chronic lung disease, chronic renal failure, peptic ulcers, dementia, ill-fitting dentures, dysphagia, malignancy, diabetes mellitus, hyperthyroidism, malabsorption, systemic infections, hospitalization)
    - Social problems (poverty, isolation, inability to shop or prepare food, alcoholism, abuse and neglect, poor knowledge of nutrition, food restrictions)
    - Psychiatric disorders (depression, schizophrenia, bereavement, anorexia nervosa, bulimia)
    - Drug effects (selective serotonin reuptake inhibitors, NSAIDs, digoxin, antibiotics, acetylcholinesterase inhibitors)

13

- **Treatment**
    - Directed at underlying cause of weight loss, which is usually multifactorial
    - Frequent meals, hand-feed, protein-calorie supplements, multivitamins, enhance food flavor
    - Among patients with psychosocial causes of malnutrition, referral to community services such as senior centers
    - "Watchful waiting" when cause is unknown after basic evaluation (25% of cases)
    - Consider enteral tube feedings if treatment would improve quality of life, remembering the importance of identifying goals of care before instituting feedings

- **Pearl**

Pay attention to the definition; many older patients have gradual weight loss over many years, and aggressive evaluation may be harmful.

Reference

Huffman GB: Evaluating and treating unintentional weight loss in the elderly. Am Fam Physician 2002;65:640.

14

Psychiatric Disorders

Alcohol Dependence

- **Essentials of Diagnosis**
  - Intoxication: Mood lability, impaired judgment, somnolence, slurred speech, ataxia, attention or memory deficits, coma
  - Symptoms of withdrawal when intake is interrupted
  - Tolerance to the effects of alcohol
  - Presence of alcohol-associated medical illnesses (eg, liver disease, neuropathy, cerebellar ataxia, pancreatitis)
  - Recurrent use resulting in multiple legal problems, hazardous situations, or failure to fulfill role obligations
  - Continued drinking despite strong medical and social contraindications and life disruptions
  - High comorbidity with depression

- **Differential Diagnosis**
  - Alcohol use secondary to psychiatric illness
  - Other sedative-hypnotic dependence or intoxication
  - Withdrawal from other substances (eg, cocaine, amphetamine)
  - Pathophysiologic disturbance such as hypoxia, hypoglycemia, stroke, central nervous system infection or neoplasm, or subdural hematoma

- **Treatment**
  - Total abstinence, not "controlled drinking," should be the goal
  - Substance abuse counseling and groups (eg, Alcoholics Anonymous)
  - Disulfiram in selected patients; naltrexone may also be of benefit, in conjunction with substance abuse counseling
  - Treat underlying depression if present

- **Pearl**

Healed rib fractures without a history of trauma suggests chronic alcoholism absent other disorders.

Reference

Maisto SA, Saitz R: Alcohol use disorders: screening and diagnosis. Am J Addict 2003;12(Suppl 1):S12. [PMID: 14972777]

Alcohol Withdrawal

- **Essentials of Diagnosis**
  - Symptoms when patient with dependence abruptly stops drinking
  - Tremor, wakefulness, psychomotor agitation, anxiety, seizures, hallucinations or delusions
  - Severe withdrawal: Disorientation, frightening visual hallucinations, marked autonomic hyperactivity (delirium tremens)

- **Differential Diagnosis**
  - Delirium secondary to other medical illness (eg, infection, hypoglycemia, hepatic disease)
  - Withdrawal from other sedative-hypnotics (eg, benzodiazepines) or opioids
  - Substance intoxication (eg, cocaine, amphetamine)
  - Anxiety disorders
  - Manic episode
  - Psychotic disorders
  - Seizure disorder

- **Treatment**
  - Benzodiazepines, with target of keeping vital signs normal
  - Haloperidol if hallucinations or delusions are present
  - Folic acid, multivitamins, and parenteral thiamin
  - Encourage hydration

- **Pearl**

The longer the period between discontinuation of alcohol and the appearance of symptoms, the worse the delirium tremens.

14

Reference

Kosten TR, O'Connor PG: Management of drug and alcohol withdrawal. N Engl J Med 2003;348:1786. [PMID: 12724485]

Bipolar Disorder

- **Essentials of Diagnosis**
  - History of manic episode: Grandiosity, decreased need for sleep, pressured speech, racing thoughts, distractibility, increased activity, excessive spending or hypersexuality
  - A single manic episode establishes the diagnosis
  - Depressive episodes may alternate with periods of mania
  - Manic episode may have psychotic component

- **Differential Diagnosis**
  - Substance intoxication and/or withdrawal (eg, cocaine, amphetamine, alcohol)
  - Medication use (eg, steroids, thyroxine, methylphenidate)
  - Infectious disease (eg, neurosyphilis, complications of HIV infection)
  - Endocrinopathies (eg, hyperthyroidism, Cushing's syndrome)
  - Central nervous system neoplasm
  - Complex partial seizures
  - Personality disorders (eg, borderline, narcissistic)

- **Treatment**
  - Mood stabilizer: Lithium, valproic acid, carbamazepine
  - Antipsychotic medication (eg, olanzapine, quetiapine) for acute mania or psychotic component
  - Lamotrigine useful for bipolar depression
  - Psychotherapy may be helpful once acute mania is controlled

- **Pearl**

14

Inexperienced clinicians seeing their first manic patient commonly diagnose hyperthyroidism.

Reference

Belmaker RH: Bipolar disorder. N Engl J Med 2004;351:476. [PMID: 15282355]

Eating Disorders

- **Essentials of Diagnosis**
  - Severe abnormalities in eating behavior
  - Includes anorexia nervosa and bulimia nervosa
  - Disturbance in perception of body shape or weight
  - Anorexia: Refusal to maintain a minimally normal body weight
  - Bulimia: Repeated binge eating, followed by compensatory behavior to prevent weight gain (eg, vomiting, use of laxatives, excessive exercise, fasting)
  - Medical sequelae include gastrointestinal disturbances, electrolyte imbalance, cardiovascular abnormalities, amenorrhea or oligomenorrhea, caries or periodontitis

- **Differential Diagnosis**
  - Major depressive disorder
  - Body dysmorphic disorder: Excessive preoccupation with an imagined defect in appearance
  - Obsessive-compulsive disorder
  - Weight loss secondary to medical illness (eg, neoplasm, gastrointestinal disease, hyperthyroidism, diabetes)

- **Treatment**
  - Psychotherapy (eg, cognitive-behavioral, interpersonal)
  - Family therapy, particularly for adolescent patients
  - Selective serotonin reuptake inhibitors (eg, fluoxetine) may be of benefit, particularly for bulimic patients
  - Medical management of associated physical sequelae
  - Consider inpatient or partial hospitalization for severe cases

14

- **Pearl**

If bulimia is suspected, examine the knuckles, teeth, and perioral skin for signs of self-induced vomiting.

Reference

Fairburn CG, Harrison PJ: Eating disorders. Lancet 2003;361:407. [PMID: 12573387]

Factitious Disorder

- **Essentials of Diagnosis**
  - Also known as Munchausen's syndrome
  - Intentional production or feigning of symptoms
  - Motivation for symptoms is unconscious, to assume the sick role
  - External incentives for symptom production are absent
  - Patient may produce symptoms in another person in order to indirectly assume the sick role (Munchausen's by proxy)
  - High correlation with personality disorders

- **Differential Diagnosis**
  - Somatoform disorders
  - Malingering
  - Organic disease producing symptoms

- **Treatment**
  - Gentle confrontation regarding diagnosis
  - Emphasis on patient's strengths
  - Empathy with patient's long history of suffering
  - Attention to building therapeutic relationship between patient and a single primary provider
  - Psychotherapy; seldom decisive
  - Many with less severe forms eventually stop or decrease self-destructive behaviors upon confrontation

- **Pearl**

When an obscure disorder eluding diagnosis develops in a patient with recent training or studies in the medical field, a factitious etiology is high on the list, if not at the top.

14

Reference

Wise MG, Ford CV: Factitious disorders. Prim Care 1999;26:315. [PMID: 10318750]

Generalized Anxiety Disorder

- **Essentials of Diagnosis**
  - Excessive, persistent worry about numerous things
  - Worry is difficult to control
  - Physiologic symptoms of restlessness, fatigue, irritability, muscle tension, sleep disturbance

- **Differential Diagnosis**
  - Endocrinopathies (eg, hyperthyroidism)
  - Pheochromocytoma
  - Medication or substance use (eg, caffeine, nicotine, amphetamine, pseudoephedrine)
  - Medication or substance withdrawal (eg, alcohol, benzodiazepines)
  - Major depressive disorder
  - Adjustment disorder
  - Other anxiety disorders (eg, obsessive-compulsive disorder)
  - Somatoform disorders
  - Personality disorders (eg, avoidant, dependent, obsessive-compulsive)

- **Treatment**
  - Psychotherapy, especially cognitive-behavioral
  - Relaxation techniques (eg, biofeedback)
  - Buspirone, paroxetine, extended-release venlafaxine, benzodiazepines

14

- **Pearl**

In patients with anxiety and depression, treat the depression first.

Reference

Fricchione G: Generalized anxiety disorder. N Engl J Med 2004;351:675. [PMID: 15306669]

Major Depressive Disorder

- ■ Essentials of Diagnosis
  - • Depressed mood or anhedonia (loss of interest or pleasure in usual activities), with hopelessness, intense feelings of sadness
  - • Poor concentration, thoughts of suicide, worthlessness, guilt
  - • Sleep or appetite disturbance (increased or decreased), malaise, psychomotor retardation or agitation
  - • Increased isolation and social withdrawal, decreased libido
  - • May have psychotic component (eg, self-deprecatory auditory hallucinations), or multiple somatic complaints
  - • Symptoms last longer than 2 weeks and impair functioning

- ■ Differential Diagnosis
  - • Bipolar disorder
  - • Adjustment disorder
  - • Dysthymic disorder: presence of some depressive symptoms for at least 2 years
  - • Bereavement
  - • Substance abuse or withdrawal
  - • Medication use (eg, steroids, interferon)
  - • Medical illness (eg, hypothyroidism, stroke, Parkinson's disease, neoplasm, polymyalgia rheumatica)
  - • Delirium or dementia
  - • Anxiety disorders (eg, generalized anxiety disorder, post-traumatic stress disorder)
  - • Psychotic disorders
  - • Personality disorders

14

- ■ Treatment
  - • Assess suicidal risk; specific plans indicate higher probability
  - • Antidepressant medications: selective serotonin reuptake inhibitors, tricyclic antidepressants, venlafaxine, nefazodone, bupropion, mirtazapine, monoamine oxidase inhibitors
  - • Psychotherapy (eg, cognitive-behavioral, interpersonal)
  - • Interventions to help with resocialization (eg, supportive groups, day treatment programs)
  - • Education of patient and family about depression
  - • Electroconvulsive therapy for refractory cases
  - • Antipsychotic medication if psychotic component present

- ■ Pearl

Ask about history of mania before starting an antidepressant; bipolar patients may develop a manic episode when treated with an antidepressant.

Reference

Remick RA: Diagnosis and management of depression in primary care: a clinical update and review. CMAJ 2002;167:1253. [PMID: 12451082]

Obsessive-Compulsive Disorder

- ■ Essentials of Diagnosis
  - Obsessions: Recurrent, distressing, intrusive thoughts
  - Compulsions: Repetitive behaviors (eg, hand washing, checking) that patient cannot resist performing
  - Patient recognizes obsessions and compulsions as excessive
  - Obsessions and compulsions cause distress and interfere with functioning

- ■ Differential Diagnosis
  - Psychotic disorders
  - Other anxiety disorders (eg, generalized anxiety disorder, phobia)
  - Major depressive disorder
  - Somatoform disorders
  - Obsessive-compulsive personality disorder: Lifelong pattern of preoccupation with orderliness and perfectionism but without presence of true obsessions or compulsions
  - Substance intoxication
  - Tic disorder (eg, Tourette's syndrome)

- ■ Treatment
  - Behavioral therapy (eg, exposure, response prevention)
  - Selective serotonin reuptake inhibitors or clomipramine

- ■ Pearl

Presence of insight is typical; its absence makes psychotic disorders more likely.

Reference

Jenike MA: Obsessive-compulsive disorder. N Engl J Med 2004;350:259. [PMID: 14724305]

14

Opioid Dependence & Withdrawal

- **Essentials of Diagnosis**
  - Intoxication: Mood lability, impaired judgment, psychomotor disturbance, attention or memory deficits, somnolence, slurred speech, miotic pupils, hallucinations, respiratory depression, coma
  - Physical dependence with tolerance
  - Continued use despite disruptions in social and occupational functioning
  - Withdrawal: Nausea, vomiting, abdominal cramps, lacrimation, rhinorrhea, dilated pupils, dysphoria, irritability, diaphoresis, insomnia, tachycardia, fever
  - Withdrawal uncomfortable but not life-threatening

- **Differential Diagnosis**
  - Alcohol or other sedative-hypnotic intoxication, dependence, or withdrawal
  - Intoxication by or withdrawal from other substances or medications
  - Medical abnormalities while intoxicated: Hypoxia, hypoglycemia, stroke, central nervous system infection or hemorrhage; during withdrawal, other gastrointestinal or infectious disease

- **Treatment**
  - Naloxone for suspected overdose with close medical observation
  - Methadone maintenance after withdrawal for selected patients
  - Buprenorphine may also be used for maintenance treatment
  - Clonidine may be helpful in alleviating the autonomic symptoms of withdrawal
  - Methadone may be used to treat acute withdrawal, but only under specific federal guidelines
  - Substance abuse counseling and groups (eg, Narcotics Anonymous)

- **Pearl**

Many opioids are prescribed in fixed-drug combinations with agents such as acetaminophen; be alert for relevant toxicities in overdose.

Reference

Fiellin DA, O'Connor PG: Office-based treatment of opioid-dependent patients. N Engl J Med 2002;347:817. [PMID: 12226153]

Panic Disorder

- **Essentials of Diagnosis**
  - Sudden, recurrent, unexpected panic attacks
  - Characterized by palpitations, tachycardia, sensation of dyspnea or choking, chest pain or discomfort, nausea, dizziness, diaphoresis, numbness, depersonalization
  - Sense of doom; fear of losing control or of dying
  - Persistent worry about future attacks
  - Change in behavior due to anxiety about being in places where an attack might occur (agoraphobia)

- **Differential Diagnosis**
  - Endocrinopathies (eg, hyperthyroidism)
  - Supraventricular tachycardia
  - Asthma, COPD exacerbation
  - Pheochromocytoma
  - Medication or substance use or withdrawal
  - Other anxiety disorders (eg, generalized anxiety disorder, post-traumatic stress disorder)
  - Major bipolar or depressive disorder
  - Somatoform disorders

- **Treatment**
  - Cognitive-behavioral therapy
  - Antidepressant medication (selective serotonin reuptake inhibitors, tricyclic antidepressants, monoamine oxidase inhibitors)
  - Benzodiazepines as adjunctive treatment
  - May have only a single attack; reassurance, education thus important early

14

- **Pearl**

In younger patients with multiple emergency room visits for cardiac complaints and negative evaluations, panic attack is the most common diagnosis.

Reference

Culpepper L: Identifying and treating panic disorder in primary care. J Clin Psychiatry 2004;65(Suppl 5):19. [PMID: 15078114]

Personality Disorders

- Three Types
  1. Odd, eccentric: Paranoid, schizoid, schizotypal personality disorders
  2. Dramatic: Borderline, histrionic, narcissistic, antisocial personality disorders
  3. Anxious, fearful: Avoidant, dependent, obsessive-compulsive personality disorders

- Essentials of Diagnosis
  - History dating from childhood or adolescence of recurrent maladaptive behavior
  - Minimal introspective ability
  - Major recurrent difficulties with interpersonal relationships
  - Enduring pattern of behavior stable over time, deviating markedly from cultural expectations
  - Increased risk of substance abuse

- Differential Diagnosis
  - Anxiety disorders
  - Major depressive disorder
  - Bipolar disorder
  - Psychotic disorders
  - Dissociative disorders
  - Substance use or withdrawal
  - Personality change due to medical illness (eg, central nervous system neoplasm, stroke)

14

- Treatment
  - Maintenance of a highly structured environment and clear, consistent interactions with the patient
  - Individual or group therapy (eg, cognitive-behavioral, interpersonal)
  - Antipsychotic medications may be required transiently in times of stress or decompensation
  - Serotonergic medications if depression or anxiety is prominent
  - Serotonergic medications or mood stabilizers if emotional lability is prominent

- Pearl

One of the most challenging therapeutic problems in all of medicine.

Reference

Sugarman P: Personality disorder in primary care. Practitioner 2000;244:400, 403, 407. [PMID: 10962831]

Phobic Disorders

■ Essentials of Diagnosis
- Includes specific and social phobias
- Persistent, irrational fear due to the presence or anticipation of an object or situation
- Exposure to the phobic object or situation results in excessive anxiety
- Avoidance of phobic object or situation
- Social phobia (social anxiety disorder): fear of humiliation or embarrassment in a performance or social situation (eg, speaking or eating in public)

■ Differential Diagnosis
- Other anxiety disorders (eg, generalized anxiety disorder, panic disorder, post-traumatic stress disorder)
- Psychotic disorders
- Personality disorders (eg, avoidant)

■ Treatment
- Behavioral therapy (eg, exposure)
- Hypnosis
- Benzodiazepines as necessary for anticipated situations that cannot be avoided (eg, flying)
- Beta-blockers for anticipated, circumscribed social phobia (performance anxiety)
- Paroxetine, sertraline for social phobia

14

■ Pearl

The most common anxiety disorder is the fear of public speaking.

Reference

Coupland NJ: Social phobia: etiology, neurobiology, and treatment. J Clin Psychiatry 2001;62(Suppl 1):25. [PMID: 11206031]

Psychotic Disorders

■ Essentials of Diagnosis

- Includes schizophrenia, schizoaffective and schizophreniform disorders, delusional disorder, brief psychotic disorder, and shared psychotic disorder
- Loss of ego boundaries, gross impairment in reality testing
- Prominent delusions or hallucinations
- May have flat or inappropriate affect and disorganized speech, thought processes, or behavior
- Brief psychotic disorder: Symptoms last less than 1 month, then resolve completely

■ Differential Diagnosis

- Major depressive or manic episode with psychotic features
- Medication or substance use (eg, steroids, levodopa, cocaine, amphetamines)
- Medication or substance withdrawal (eg, alcohol)
- Heavy metal toxicity
- Psychotic symptoms associated with dementia
- Delirium
- Complex partial seizures
- Central nervous system neoplasm
- Multiple sclerosis
- Systemic lupus erythematosus
- Endocrinopathies (eg, hypercalcemia, Cushing's syndrome)
- Infectious disease (eg, neurosyphilis)
- Acute intermittent porphyria
- Personality disorders (eg, paranoid, schizoid, schizotypal)

14

■ Treatment

- Antipsychotic medications: Atypical agents (risperidone, olanzapine, quetiapine, clozapine, ziprasidone, aripiprazole) less likely to cause extrapyramidal symptoms
- Attempt to stabilize living situation and provide structured environment
- Psychotherapy may be effective for brief psychotic disorder after episode resolves
- Behavioral therapy (eg, skills training)

■ Pearl

The presence of hallucinations or delusions means psychosis; whether it is organic or functional in origin is determined next.

Reference

Ferran E Jr, Barron C, Chen T: Psychosis. West J Med 2002;176:263. [PMID: 12208835]

Sexual Dysfunction

■ Essentials of Diagnosis

- Includes hypoactive sexual desire disorder, sexual aversion disorder, female sexual arousal disorder, male erectile disorder, orgasmic disorder, premature ejaculation
- Persistent disturbance in the phases of the sexual response cycle (eg, absence of desire, arousal, or orgasm)
- Causes significant distress or interpersonal difficulty
- Conditioning may cause or exacerbate dysfunction

■ Differential Diagnosis

- Underlying medical condition (eg, chronic illness, various hormone deficiencies, diabetes mellitus, hypertension, peripheral vascular disease, pelvic pathology)
- Medication (eg, selective serotonin reuptake inhibitors, numerous antihypertensives) or substance use (eg, alcohol)
- Depression

■ Treatment

- Encourage increased communication with sexual partner
- Decrease performance anxiety via sensate focus, relaxation exercises
- Sex or couples therapy, especially if life or relationship stressors are present
- Estrogen replacement in women or testosterone replacement in men if levels are low
- Erectile dysfunction in men: Consider oral medication (eg, sildenafil, vardenafil, tadalafil), alprostadil pellet or injection, vacuum device, penile implant
- Premature ejaculation: Selective serotonin reuptake inhibitors may help

14

■ Pearl

Sexual dysfunction is often undiagnosed in women; relevant inquiries should be made if there are ill-defined and poorly explained somatic symptoms.

Reference

Heiman JR: Sexual dysfunction: overview of prevalence, etiological factors, and treatments. J Sex Res 2002;39:73. [PMID: 12476261]

Somatoform Disorders (Psychosomatic Disorders)

- ■ Essentials of Diagnosis
    - Includes conversion, somatization, pain disorder with psychologic factors, hypochondriasis, and body dysmorphic disorder
    - Symptoms may involve one or more organ systems and are unintentional
    - Subjective complaints exceed objective findings
    - Symptom development may correlate with psychosocial stress, and symptoms are real to the patient

- ■ Differential Diagnosis
    - Major depressive disorder
    - Anxiety disorders (eg, generalized anxiety disorder)
    - Psychotic disorders
    - Factitious disorder
    - Malingering
    - Organic disease producing symptoms

- ■ Treatment
    - Attention to building therapeutic relationship between patient and a single primary provider
    - Acknowledgment that patient's distress is real
    - Avoidance of confrontation regarding reality of the symptoms
    - Follow-up visits at regular intervals
    - Focus on patient's level of functioning
    - Empathy regarding patient's psychosocial difficulties
    - Continued vigilance about organic disease
    - Psychotherapy, especially group cognitive-behavioral
    - Biofeedback; hypnosis

14

- ■ Pearl

Table 14-1. Somatoform disorders

| | | Symptom Production | |
		Unconscious	Conscious
Motivation	Unconscious	Somatoform disorders	Factitious disorders
	Conscious	Not applicable	Malingering

Reference

Mayou R, Farmer A: Functional somatic symptoms and syndromes. BMJ 2002;325:265. [PMID: 12153926]

Stress Disorders

- **Essentials of Diagnosis**
  - Includes acute stress disorder and post-traumatic stress disorder
  - Exposure to a traumatic event
  - Intrusive thoughts, nightmares, flashbacks
  - Mental distress or physiologic symptoms or signs (eg, tachycardia, diaphoresis) when exposed to stimuli that cue the trauma
  - Avoidance of thoughts, feelings, or situations associated with the trauma
  - Isolation, detachment from others, emotional numbness
  - Sleep disturbance, irritability, hypervigilance, startle response, poor concentration
  - Comorbid depression and substance abuse common

- **Differential Diagnosis**
  - Other anxiety disorders (eg, panic disorder, generalized anxiety disorder)
  - Major depressive disorder
  - Adjustment disorder
  - Psychotic disorders
  - Substance use or withdrawal
  - Neurologic syndrome secondary to head trauma

- **Treatment**
  - Individual and group psychotherapy
  - Cognitive-behavioral therapy
  - Antidepressant medication (selective serotonin reuptake inhibitors, tricyclic antidepressants, phenelzine)

14

- **Pearl**

Consider this diagnosis in any patient with a wide array of symptoms and a history of trauma including rape, combat, or physical or sexual abuse.

Reference

Grinage BD: Diagnosis and management of post-traumatic stress disorder. Am Fam Physician 2003;68:2401. [PMID: 14705759]

Dermatologic Disorders

Acanthosis Nigricans

- **Essentials of Diagnosis**
  - Symmetric velvety hyperpigmented plaques on axillae, groin, and neck; the face, umbilicus, inner thighs, anus, flexor surfaces of elbows and knees, and mucosal surfaces may also be affected
  - Associated with insulin-resistant states such as obesity
  - Laboratory evaluation of testosterone and dehydroepiandrosterone sulfate (DHEAS) levels in women with the type A syndrome of insulin resistance
  - Patients with the type B syndrome have acanthosis nigricans and insulin resistance secondary to anti–insulin receptor autoantibodies generated by autoimmune diseases
  - Associated with some drugs (testosterone, nicotinic acid, oral contraceptives, corticosteroids)
  - Widespread lesions or disease occurring in a nonobese patient arouse suspicion of malignant acanthosis nigricans associated with adenocarcinomas of the stomach, lung, and breast
  - Work-up for malignancy if palmar involvement present

- **Differential Diagnosis**
  - Confluent and reticulated papillomatosis (Gougerot-Carteaud syndrome)
  - Epidermal nevus
  - Dowling-Degos disease

- **Treatment**
  - Weight loss for obese patients
  - Malignant form often responds to treatment of the causal tumor

- **Pearl**

A harbinger of impending diabetes before fasting glucose levels are elevated.

Reference

Hermanns-Le T, Scheen A, Pierard GE: Acanthosis nigricans associated with insulin resistance: pathophysiology and management. Am J Clin Dermatol 2004;5:199. [PMID: 15186199]

Acne Vulgaris

- ■ Essentials of Diagnosis
  - • Often occurs at puberty, though onset may be delayed until the third or fourth decade
  - • Open and closed comedones the hallmarks
  - • Severity varies from comedonal to papular or pustular inflammatory acne to cysts or nodules
  - • Face, neck, upper chest, and back may be affected
  - • Pigmentary changes and severe scarring can occur

- ■ Differential Diagnosis
  - • Acne rosacea, perioral dermatitis, gram-negative folliculitis, tinea faciei, and pseudofolliculitis
  - • Trunk lesions may be confused with staphylococcal folliculitis, miliaria, or eosinophilic folliculitis
  - • May be induced by topical, inhaled, or systemic steroids, oily topical products, and anabolic steroids
  - • Foods neither cause nor exacerbate acne
  - • In women with resistant acne, hyperandrogenism should be considered; may be accompanied by hirsutism and irregular menses

- ■ Treatment
  - • Improvement usually requires 4–6 weeks
  - • Topical retinoids very effective for comedonal acne but usefulness limited by irritation
  - • Topical benzoyl peroxide agents
  - • Topical antibiotics (clindamycin combined with benzoyl peroxide) effective against comedones and mild inflammatory acne
  - • Oral antibiotics (tetracycline, doxycycline, minocycline) for moderate inflammatory acne; erythromycin is an alternative when tetracyclines are contraindicated
  - • Low-dose oral contraceptives containing a nonandrogenic progestin can be effective in women
  - • Diluted intralesional corticosteroids effective in reducing highly inflammatory papules and cysts
  - • Oral isotretinoin useful in some who fail antibiotic therapy; pregnancy prevention and monitoring essential
  - • Surgical and laser techniques available to treat scarring

15

- ■ Pearl

Don't waste time continuing failing therapies in scarring acne—treat aggressively to prevent further scars.

Reference

Haider A, Shaw JC: Treatment of acne vulgaris. JAMA 2004;292:726. [PMID: 15304471]

Actinic Keratosis (Solar Keratosis)

■ Essentials of Diagnosis

- Most common in fair-skinned individuals and in organ transplant recipients and other immunocompromised patients
- Discrete keratotic, scaly papules; red, pigmented, or skin-colored
- Found on the face, ears, scalp, dorsal hands, and forearms
- Induced by chronic sun exposure
- Lesions may become hypertrophic or develop a cutaneous horn
- Lower lip actinic keratosis (actinic cheilitis) presents as diffuse, slight scaling of the entire lip
- Some develop into squamous cell carcinoma

■ Differential Diagnosis

- Squamous cell carcinoma
- Bowen's disease (squamous cell carcinoma in-situ)
- Seborrheic keratosis
- Discoid lupus erythematosus

■ Treatment

- Cryotherapy standard when limited number of sites present
- Topical fluorouracil or imiquimod effective for extensive disease; usually causes a severe inflammatory reaction
- Laser therapy for severe actinic cheilitis
- Biopsy atypical lesions or those that do not respond to therapy
- Sun protection, sunscreen use

■ Pearl

In patients with facial pain, check for a history of actinic keratosis; when these lesions become carcinomas, they can invade the local sheath of the fifth cranial nerve and produce this symptom.

15

Reference

Fu W, Cockerell CJ: The actinic (solar) keratosis: a 21st-century perspective. Arch Dermatol 2003;139:66. [PMID: 12533168]

Allergic Contact Dermatitis

- ■ Essentials of Diagnosis
  - Erythema, edema, and vesicles in an area of contact with suspected agent
  - Weeping, crusting, or secondary infection may follow
  - Intense pruritus
  - Pattern of eruption may be diagnostic (eg, linear streaked vesicles in poison oak or ivy)
  - History of previous reaction to suspected contactant, though patients may be exposed to allergens for years before developing hypersensitivity
  - Patch testing usually positive
  - Common allergens include nickel, plants, neomycin, topical anesthetics, fragrances, preservatives, hair dyes, textile dyes, nail care products, adhesives, and constituents of rubber and latex products

- ■ Differential Diagnosis
  - Nonallergic (irritant) contact dermatitis
  - Scabies
  - Impetigo
  - Dermatophytid reaction
  - Atopic dermatitis
  - Seborrheic dermatitis

- ■ Treatment
  - Identify and avoid contactant
  - Topical corticosteroids for localized involvement
  - Wet compresses with aluminum acetate solutions for weeping lesions
  - Systemic corticosteroids for acute, severe cases; tapering may require 2–3 weeks to avoid rebound
  - Antihistaminic ointments should be avoided because of their sensitization potential

15

- ■ Pearl

If the agent can be aerosolized, as with Rhus *(poison oak and ivy), noncardiogenic pulmonary edema may result (eg, a campfire burning* Rhus *branches).*

Reference

Belsito DV: The diagnostic evaluation, treatment, and prevention of allergic contact dermatitis in the new millennium. J Allergy Clin Immunol 2000;105:409. [PMID: 10719287]

Alopecia Areata

- **Essentials of Diagnosis**
  - Usually occurs without associated disease, but patients with alopecia areata have an increased incidence of atopic dermatitis, Down's syndrome, lichen planus, vitiligo, autoimmune thyroiditis, and systemic lupus erythematosus
  - Rapid and complete hair loss in one or several round or oval patches
  - Occurs on the scalp or in the beard, eyebrows, or eyelashes; other hair-bearing areas less frequently affected
  - Short broken hairs on patch periphery
  - During active disease, telogen hairs near the patches easily pulled; gray hairs spared
  - The patches show preservation of follicles and normal scalp
  - Some patients have nail pitting
  - Some progress to total loss of scalp hair (alopecia totalis); a few lose all body hair (alopecia universalis)
  - Biopsy with horizontal sectioning if diagnosis unclear

- **Differential Diagnosis**
  - Tinea capitis
  - Discoid lupus erythematosus, early lesions
  - Lichen planopilaris, early lesions
  - Secondary syphilis
  - Trichotillomania
  - Metastatic or cutaneous malignancy
  - Loose anagen syndrome
  - Androgenic alopecia

- **Treatment**
  - Course is variable: Some patches regrow spontaneously, others resist therapy
  - Intralesional steroid injections for regrowth
  - Topical anthralin, corticosteroids, or minoxidil, contact sensitization with squaric acid, and psoralen plus UVA
  - Psychologic stress can be devastating; emotional support and patient education essential

15

- **Pearl**

Spontaneous recovery is common in patients with limited disease who are postpubertal at onset.

Reference

Bertolino AP: Alopecia areata. A clinical overview. Postgrad Med 2000;107:81,89. [PMID: 10887448]

Androgenetic Alopecia (Common Baldness)

- Essentials of Diagnosis
  - Genetic predisposition plus excessive androgen response
  - Men in third and fourth decades: Gradual loss of hair, chiefly from vertex and frontotemporal regions; rate variable
  - Women: Diffuse hair loss throughout the mid scalp, sparing frontal hairline
  - Appropriate laboratory work-up for women with signs of hyperandrogenism (hirsutism, acne, abnormal menses)
  - Hair pull test may show a normal or increased number of telogen hairs; hair shafts narrow but not fragile

- Differential Diagnosis
  - Telogen effluvium
  - Alopecia induced by hypothyroidism
  - Alopecia induced by iron deficiency
  - Secondary syphilis
  - Trichotillomania
  - Tinea capitis
  - Alopecia areata in evolution

- Treatment
  - Early topical minoxidil effective in most with limited disease
  - Oral finasteride prevents further loss and increases hair counts (except on the temples); contraindicated in women of childbearing potential; lacks efficacy in postmenopausal women
  - Wigs or interwoven hair for cosmetic purposes
  - Hair transplantation with minigrafts
  - Women with hyperandrogenism may respond to antiandrogen therapies

15

- Pearl

Anxious patients with this condition support an enormous market for uninvestigated—and ineffective—products.

Reference

Springer K, Brown M, Stulberg DL: Common hair loss disorders. Am Fam Physician 2003;68:93. [PMID: 12887115]

Atopic Dermatitis (Atopic Eczema)

- **Essentials of Diagnosis**
  - Pruritic, exudative, or lichenified eruption on face, neck, upper trunk, wrists, hands, antecubital and popliteal folds
  - Involves face and extensor surfaces more typically in infants
  - Personal or family history of allergies or asthma
  - Recurring; remission possible in adolescence
  - Peripheral eosinophilia, increased serum IgE—not needed for diagnosis

- **Differential Diagnosis**
  - Seborrheic dermatitis
  - Contact dermatitis
  - Scabies
  - Impetigo
  - Eczema herpeticum may be superimposed on atopic dermatitis
  - Eczematous dermatitis may be presenting feature of immunodeficiency syndromes in infants

- **Treatment**
  - Avoidance of anything that dries or irritates skin
  - Frequent emollients
  - Topical corticosteroids
  - Topical tacrolimus and pimecrolimus are effective but expensive alternatives to steroids
  - Phototherapy sometimes helpful
  - Sedative antihistamines relieve pruritus
  - Atopic patients frequently colonized with staphylococci; systemic antibiotics helpful in flares
  - Systemic steroids, cyclosporine in highly selected cases
  - Dietary restrictions may be of benefit in limited cases when specific food allergies are implicated

15

- **Pearl**

While RAST testing is useful to exclude food allergies, positive results correlate poorly with food challenges.

Reference

Leung DY, Boguniewicz M, Howell MD, Nomura I, Hamid QA: New insights into atopic dermatitis. J Clin Invest 2004;113:651. [PMID: 14991059]

Basal Cell Carcinoma

- **Essentials of Diagnosis**
    - Dome-shaped semitranslucent papule with overlying telangiectases, or a plaque of such nodules around a central depression; central area may crust or ulcerate
    - Most occur on head and neck, but the trunk and extremities also affected
    - Pigmented, cystic, sclerotic, and superficial clinical variants
    - Immunosuppressive medications increase frequency and aggressiveness; patients with albinism or xeroderma pigmentosum or exposed to radiation therapy or arsenic also at increased risk
    - Chronic, local spread typical; metastasis rare
    - Biopsy critical for diagnosis

- **Differential Diagnosis**
    - Squamous cell carcinoma
    - Actinic keratosis
    - Seborrheic keratosis
    - Paget's disease
    - Melanoma
    - Nevus
    - Psoriasis
    - Nevoid basal cell carcinoma syndrome

- **Treatment**
    - Simple excision with histologic examination of margins
    - Curettage with electrodesiccation in superficial lesions of trunk or small nodular tumors in select locations
    - Mohs microsurgery with immediate mapping of margins for lesions with aggressive histology, recurrences, or in areas where tissue conservation is important
    - Ionizing radiation is an alternative
    - Sun protection, regular sunscreen use, regular skin screening

15

- **Pearl**

An extremely common malignancy, with millions of cases annually worldwide.

Reference

Wong CS, Strange RC, Lear JT: Basal cell carcinoma. BMJ 2003;327:794. [PMID: 14525881]

Bullous Drug Reactions (Erythema Multiforme Major, Stevens-Johnson Syndrome, and Toxic Epidermal Necrolysis)

- ■ Essentials of Diagnosis
  - Flu-like symptoms frequently precede eruption
  - Initial lesions erythematous and macular; may become targetoid, form bullae, or desquamate
  - Two or more mucosal surfaces (oral, conjunctival, anogenital) usually affected; gastrointestinal tract or respiratory tract involved in severe cases
  - Skin biopsies confirm diagnosis
  - Stevens-Johnson syndrome: < 10% of body surface involvement; toxic epidermal necrolysis: > 30% of body surface involvement
  - Sulfonamide drugs, phenytoin, carbamazepine, phenobarbital, penicillins, allopurinol, NSAIDs, and bupropion are frequent offenders
  - In anticonvulsant hypersensitivity reactions, hepatitis, nephritis, or pneumonitis may occur

- ■ Differential Diagnosis
  - Generalized bullous fixed drug eruption
  - Staphylococcal scalded skin syndrome
  - Infection-induced erythema multiforme major (most frequently associated with *Mycoplasma pneumoniae* infection)
  - Early disease may be confused with morbilliform drug eruptions or erythema multiforme minor
  - Bullous pemphigoid and pemphigus vulgaris
  - Graft-versus-host disease

- ■ Treatment
  - Discontinuation of provocative agent
  - Extensive involvement may require transfer to a burn unit for fluid and electrolyte management
  - Antibiotics
  - Systemic corticosteroids are controversial
  - Wet dressings, oral and ophthalmologic care, pain relief
  - Intravenous immunoglobulin should be given early in severe cases

15

- ■ Pearl

Beware of rechallenge with phenytoin, carbamazepine, or phenobarbital in any patient with anticonvulsant hypersensitivity given cross-reactivity; valproic acid is the alternative.

Reference

Bachot N, Roujeau JC: Differential diagnosis of severe cutaneous drug eruptions. Am J Clin Dermatol 2003;4:561. [PMID: 12862499]

Bullous Pemphigoid

■ Essentials of Diagnosis

- Age at onset seventh or eighth decade, though also occurs in young children
- Caused by autoantibodies to two specific components of the hemidesmosome
- Occasionally drug-induced (penicillamine, furosemide, captopril, enalapril, penicillin, sulfasalazine, nalidixic acid)
- Large, tense blisters that rupture, leaving denuded areas which heal without scarring
- Erythematous patches and urticarial plaques even in the absence of bullae
- Predilection for groin, axillae, flexor forearms, thighs, and shins; may occur anywhere; some have oral involvement
- Frequently pruritic
- Diagnosis by lesional biopsy, perilesional direct immunofluorescence, and indirect immunofluorescence

■ Differential Diagnosis

- Epidermolysis bullosa acquisita
- Cicatricial pemphigoid
- Herpes gestationis
- Linear IgA dermatosis
- Dermatitis herpetiformis

■ Treatment

- Prednisone initially
- Nicotinamide plus tetracycline are steroid sparing
- Aggressive immunosuppression may be required (azathioprine, low-dose methotrexate, or mycophenolate mofetil); monitor patients for side effects and infections
- Topical steroids for localized mild disease that breaks through medical treatment
- Pemphigoid usually self-limited, lasting months to years

15

■ Pearl

Underappreciated as a side effect of ACE inhibitors.

Reference

Fontaine J, Joly P, Roujeau JC: Treatment of bullous pemphigoid. J Dermatol 2003;30:83. [PMID: 12692373]

Common Warts (Verrucae Vulgaris)

- **Essentials of Diagnosis**
  - Scaly, rough, spiny papules or plaques
  - Most frequently seen on hands, may occur anywhere on skin
  - Caused by human papillomavirus

- **Differential Diagnosis**
  - Actinic keratosis
  - Squamous cell carcinoma
  - Seborrheic keratosis
  - Acrochordon (skin tag)
  - Nevus
  - Molluscum contagiosum
  - Verrucous zoster in HIV-infected patients
  - Extensive warts suggest epidermodysplasia verruciformis, HIV infection, or lymphoproliferative disorders

- **Treatment**
  - Avoid aggressive treatment in young children; spontaneous resolution is common
  - Cryotherapy
  - Patient-applied salicylic acid products
  - Office-applied cantharidin
  - Curettage and electrodesiccation
  - Pulsed dye laser therapy
  - Sensitization with squaric acid in resistant cases
  - Intralesional bleomycin
  - Oral cimetidine has low efficacy but may be a useful adjunct
  - Topical imiquimod less effective in common warts than genital warts

15

- **Pearl**

The first tumor of Homo sapiens *proved to be caused by a virus.*

Reference

Gibbs S, Harvey I, Sterling J, Stark R: Local treatments for cutaneous warts: systematic review. BMJ 2002;325:461. [PMID: 12202325]

Cutaneous Candidiasis

■ Essentials of Diagnosis
- Candidal intertrigo causes superficial denuded, pink to beefy-red patches that may be surrounded by tiny satellite pustules in genitocrural, subaxillary, gluteal, interdigital, and submammary areas
- Oral candidiasis shows grayish white plaques that scrape off to reveal a raw, erythematous base
- Oral candidiasis more common in elderly, debilitated, malnourished, diabetic, or HIV-infected patients as well as those taking antibiotics, systemic steroids, or chemotherapy
- Angular cheilitis (perlèche) sometimes due to *Candida*
- Perianal candidiasis may cause pruritus ani
- Candidal paronychia causes thickening and erythema of the nail fold and occasional discharge of thin pus

■ Differential Diagnosis
- Candidal intertrigo: Dermatophytosis, bacterial skin infections, seborrheic dermatitis, contact dermatitis, deep fungal infection, inverse psoriasis, erythrasma, eczema
- Oral candidiasis: Lichen planus, leukoplakia, geographic tongue, herpes simplex infection, erythema multiforme, pemphigus
- Candidal paronychia: Acute bacterial paronychia, paronychia associated with hypoparathyroidism, celiac disease, acrodermatitis enteropathica, or reactive arthritis
- Chronic mucocutaneous candidiasis

■ Treatment
- Control exacerbating factors (eg, hyperglycemia in diabetics, chronic antibiotic use, estrogen-dominant oral contraceptives, systemic steroids, ill-fitting dentures, malnutrition)
- Treat localized skin disease with topical azoles or polyenes
- Soaks with aluminum acetate solutions for raw, denuded lesions
- Fluconazole or itraconazole for systemic therapy
- Nystatin suspension or clotrimazole troches for oral disease
- Treat chronic paronychia with topical imidazoles or 4% thymol in chloroform
- Avoid chronic water exposure

■ Pearl

Look for adjacent pustules and the absence of much scale; it helps differentiate candidal intertrigo from tinea cruris.

Reference

Loo DS: Cutaneous fungal infections in the elderly. Dermatol Clin 2004;22:33. [PMID: 15018008]

15

Cutaneous Kaposi's Sarcoma

- **Essentials of Diagnosis**
  - Vascular neoplasm presenting with one or several red to purple macules which progress to papules or nodules
  - Classic form occurs on legs of elderly men of Mediterranean, East European, or Jewish descent
  - African endemic form cutaneous and locally aggressive in young adults or lymphadenopathic and fatal in children
  - AIDS-associated form shows cutaneous lesions on head, neck, trunk, and mucous membranes; may progress to nodal, pulmonary, and gastrointestinal involvement
  - The form associated with iatrogenic immunosuppression can mimic either classic or AIDS-associated type
  - Human herpesvirus 8 the causative agent in all types
  - Skin biopsy for diagnosis

- **Differential Diagnosis**
  - Dermatofibroma
  - Bacillary angiomatosis
  - Pyogenic granuloma
  - Prurigo nodularis
  - Blue nevus
  - Melanoma
  - Cutaneous lymphoma

- **Treatment**
  - In AIDS-associated cases, combination antiretroviral therapy—increasing CD4 counts—is the treatment of choice
  - Intralesional vincristine or interferon, radiation therapy, cryotherapy, alitretinoin gel, laser ablation, or excision
  - Systemic therapy with liposomal doxorubicin or other cytotoxic drugs in certain cases with rapid progression or visceral involvement

15

- **Pearl**

The first alert to the HIV epidemic was a New York dermatologist reporting two cases of atypical Kaposi's sarcoma to the Centers for Disease Control; a single physician giving thought to a patient's problem can still make a difference.

Reference

Von Roenn JH: Clinical presentations and standard therapy of AIDS-associated Kaposi's sarcoma. Hematol Oncol Clin North Am 2003;17:747. [PMID: 12852654]

Cutaneous T Cell Lymphoma (Mycosis Fungoides)

- ■ Essentials of Diagnosis
  - • Early stage: Erythematous 1- to 5-cm patches, sometimes pruritic, on lower abdomen, buttocks, upper thighs, and in women, breasts
  - • Middle stages: Infiltrated, erythematous, scaly plaques
  - • Advanced stages: Skin tumors, erythroderma, lymphadenopathy, or visceral involvement
  - • Skin biopsy critical; serial biopsies may be required to confirm diagnosis
  - • CD4:CD8 ratios, tests to detect clonal rearrangement of the T-cell receptor gene

- ■ Differential Diagnosis
  - • Psoriasis
  - • Drug eruption
  - • Eczematous dermatoses
  - • Leprosy
  - • Tinea corporis
  - • Other lymphoreticular malignancies

- ■ Treatment
  - • Treatment depends on stage of disease
  - • Early and aggressive therapy may control cutaneous lesions—not shown to prevent progression
  - • High-potency corticosteroids, mechlorethamine, or carmustine (BCNU) topically
  - • Phototherapy (psoralen plus UVA) in early stages
  - • Total skin electron beam radiation, photophoresis, systemic chemotherapy, retinoids, and alpha interferon for advanced disease
  - • Denileukin diftitox (diphtheria toxin fused to recombinant IL-2)

15

- ■ Pearl

Be careful of the uncharacterized chronic skin eruption; this may be the diagnosis.

Reference

Girardi M, Heald PW, Wilson LD: The pathogenesis of mycosis fungoides. N Engl J Med 2004;350:1978. [PMID: 15128898]

Diffuse Pruritus

- ■ Essentials of Diagnosis
  - • May be idiopathic, but work-up needed to rule out internal causes
  - • Excoriations are an objective sign of pruritus, but not always present

- ■ Differential Diagnosis
  - • Hepatic disease, especially cholestatic
  - • Hepatitis C with or without liver dysfunction
  - • Uremia
  - • Hypothyroidism or hyperthyroidism
  - • Intestinal parasites
  - • Polycythemia vera
  - • Lymphomas, leukemias, myeloma, other malignancies
  - • Neuropsychiatric diseases (anorexia nervosa, delusions of parasitosis)
  - • Scabies or other infestations

- ■ Treatment
  - • Sedative antihistamines for symptomatic relief
  - • Topical menthol lotions
  - • Aspirin for pruritus of polycythemia vera
  - • Cholestyramine, naloxone, prednisone, and colchicine helpful in some with hepatobiliary pruritus
  - • Optimization of dialysis, erythropoietin (epoetin alfa), emollients, cholestyramine, phosphate binders, and phototherapy helpful in some with uremic pruritus

- ■ Pearl

Excoriations spare areas out of the patient's reach, such as the "butterfly zone" on the back, and show that the pruritus is primary.

15

Reference

Yosipovitch G, Greaves MW, Schmelz M: Itch. Lancet 2003;361:690. [PMID: 12606187]

Discoid (Chronic Cutaneous) Lupus Erythematosus

- **Essentials of Diagnosis**
  - Dull red macules or papules developing into sharply demarcated hyperkeratotic plaques with follicular plugs
  - Lesions heal from the center with atrophy, dyspigmentation, and telangiectasias
  - Localized lesions most common on scalp, nose, cheeks, ears, lower lip, and neck
  - Scalp lesions cause scarring alopecia
  - Generalized disease involves trunk and upper extremities
  - Abnormal serologies, leukopenia, and albuminuria identify DLE patients likely to progress; children with DLE more likely to progress
  - Skin biopsy for diagnosis; direct immunofluorescence

- **Differential Diagnosis**
  - Seborrheic dermatitis
  - Rosacea
  - Lupus vulgaris (cutaneous tuberculosis)
  - Sarcoidosis
  - Bowen's disease (squamous cell carcinoma in-situ)
  - Polymorphous light eruption
  - Tertiary syphilis
  - Lichen planopilaris of the scalp

- **Treatment**
  - Screen for systemic disease with history, physical, and laboratory tests
  - Aggressive sun protection, including a high-SPF sunscreen
  - Potent topical corticosteroids or intralesional steroids for localized lesions
  - Systemic therapy with antimalarials; monitor laboratory studies; ophthalmologic consultation every 6 months
  - Thalidomide in resistant cases; pregnancy prevention and monitoring for side effects critical

- **Pearl**

Does not progress to SLE, but SLE does progress to it.

Reference

Fabbri P, Cardinali C, Giomi B, Caproni M: Cutaneous lupus erythematosus: diagnosis and management. Am J Clin Dermatol 2003;4:449. [PMID: 12814335]

15

Erysipelas & Cellulitis

- **Essentials of Diagnosis**
  - Cellulitis: An acute infection of the subcutaneous tissue, most frequently caused by *Streptococcus pyogenes* or *Staphylococcus aureus*
  - Erythema, edema, tenderness are the hallmarks of cellulitis; vesicles, exudation, purpura, necrosis may follow
  - Lymphangitic streaking may be seen
  - Demarcation from uninvolved skin indistinct
  - Erysipelas: Involves superficial dermal lymphatics
  - Erysipelas characterized by a warm, red, tender, edematous plaque with a sharply demarcated, raised, indurated border; classically occurs on the face
  - Both erysipelas and cellulitis require a portal of entry
  - Recurrence seen in lymphatic damage or venous insufficiency
  - A prodrome of malaise, fever, and chills may accompany either entity

- **Differential Diagnosis**
  - Acute contact dermatitis
  - Scarlet fever
  - Lupus erythematosus
  - Erythema nodosum
  - Early necrotizing fasciitis or clostridial gangrene
  - Underlying osteomyelitis
  - Evolving herpes zoster
  - Fixed drug eruption
  - Venous thrombosis
  - Beriberi

15

- **Treatment**
  - Appropriate systemic antibiotics
  - Local wound care and elevation

- **Pearl**

Look for tinea pedis as a portal of entry in patients with leg cellulitis.

Reference

Bonnetblanc JM, Bedane C: Erysipelas: recognition and management. Am J Clin Dermatol 2003;4:157. [PMID: 12627991]

Erythema Multiforme Minor

- ■ Essentials of Diagnosis
  - • Uniformly associated with herpes simplex infection (orolabial more than genital)
  - • Episodes follow orolabial herpes by 1–3 weeks and may recur with succeeding outbreaks
  - • Early sharply demarcated erythematous papules which become edematous
  - • Later "target" lesions with three zones: Central duskiness that may vesiculate; edematous, pale ring; and surrounding erythema
  - • Dorsal hands, dorsal feet, palms, soles, and extensor surfaces most frequently affected, with few to hundreds of lesions
  - • Mucosal involvement (usually oral) in 25%
  - • Biopsies often diagnostic

- ■ Differential Diagnosis
  - • Stevens-Johnson in evolution
  - • Pemphigus vulgaris
  - • Bullous pemphigoid
  - • Urticaria
  - • Acute febrile neutrophilic dermatosis (Sweet's syndrome)

- ■ Treatment
  - • Chronic suppressive antiherpetic therapy prevents 90% of recurrences
  - • Facial and lip sunscreens may also decrease recurrences by limiting herpes outbreaks
  - • Episodes usually self-limited (resolving in 1–4 weeks) and do not require therapy
  - • Systemic corticosteroids discouraged

15

- ■ Pearl

Even when a history of herpes cannot be elicited, empiric antivirals may prevent recurring target lesions.

Reference

Nikkels AF, Pierard GE: Treatment of mucocutaneous presentations of herpes simplex virus infections. Am J Clin Dermatol 2002;3:475. [PMID: 12180895]

Erythema Nodosum

- **Essentials of Diagnosis**
  - A reactive inflammation of the subcutis associated with infections (streptococcal, tuberculous, *Yersinia, Salmonella, Shigella,* systemic fungal infections), drugs (oral contraceptives, sulfonamides, bromides), sarcoidosis, and inflammatory bowel disease
  - Symmetric, erythematous, tender plaques or nodules 1–10 cm in diameter on anterior shins
  - Lesions also seen on upper legs, neck, and arms
  - Onset accompanied by malaise, leg edema, and arthralgias
  - Lesions flatten over a few days leaving a violaceous patch, then heal without atrophy or scarring
  - All lesions generally resolve within 6 weeks
  - Chronic form with prolonged course not associated with underlying diseases
  - Deep skin biopsy for diagnosis

- **Differential Diagnosis**
  - Erythema induratum or nodular vasculitis (secondary to tuberculosis)
  - Poststeroid panniculitis
  - Lupus panniculitis
  - Erythema multiforme
  - Syphilis
  - Subcutaneous fat necrosis associated with pancreatitis

- **Treatment**
  - Treat underlying causes
  - Bed rest, gentle support hose; avoid vigorous exercise
  - NSAIDs
  - Potassium iodide
  - Intralesional steroids in persistent cases
  - Systemic steroids in severe cases; contraindicated when the underlying cause is infectious

15

- **Pearl**

Persistent lesions should prompt a work-up for subclinical tuberculosis.

Reference

Requena L, Requena C: Erythema nodosum. Dermatol Online J 2002;8:4. [PMID: 12165214]

Exfoliative Dermatitis (Erythroderma)

- **Essentials of Diagnosis**
  - Erythema and scaling over most of the body
  - Itching, malaise, fever, chills, lymphadenopathy, weight loss
  - Preexisting dermatosis causes more than half of cases
  - Skin biopsy to identify cause
  - Leukocyte gene rearrangement studies if Sézary syndrome suspected and biopsies nondiagnostic

- **Differential Diagnosis**
  - Erythrodermic psoriasis
  - Pityriasis rubra pilaris
  - Drug eruption
  - Atopic dermatitis
  - Contact dermatitis
  - Severe seborrheic dermatitis
  - Sézary syndrome of cutaneous T-cell lymphoma
  - Hodgkin's disease

- **Treatment**
  - Soaks and emollients
  - Midpotency topical steroids, possibly under occlusive suit
  - Hospitalization may be required
  - Specific systemic therapies
  - Discontinue offending agent in drug-induced cases
  - Antibiotics for secondary bacterial infections

- **Pearl**

  Unexplained erythroderma in a middle-aged person raises the index of suspicion for a visceral malignancy.

15

Reference

Sehgal VN, Srivastava G, Sardana K: Erythroderma/exfoliative dermatitis: a synopsis. Int J Dermatol 2004;43:39. [PMID: 14693020]

Fixed Drug Eruption

■ **Essentials of Diagnosis**

- Lesions recur at the same site with each repeat exposure to the causative medication
- From one to six lesions
- Oral, genital, facial, and acral lesions most common
- Lesions begin as erythematous, edematous, round, sharply demarcated patches or plaques
- May evolve to become targetoid, bullous, or erosive
- Postinflammatory hyperpigmentation common
- Offending agents: NSAIDs, sulfonamides, barbiturates, tetracyclines, erythromycin, and laxatives with phenolphthalein

■ **Differential Diagnosis**

- Bullous pemphigoid
- Erythema multiforme
- Sweet's syndrome (acute febrile neutrophilic dermatosis)
- Residual hyperpigmentation can appear similar to pigmentation left behind by numerous other inflammatory disorders
- The differential of genital lesions includes psoriasis, lichen planus, and syphilis

■ **Treatment**

- Avoidance of the causative agent
- Symptomatic care of lesions

■ **Pearl**

An often overlooked source of penile erosions.

Reference

Lee AY: Fixed drug eruptions. Incidence, recognition, and avoidance. Am J Clin Dermatol 2000;1:277. [PMID: 11702319]

15

Folliculitis, Furuncles, & Carbuncles

- **Essentials of Diagnosis**
  - Folliculitis: Thin-walled pustules at follicular orifices, particularly extremities, scalp, face, and buttocks; develop in crops and heal in a few days
  - Furuncle: Acute, round, tender, circumscribed, perifollicular abscess; most undergo central necrosis and rupture with purulent discharge
  - Carbuncle: Two or more confluent furuncles
  - Classic folliculitis caused by *S aureus*

- **Differential Diagnosis**
  - Pseudofolliculitis barbae
  - Acne vulgaris and acneiform drug eruptions
  - Pustular miliaria (heat rash)
  - Fungal folliculitis
  - Herpes folliculitis
  - Hot tub folliculitis caused by *Pseudomonas*
  - Gram-negative folliculitis (in acne patients on long-term antibiotic therapy)
  - Eosinophilic folliculitis (AIDS patients)
  - Nonbacterial folliculitis (occlusion or oil-induced)
  - Hidradenitis suppurativa of axillae or groin
  - Dissecting cellulitis of scalp

- **Treatment**
  - Thorough cleansing with antibacterial soaps
  - Mupirocin ointment in limited disease
  - Oral antibiotics (dicloxacillin or cephalexin) for more extensive involvement
  - Warm compresses and systemic antibiotics for furuncles and carbuncles
  - Culture for methicillin-resistant strains in unresponsive lesions
  - Avoid incision and drainage with acutely inflamed lesions; may be helpful when furuncle becomes localized and fluctuant
  - Culture anterior nares in recurrent cases to rule out *S aureus* carriage; if positive, consider applying mupirocin to nares and oral rifampin.

15

- **Pearl**

The staphylococcal infections are most common in HIV-infected patients, diabetics, alcoholics, and dialysis patients.

Reference

Stulberg DL, Penrod MA, Blatny RA: Common bacterial skin infections. Am Fam Physician 2002;66:119. [PMID: 12126026]

Genital Warts (Condylomata Acuminata)

■ Essentials of Diagnosis

- Gray, yellow, or pink lobulated multifocal papules
- Occur on the penis, vulva, cervix, perineum, crural folds, or peri-anal area; also may be intraurethral or intra-anal
- Caused by human papillomavirus; sexually transmitted
- Increased risk of progression to cervical cancer, anal cancer, or bowenoid papulosis in certain HPV subtypes
- Children with genital warts should be evaluated for sexual abuse, but childhood infection can also be acquired via perinatal vertical transmission or digital autoinoculation

■ Differential Diagnosis

- Psoriasis
- Lichen planus
- Bowenoid papulosis and squamous cell carcinoma
- Seborrheic keratosis
- Pearly penile papules (circumferential around base of glans)
- Acrochordon (skin tag)
- Secondary syphilis (condyloma latum)

■ Treatment

- Treatment may remove lesions but has not been shown to reduce transmission or prevent progression to cancer
- Cryotherapy, topical podophyllum resin, topical trichloroacetic acid, electrofulguration, and carbon dioxide laser; plume generated by lasers or electrofulguration is potentially infectious to health care personnel
- Topical imiquimod; women have a higher response rate than men
- Pap smear for women with genital warts and female sexual partners of men with genital warts
- Biopsy suspicious lesions; HIV-infected patients with genital warts are at increased risk of HPV-induced carcinomas

15

■ Pearl

Subclinical disease, common and impossible to eradicate, is neither investigated nor treated.

Reference

Gunter J: Genital and perianal warts: new treatment opportunities for human papillomavirus infection. Am J Obstet Gynecol 2003;189(3 Suppl):S3. [PMID: 14532897]

Granuloma Annulare

- **Essentials of Diagnosis**
  - White or red flat-topped, asymptomatic papules that spread with central clearing to form annular plaques; cause unknown
  - May coalesce, then involute spontaneously
  - Predilection for dorsum of fingers, hands, or feet; elbows or ankles also favored sites
  - Generalized form sometimes associated with diabetes; subcutaneous form most common in children
  - Skin biopsy secures diagnosis

- **Differential Diagnosis**
  - Necrobiosis lipoidica
  - Tinea corporis
  - Erythema migrans (Lyme disease)
  - Sarcoidosis
  - Secondary syphilis
  - Erythema multiforme
  - Subacute cutaneous lupus erythematosus
  - Annular lichen planus
  - Leprosy (Hansen's disease)
  - Rheumatoid nodules (subcutaneous form)

- **Treatment**
  - None required in mild cases; 75% of patients with localized disease clear in 2 years
  - Intralesional or potent topical corticosteroids effective for limited disease
  - Prednisone contraindicated due to relapse upon withdrawal
  - Anecdotal success with dapsone, nicotinamide, potassium iodide, systemic retinoids, antimalarials, and psoralen plus UVA (PUVA)

15

- **Pearl**

Consider HIV infection in generalized granuloma annulare.

Reference

Hsu S, Le EH, Khoshevis MR: Differential diagnosis of annular lesions. Am Fam Physician 2001;64:289. [PMID: 11476274]

Herpes Simplex

- ■ Essentials of Diagnosis
  - Orolabial herpes: Initial infection usually asymptomatic; gingivostomatitis may occur
  - Recurrent grouped blisters on erythematous base (cold sore or fever blister); lips most frequently involved
  - UV exposure a common trigger
  - Genital herpes: Primary infection presents as systemic illness with grouped blisters and erosions on penis, rectum, or vagina
  - Recurrences common, present with painful grouped vesicles; active lesions infectious; asymptomatic shedding also occurs
  - A prodrome of tingling, itching, or burning
  - More severe and persistent in immunocompromised patients
  - Eczema herpeticum is diffuse, superimposed upon a preexisting inflammatory dermatosis
  - Herpetic whitlow; infection of fingers or hands
  - Tzanck smears, fluorescent antibody tests, viral cultures, and skin biopsies diagnostic

- ■ Differential Diagnosis
  - Impetigo
  - Zoster
  - Syphilis, chancroid, lymphogranuloma venereum, or granuloma inguinale
  - Oral aphthosis, coxsackievirus infection (herpangina), erythema multiforme, pemphigus, or primary HIV infection

- ■ Treatment
  - Sunblock to prevent orolabial recurrences
  - Early acute intermittent therapy with acyclovir, famciclovir, or valacyclovir
  - Prophylactic suppressive therapy for patients with frequent recurrences
  - Short-term prophylaxis before intense sun exposure, dental procedures, and laser resurfacing for patients with recurrent orolabial disease
  - Suppressive therapy for immunosuppressed patients
  - IV foscarnet for resistance in severely immunosuppressed

15

- ■ Pearl

Think of genital herpes in chronic heel pain—the virus lives in the sacral ganglion and refers pain to that site.

Reference

Brady RC, Bernstein DI: Treatment of herpes simplex virus infections. Antiviral Res 2004;61:73. [PMID: 14670580]

Leg Ulcers from Venous Insufficiency

- **Essentials of Diagnosis**
  - Occurs in patients with signs of venous insufficiency
  - Irregular ulcerations, often on medial aspect of lower legs; fibrinous eschar at the base
  - Light rheography to assess venous insufficiency
  - Measurement of the ankle-brachial index to eliminate arterial component
  - Atypical or persistent ulcers should be biopsied to rule out other causes

- **Differential Diagnosis**
  - Arterial insufficiency
  - Pyoderma gangrenosum
  - Diabetic neuropathy and microangiopathy
  - Vasculitis
  - Cryoglobulins
  - Infection (mycobacteria, fungi)
  - Trauma
  - Sickle cell anemia or thalassemia
  - Neoplasm (eg, basal cell or squamous cell carcinoma, melanoma, lymphoma)

- **Treatment**
  - Clean ulcer base, remove eschar regularly
  - Topical antibiotics (metronidazole) reduce bacterial growth and odor; topical steroids when inflammation is present
  - Cover ulcer with occlusive permeable biosynthetic dressing
  - Compression therapy with Unna's boot or elastic bandage essential
  - Becaplermin (recombinant platelet-derived growth factor) in diabetics with refractory ulcers
  - Cultured epidermal cell grafts or bilayered skin substitutes in highly refractory ulcers
  - Compression stockings to reduce edema and risk of further ulcerations

15

- **Pearl**

About 90% of all leg ulcers result from chronic venous insufficiency, but be alert for the other causes.

Reference

Valencia IC, Falabella A, Kirsner RS, Eaglstein WH: Chronic venous insufficiency and venous leg ulceration. J Am Acad Dermatol 2001;44:401; quiz 422. [PMID: 11209109]

Lichen Planus

■ Essentials of Diagnosis

- Small pruritic, violaceous, polygonal, flat-topped papules; may show white streaks (Wickham's striae) on surface
- On flexor wrists, dorsal hands, trunk, thighs, shins, ankles, glans penis
- Oral mucosa frequently affected with ulcers or reticulated white patches
- Vulvovaginal and perianal lesions show leukoplakia or erosions
- Scalp involvement (lichen planopilaris) causes scarring alopecia
- Nail changes infrequent but can include pterygium
- Trauma may induce additional lesions (Koebner phenomenon)
- Linear, annular, and hypertrophic variants
- Skin biopsy when diagnosis not clear

■ Differential Diagnosis

- Lichenoid drug eruption
- Pityriasis rosea
- Psoriasis
- Secondary syphilis
- Mucosal lesions: Lichen sclerosus, candidiasis, erythema multiforme, leukoplakia, pemphigus vulgaris, bullous pemphigoid
- Discoid lupus erythematosus

■ Treatment

- Topical or intralesional steroids for limited cutaneous or mucosal lesions
- Systemic corticosteroids, psoralen plus UVA, oral isotretinoin, low-molecular-weight heparin for generalized disease
- Cyclosporine for severe cases
- Monitor for malignant transformation to squamous cell carcinoma in erosive mucosal disease
- Aggressive management to avoid debilitating scarring in vulvar lichen planus

15

■ Pearl

Hepatitis C infection is more common in lichen planus patients; obtain the antibody in these patients.

Reference

Katta R: Lichen planus. Am Fam Physician 2000;61:3319, 3327. [PMID: 10865927]

Lichen Simplex Chronicus & Prurigo Nodularis

- **Essentials of Diagnosis**
  - Chronic, severe, localized itching
  - Lichen simplex chronicus: Well-circumscribed, erythematous plaques with accentuated skin markings, often on the extremities and posterior neck
  - Prurigo nodularis: Multiple pea-sized firm, erythematous or brownish, dome-shaped, excoriated nodules, typically on the extremities

- **Differential Diagnosis**
  - Lichen simplex chronicus: Secondary phenomenon in atopic dermatitis, stasis dermatitis, insect bite reactions, contact dermatitis, or pruritus of other cause
  - Lesions of psoriasis, cutaneous lymphoma, lichen planus, and tinea corporis may resemble lichen simplex chronicus
  - Prurigo nodularis: Associated with HIV disease, renal failure, hepatic diseases (especially hepatitis), atopic dermatitis, anemia, emotional stress, pregnancy, and gluten enteropathy
  - Prurigo nodularis: Similar to hypertrophic lichen planus and scabietic nodules

- **Treatment**
  - Avoid scratching involved areas—occlusion with steroid tape, semipermeable dressings, or even Unna's boots may be of value
  - Intralesional steroids or topical superpotent steroids helpful in treating individual lesions
  - Oral antihistamines of limited benefit
  - Phototherapy, isotretinoin, topical calcipotriene, and oral cyclosporine are alternatives
  - Thalidomide in recalcitrant, severe prurigo nodularis; pregnancy prevention and monitoring for side effects are critical

15

- **Pearl**

These lesions are a response to chronic rubbing or picking; typically, no specific cause is suggested by the morphology.

Reference

Moses S: Pruritus. Am Fam Physician 2003;68:1135. [PMID: 14524401]

Malignant Melanoma

■ **Essentials of Diagnosis**

- Higher incidence in those with fair skin, blue eyes, blond or red hair, blistering sunburns, chronic sun exposure, family history, immunodeficiency, many nevi, dysplastic nevi, giant congenital nevus, and certain genetic diseases such as xeroderma pigmentosum
- ABCD warning signs: Asymmetry, Border irregularity, Color variegation, and Diameter over 6 mm
- Clinical characteristics vary depending on subtype and location
- Early detection is critical; advanced-stage disease has high mortality
- Epiluminescence microscopy to identify high-risk lesions
- Biopsies for diagnosis must be deep enough to permit measurement of thickness; partial biopsies should be avoided

■ **Differential Diagnosis**

- Seborrheic keratosis
- Basal cell carcinoma, pigmented type
- Nevus (ordinary melanocytic nevus, dysplastic nevus)
- Solar lentigo
- Pyogenic granuloma
- Kaposi's sarcoma
- Pregnancy-associated darkening of nevi

■ **Treatment**

- For localized disease, prognosis determined by histologic features
- Appropriate staging work-up including history, physical examination, laboratory tests, and scans to evaluate for metastatic spread
- Sentinel lymph node biopsy in selected cases; lymph node dissection if evidence of lymphatic disease
- Reexcision with appropriate margins determined by histologic characteristics of the tumor
- Adjuvant therapy for high risk
- Close follow-up

15

■ **Pearl**

When a mole is suspicious or changing, it belongs in formalin.

Reference

Tsao H, Atkins MB, Sober AJ: Management of cutaneous melanoma. N Engl J Med 2004;351:998. [PMID: 15342808]

Melasma (Chloasma Faciei)

- **Essentials of Diagnosis**
    - Most frequently seen in women during pregnancy or menopause—also associated with oral contraceptives and phenytoin use
    - Well-demarcated symmetric brown patches with irregular borders
    - Typically on cheeks and forehead, but may also involve nipples, genitals, or forearms
    - Exacerbated by sun exposure

- **Differential Diagnosis**
    - Postinflammatory hyperpigmentation
    - Contact photodermatitis from perfumes
    - Exogenous ochronosis (from hydroquinones, phenol, or resorcinol)
    - Drug-induced hyperpigmentation (minocycline, gold, etc)

- **Treatment**
    - Sun protection, including broad-spectrum sunscreen with UVA coverage
    - Bleaching creams with hydroquinone moderately effective, sometimes combined with topical retinoids and mild topical steroid (contraindicated during pregnancy or lactation)

- **Pearl**

Pregnancy-induced melasma clears within months; medication-induced disease persists for years.

Reference

Stulberg DL, Clark N, Tovey D: Common hyperpigmentation disorders in adults: Part II. Melanoma, seborrheic keratoses, acanthosis nigricans, melasma, diabetic dermopathy, tinea versicolor, and postinflammatory hyperpigmentation. Am Fam Physician 2003;68:1963. [PMID: 14655805]

15

Molluscum Contagiosum

- **Essentials of Diagnosis**
  - Smooth, firm, dome-shaped, pearly papules; characteristic central umbilication and white core
  - Sexually transmitted in immunocompetent adults; usually with less than 20 lesions; on lower abdomen, upper thighs, and penile shaft
  - Frequently generalized in young children
  - Patients with AIDS, particularly those with a CD4 count of less than 100/μL, are at highest risk; large lesions on face and genitalia
  - Patients with malignancies, sarcoidosis, extensive atopic dermatitis, or history of diffuse topical steroid use are also predisposed

- **Differential Diagnosis**
  - Warts
  - Varicella
  - Bacterial infection
  - Basal cell carcinoma
  - Lichen planus

- **Treatment**
  - Avoid aggressive treatment in young children; possible therapies for children include topical tretinoin or imiquimod, or continuous application of occlusive tape
  - Cryotherapy, curettage, or a topical agent (eg, podophyllotoxin) for adults with genital disease
  - Antiretroviral therapies resulting in increasing CD4 counts are most effective for HIV-infected patients

- **Pearl**

Cutaneous cryptococcal infection may mimic molluscum lesions in patients with AIDS.

15

Reference

Stulberg DL, Hutchinson AG: Molluscum contagiosum and warts. Am Fam Physician 2003;67:1233. [PMID: 12674451]

Morbilliform Drug Eruption

- **Essentials of Diagnosis**
  - Erythema, small papules
  - Occurs within first 2 weeks of drug treatment; may appear later
  - Pruritus prominent
  - Eruption symmetric, beginning proximally and then generalizing
  - Ampicillin, amoxicillin, allopurinol, and trimethoprim-sulfamethoxazole most common causes
  - Amoxicillin eruptions more frequent in patients with infectious mononucleosis; sulfonamide rashes common in HIV-infected patients

- **Differential Diagnosis**
  - Viral exanthems
  - Early stages of erythema multiforme major or drug hypersensitivity syndrome
  - Scarlet fever
  - Toxic shock syndrome
  - Acute graft-versus-host disease

- **Treatment**
  - Discontinue offending agent unless this represents a greater risk to the patient than the eruption
  - Topical corticosteroids and oral antihistamines
  - Avoid rechallenge in complex exanthems and with certain antiretroviral medications

- **Pearl**

It's not only prescription drugs that cause this condition; many patients do not consider over-the-counter agents to be "drugs."

15

Reference

Bigby M: Rates of cutaneous reactions to drugs. Arch Dermatol 2001;137:765. [PMID: 11405768]

Nevi (Congenital Nevi, Acquired Nevi)

- **Essentials of Diagnosis**

  - Common acquired nevi have homogeneous surfaces and color patterns, smooth and sharp borders, and are round or oval in shape
  - Color may vary from flesh-colored to brown
  - Flat or raised depending on the subtype or stage of evolution
  - Excisional biopsy to rule out melanoma in changing nevi or those with ABCD warning signs (see Malignant Melanoma)
  - Congenital nevi darkly pigmented; sometimes hairy papules or plaques that may be present at birth
  - Large congenital nevi (those whose longest diameter will be greater than 20 cm in adulthood) are at increased risk for melanoma; when found on head, neck, or posterior midline, associated with underlying leptomeningeal melanocytosis

- **Differential Diagnosis**

  - Dysplastic nevus
  - Melanoma
  - Lentigo simplex
  - Solar lentigo
  - Dermatofibroma
  - Basal cell carcinoma
  - Molluscum contagiosum
  - Blue nevus
  - Café au lait spot
  - Epidermal nevus
  - Becker's nevus

- **Treatment**

  - Excision of bothersome nevi, and those at high risk of developing melanoma
  - Biopsy suspicious lesions
  - Partial biopsies of suspicious lesions should be avoided when excisional biopsies feasible
  - Head or spinal scans in children with large congenital nevi occurring on the head, neck, or posterior midline

15

- **Pearl**

Any nevus you aren't certain about should be considered melanoma until proved otherwise.

Reference

Marghoob AA: Congenital melanocytic nevi. Evaluation and management. Dermatol Clin 2002;20:607, viii. [PMID: 12380048]

Nummular Eczema

- ■ Essentials of Diagnosis
  - • Middle-aged and older men most frequently affected
  - • Discrete coin-shaped, crusted, erythematous, 1- to 5-cm plaques that may contain vesicles
  - • Usually begins on lower legs, dorsal hands, or extensor surfaces of arms, but may spread to involve all extremities and the trunk over several months
  - • Pruritus often severe

- ■ Differential Diagnosis
  - • Tinea corporis
  - • Psoriasis
  - • Xerotic dermatitis
  - • Impetigo
  - • Contact dermatitis

- ■ Treatment
  - • Avoidance of agents capable of drying or irritating skin (hot or frequent baths, extensive soaping, etc)
  - • Frequent emollients
  - • Topical corticosteroids (potency appropriate to location and severity) applied twice daily and tapered as tolerated
  - • Topical tacrolimus and pimecrolimus are effective but expensive alternatives to steroids
  - • Topical tar preparations
  - • Phototherapy may be helpful in severe cases
  - • Sedative antihistamines to relieve pruritus, given at bedtime
  - • Antibiotics when signs of impetiginization are present (fissures, crusts, erosions, or pustules)
  - • Systemic steroids only in highly selected, refractory cases

15

- ■ Pearl

If it scales, scrape it; KOH preparation should always be examined to rule out tinea corporis.

Reference

Aoyama H, Tanaka M, Hara M, Tabata N, Tagami H: Nummular eczema: An addition of senile xerosis and unique cutaneous reactivities to environmental aeroallergens. Dermatology 1999;199:135. [PMID: 10559579]

Onychomycosis (Tinea Unguium)

- **Essentials of Diagnosis**
  - Yellowish discoloration, piling up of subungual keratin, friability, and separation of the nail plate
  - May show only overlying white scale if superficial
  - Nail shavings for immediate microscopic examination, culture, or histologic examination with periodic acid-Schiff stain to establish diagnosis; repeated sampling may be required

- **Differential Diagnosis**
  - Candidal onychomycosis shows erythema, tenderness, swelling of the nail fold (paronychia)
  - Psoriasis
  - Lichen planus
  - Allergic contact dermatitis from nail polish
  - Contact urticaria from foods or other sensitizers
  - Nail changes associated with reactive arthritis (Reiter's), Darier's disease, crusted scabies

- **Treatment**
  - Antifungal creams not effective; topical ciclopirox lacquer approved but has very low efficacy
  - Oral terbinafine and itraconazole effective in many
  - Establish diagnosis before initiating therapy
  - Adequate informed consent critical; patients must decide if benefits of oral therapy outweigh risks
  - Weekly prophylactic topical antifungals to suppress tinea pedis may prevent tinea unguium recurrences

- **Pearl**

A difficult disorder to treat, and nearly impossible to eradicate.

15

Reference

Mahoney JM, Bennet J, Olsen B: The diagnosis of onychomycosis. Dermatol Clin 2003;21:463. [PMID: 12956198]

Pediculosis

■ **Essentials of Diagnosis**
- Three types of lice (*Pediculus humanus*), each with a predilection for certain body parts
- Dermatitis caused by inflammatory response to louse saliva
- Pediculosis capitis (head lice): Intense scalp pruritus, presence of nits, possible secondary impetigo and cervical lymphadenopathy; most common in children, rare in blacks
- Pediculosis corporis (body lice): Rarely found on skin, causes generalized pruritus, erythematous macules or urticarial wheals, excoriations and lichenification; homeless persons and those living in crowded conditions most frequently affected
- Pediculosis pubis (crabs): Usually sexually transmitted; generally limited to pubic area, axillae, and eyelashes; lice may be observed on skin and nits on hairs; maculae ceruleae (blue macules) may be seen
- Body lice can transmit trench fever, relapsing fever, and epidemic typhus

■ **Differential Diagnosis**
- Head lice: Impetigo, hair casts, seborrheic dermatitis
- Body lice: Scabies, urticaria, impetigo, dermatitis herpetiformis
- Pubic lice: Scabies, anogenital pruritus, eczema

■ **Treatment**
- Head lice: Topical permethrins with interval removal of nits and retreatment in 1 week
- Pyrethrins available over the counter; resistance common
- Treat household contacts
- Body lice: Launder clothing and bedding (at least 30 minutes at 150°F in dryer, or iron pressing of wool garments); patient should then bathe; no pesticides required
- Pubic lice: Treatment is same as for head lice; eyelash lesions treated with thick coating of petrolatum maintained for 1 week; recurrence is more common in HIV-infected patients

15

■ **Pearl**
Severe body lice infestation may cause iron deficiency; search for them if other sources of blood loss have been excluded.

Reference

Ko CJ, Elston DM: Pediculosis. J Am Acad Dermatol 2004;50:1; quiz 13. [PMID: 14699358]

Pemphigus Vulgaris

- **■ Essentials of Diagnosis**
  - Presents in fifth or sixth decade
  - Caused by autoantibodies to desmogleins; occasionally drug-induced (penicillamine, captopril)
  - Thin-walled, fragile blisters; rupture to form painful erosions that crust and heal slowly without scarring
  - Often initially presents with oral involvement
  - Scalp, face, neck, axillae, and groin common sites; esophagus, trachea, conjunctiva, and other mucosal surfaces may also be involved
  - Lateral pressure applied to perilesional skin induces more blistering (Nikolsky's sign)
  - Diagnosis by lesional biopsy of intact blisters, perilesional direct immunofluorescence, indirect immunofluorescence

- **■ Differential Diagnosis**
  - Paraneoplastic pemphigus (usually associated with lymphomas and leukemias)
  - Pemphigus foliaceus
  - Fogo selvagem (endemic Brazilian pemphigus)
  - Bullous pemphigoid
  - Erythema multiforme, Stevens-Johnson syndrome, toxic epidermal necrolysis
  - Linear IgA dermatosis
  - Epidermolysis bullosa acquisita
  - Patients presenting with only oral lesions may be misdiagnosed with aphthous stomatitis, erythema multiforme, herpes simplex, lichen planus, or cicatricial pemphigoid

- **■ Treatment**
  - Viscous lidocaine and antibiotic rinses for oral erosions
  - Early and aggressive systemic therapy required; mortality high in untreated patients
  - High doses of oral prednisone combined with another immunosuppressive (azathioprine or mycophenolate mofetil)
  - Monitor for side effects and infections
  - Plasmapheresis, intravenous immune globulin, and intramuscular gold are alternatives

15

- **■ Pearl**

Don't forget the oral presentation; this very closely resembles less serious conditions.

Reference

Fellner MJ, Sapadin AN: Current therapy of pemphigus vulgaris. Mt Sinai J Med 2001;68(4-5):268. [PMID: 11514914]

Photosensitive Drug Eruption

- **Essentials of Diagnosis**
  - Morphology variable; photodistribution critical to diagnosis
  - Phototoxic reactions resemble sunburn; related to dose of both medication and UV radiation; tetracyclines, amiodarone, and NSAIDs common causes
  - Photoallergic reactions typically red, scaly, pruritic; immune-related; often slow to develop; thiazides, sulfonamide antibiotics, and oral hypoglycemic agents common causes
  - Pseudoporphyria caused by naproxen, tetracyclines, furosemide, dapsone, and other medications
  - Photodistributed lichenoid reactions most frequently due to thiazides, quinidine, NSAIDs

- **Differential Diagnosis**
  - Porphyria cutanea tarda or other porphyrias
  - Lupus erythematosus or dermatomyositis
  - Photoallergic or phototoxic contact dermatitis from fragrances, sunscreens, or furocoumarins in many plants
  - HIV-associated photosensitivity
  - Polymorphous light eruption or other idiopathic photosensitivity disorders
  - Pellagra
  - Xeroderma pigmentosum or other genetic photosensitivity disorders

- **Treatment**
  - Avoidance of the causative agent
  - Sun avoidance, protection with broad-spectrum sunscreens containing physical blockers
  - Soothing local measures or topical corticosteroids

- **Pearl**

UVA radiation is the most common trigger; make sure sunscreens block this.

Reference

Nigen S, Knowles SR, Shear NH: Drug eruptions: approaching the diagnosis of drug-induced skin diseases. J Drugs Dermatol 2003;2:278. [PMID: 12848112]

Pityriasis Rosea

■ Essentials of Diagnosis

- Oval, salmon-colored, symmetric papules with long axis following cleavage lines
- Lesions show "collarette of scale" at periphery
- Trunk most frequently involved; sun-exposed areas often spared
- A "herald" patch precedes eruption by 1–2 weeks; some patients report prodrome of constitutional symptoms
- Pruritus common but usually mild
- Variations in mode of onset, morphology, distribution, and course are common
- Attempts to isolate infective agent have been disappointing

■ Differential Diagnosis

- Secondary syphilis
- Tinea corporis
- Seborrheic dermatitis
- Tinea versicolor
- Viral exanthem
- Drug eruption
- Psoriasis

■ Treatment

- Usually none required; most cases resolve spontaneously in 3–10 weeks
- Topical steroids or oral antihistamines for pruritus
- UVB phototherapy may expedite involution of lesions
- Short course of systemic corticosteroids in selected severe cases

■ Pearl

As in all similar rashes: RPR.

Reference

Stulberg DL, Wolfrey J: Pityriasis rosea. Am Fam Physician 2004;69:87. [PMID: 14727822]

15

Psoriasis

- ■ Essentials of Diagnosis
  - Silvery scales on bright red, well-demarcated plaques most commonly on knees, elbows, and scalp
  - Pitted nails or onychodystrophy
  - Pinking of intergluteal folds
  - Pruritus mild or absent
  - Associated with psoriatic arthritis
  - Lesions may be induced at sites of injury (Koebner phenomenon)
  - Many variants

- ■ Differential Diagnosis
  - Cutaneous candidiasis
  - Tinea corporis
  - Nummular eczema
  - Seborrheic dermatitis
  - Pityriasis rosea
  - Secondary syphilis
  - Pityriasis rubra pilaris
  - Nail findings may mimic onychomycosis
  - Cutaneous features of reactive arthritis (Reiter's syndrome) may mimic psoriasis
  - Plaque stage of cutaneous T-cell lymphoma may mimic psoriasis

- ■ Treatment
  - Topical steroids, calcipotriene, tar preparations, anthralin, salicylic acid, or tazarotene
  - Tar shampoos, topical steroids, calcipotriene, keratolytic agents, or intralesional steroids for scalp lesions
  - Phototherapy (UVB, psoralen plus UVA, or the Goeckerman regimen) for widespread disease
  - In selected severe cases, systemic methotrexate, cyclosporine, acitretin, alefacept, efalizumab, etanercept, infliximab, or adalimumab

- ■ Pearl

Be careful of systemic steroids in psoriasis; rebound or induction of pustular psoriasis may occur.

Reference

Lebwohl M: Psoriasis. Lancet 2003;361:1197. [PMID: 12686053]

15

Pyoderma Gangrenosum

- **Essentials of Diagnosis**
  - Often chronic and recurrent; may be accompanied by a polyarticular arthritis
  - Associated with inflammatory bowel disease and lymphoproliferative disorders; also seen with hepatitis B or C, HIV infection, systemic lupus erythematosus, pregnancy, and other conditions
  - Up to half of cases idiopathic
  - Lesions begin as inflammatory pustules, sometimes at a trauma site
  - Erythematous halo enlarges, then ulcerates
  - Ulcers painful with ragged, undermined, violaceous borders; bases appear purulent
  - Ulcers heal slowly, form atrophic scars
  - Diagnosis of exclusion; biopsies with special stains and cultures to rule out infections (mycobacterial, fungal, tertiary syphilis, gangrene, amebiasis)

- **Differential Diagnosis**
  - Folliculitis, insect bites, or Sweet's syndrome (acute febrile neutrophilic dermatosis)
  - Ulcers secondary to underlying infection
  - Ulcers secondary to underlying neoplasm
  - Factitious ulcerations from injected substances
  - Vasculitis (especially Wegener's granulomatosis)
  - Coumadin necrosis

- **Treatment**
  - Treat inflammatory bowel disease when present
  - Local compresses, occlusive dressings, potent topical steroids, intralesional steroids, or topical tacrolimus
  - High-dose systemic steroids in widespread disease; if control is not established or if a steroid taper is unsuccessful, a steroid-sparing agent (cyclosporine, mycophenolate mofetil, etc) is added
  - Dapsone, sulfasalazine, and clofazimine also steroid-sparing

15

- **Pearl**

Its reappearance in inflammatory bowel disease may indicate an imminent enteric relapse.

Reference

Wollina U: Clinical management of pyoderma gangrenosum. Am J Clin Dermatol 2002;3:149. [PMID: 11978136]

Rosacea

- **Essentials of Diagnosis**
  - A chronic disorder of the mid-face in middle-aged and older people
  - History of flushing evoked by hot beverages, alcohol, or sunlight
  - Erythema, sometimes persisting for hours or days after flushing episodes
  - Telangiectases become more prominent over time
  - Many patients have acneiform papules and pustules
  - Some advanced cases show large inflammatory nodules and nasal sebaceous hypertrophy (rhinophyma)

- **Differential Diagnosis**
  - Acne vulgaris
  - Seborrheic dermatitis
  - Lupus erythematosus
  - Dermatomyositis
  - Carcinoid syndrome
  - Topical steroid-induced rosacea
  - Polymorphous light eruption
  - *Demodex* (mite) folliculitis in HIV-infected patients
  - Perioral dermatitis

- **Treatment**
  - Treatment is suppressive and chronic
  - Topical metronidazole and oral tetracyclines effective against papulopustular disease
  - Daily sunscreen use and avoidance of flushing triggers may slow progression
  - Oral isotretinoin can produce dramatic improvement in resistant cases, but relapse common
  - Laser therapy may obliterate telangiectases
  - Surgery in severe rhinophyma

- **Pearl**

Watch for ocular symptoms—blepharitis, conjunctivitis, or even keratitis occur in a majority.

Reference

van Zuuren EJ, Graber MA, Hollis S, Chaudhry M, Gupta AK: Interventions for rosacea. Cochrane Database Syst Rev 2004;1:CD003262. [PMID: 14974010]

15

Scabies

- **Essentials of Diagnosis**
  - Caused by *Sarcoptes scabiei* mite
  - Pruritogenic papular eruption favoring finger webs, wrists, antecubital fossae, axillae, lower abdomen, genitals, buttocks, and nipples
  - Itching usually worse at night
  - Face and scalp are spared (except in children and the immunosuppressed)
  - Burrows appear as short, slightly raised, wavy lines in skin, sometimes with vesicles
  - Secondary eczematization, impetigo, and lichenification in long-standing infestation
  - Red nodules on penis or scrotum
  - A crusted form in institutionalized, HIV-infected, or malnourished individuals
  - Burrow scrapings permit microscopic confirmation of mites, ova, or feces; many cases diagnosed on clinical grounds

- **Differential Diagnosis**
  - Atopic dermatitis
  - Papular urticaria
  - Insect bites
  - Dermatitis herpetiformis
  - Pediculosis corporis
  - Pityriasis rosea

- **Treatment**
  - Permethrin 5% cream applied from the neck down for 8 hours; clothing and bed linens laundered thoroughly; repeat therapy in 1 week
  - Lindane used infrequently because of potential toxicity
  - Oral ivermectin in refractory cases, institutional epidemics, or immunosuppressed patients
  - Treat all household and sexual contacts
  - Persistent postscabietic pruritic papules may require topical or intralesional corticosteroids

15

- **Pearl**

Persistent pruritus for weeks after treatment is common; it does not invariably mean treatment failure.

Reference

Huynh TH, Norman RA: Scabies and pediculosis. Dermatol Clin 2004;22:7. [PMID: 15018005]

Seborrheic Dermatitis & Dandruff

- ■ Essentials of Diagnosis
  - • Loose, dry, moist, or greasy scales with or without underlying crusted, pink or yellow-brown plaques
  - • Predilection for scalp, eyebrows, eyelids, nasolabial creases, lips, ears, presternal area, axillae, umbilicus, groin, and gluteal crease
  - • Infantile form on scalp known as cradle cap

- ■ Differential Diagnosis
  - • Psoriasis
  - • Impetigo
  - • Atopic dermatitis
  - • Contact dermatitis
  - • Pityriasis rosea
  - • Tinea versicolor
  - • Pediculosis capitis (head lice)

- ■ Treatment
  - • Selenium sulfide, tar, zinc, or ketoconazole shampoos
  - • Topical corticosteroids
  - • Topical ketoconazole cream
  - • Systemic corticosteroids and antibiotics in selected generalized or severe cases
  - • Patient should be aware that chronic therapy is required to suppress this condition

- ■ Pearl

Seborrheic dermatitis is ubiquitous at presentation in Parkinson's disease and often in severe HIV infection.

Reference

Gupta AK, Madzia SE, Batra R: Etiology and management of seborrheic dermatitis. Dermatology 2004;208:89. [PMID: 15056994]

15

Seborrheic Keratosis

- **Essentials of Diagnosis**
  - Age at onset generally fourth to fifth decades
  - Oval, raised, brown to black, warty, "stuck on"-appearing, well-demarcated papules or plaques; greasy hyperkeratotic scale may be present
  - Usually multiple; some patients have hundreds
  - Chest and back most frequent sites; scalp, face, neck, and extremities also involved
  - Rapid eruptive appearance of numerous lesions (Leser-Trélat sign) may signify internal malignancy

- **Differential Diagnosis**
  - Melanoma
  - Actinic keratosis
  - Nevus
  - Verruca vulgaris
  - Solar lentigo
  - Basal cell carcinoma, pigmented type
  - Squamous cell carcinoma
  - Dermatosis papulosa nigra in dark-skinned patients; numerous small papules on face, neck, and upper chest
  - Stucco keratosis shows hyperkeratotic, gray, verrucous, exophytic papules on the extremities, can be easily scraped off

- **Treatment**
  - Seborrheic keratoses do not require therapy
  - Cryotherapy or curettage effective in removal, may leave dyspigmentation
  - Electrodesiccation and laser therapy

15

- **Pearl**

A public health menace this is not, but look closely at all such lesions to exclude cutaneous malignancies.

Reference

Elgart GW: Seborrheic keratoses, solar lentigines, and lichenoid keratoses. Dermatoscopic features and correlation to histology and clinical signs. Dermatol Clin 2001;19:347. [PMID: 11556243]

Squamous Cell Carcinoma

- **Essentials of Diagnosis**
  - Chronic UV exposure, certain HPV infections, radiation exposure, long-standing scars, certain HIV infections, and chronic immunosuppression predispose
  - Immunosuppressed transplant patients have 250 times the baseline risk
  - Patients with albinism, xeroderma pigmentosum, and epidermodysplasia verruciformis at increased risk
  - Hyperkeratotic, firm, indurated, red or skin-colored papule, plaque, or nodule, most commonly in sun-damaged skin
  - May ulcerate and form crust; many arise in actinic keratoses
  - Lesions confined to the epidermis are squamous cell carcinoma in-situ or Bowen's disease; all others are considered invasive
  - Metastasis infrequent but devastating; lesions on lip or in scars and those with subcutaneous or perineural involvement are at higher risk
  - Regional lymphatics primary route of spread
  - Skin biopsies usually diagnostic

- **Differential Diagnosis**
  - Keratoacanthoma (a rapidly growing and sometimes self-involuting variant of squamous cell carcinoma)
  - Actinic keratosis, hypertrophic form
  - Basal cell carcinoma
  - Verruca vulgaris
  - Chronic nonhealing ulcers due to other causes (venous stasis, infection, etc)

- **Treatment**
  - Simple excision with histologic examination of margins
  - Mohs microsurgery with immediate mapping of margins for high-risk lesions or in areas where tissue conservation is important
  - Curettage and electrodesiccation in small in-situ lesions
  - Ionizing radiation
  - Evaluate patients with aggressive lesions or perineural involvement on histologic examination for metastatic disease
  - Prophylactic radiotherapy in high-risk lesions
  - Regular screening examinations and sun protection

- **Pearl**

The main reason to treat all actinic keratoses; preventing this.

Reference

Sanderson RJ, Ironside JA: Squamous cell carcinomas of the head and neck. BMJ 2002;325:822. [PMID: 12376446]

Tinea Corporis (Ringworm)

■ Essentials of Diagnosis
- Single or multiple circular, sharply circumscribed, erythematous, scaly plaques with elevated borders and central clearing
- Frequently involves neck, extremities, or trunk
- A deep, pustular form affecting the follicles (Majocchi's granuloma) may occur
- Other types affect face (tinea faciei), hands (tinea manuum), feet (tinea pedis), and groin (tinea cruris)
- Skin scrapings for microscopic examination or culture establish diagnosis
- Widespread tinea may be presenting sign of HIV infection

■ Differential Diagnosis
- Pityriasis rosea
- Impetigo
- Nummular dermatitis
- Seborrheic dermatitis
- Psoriasis
- Granuloma annulare
- Secondary syphilis
- Subacute cutaneous lupus erythematosus

■ Treatment
- One or two uncomplicated lesions usually respond to topical antifungals (allylamines or azoles)
- A low-potency steroid cream during initial days of therapy may decrease inflammation
- Oral griseofulvin, itraconazole, or terbinafine are effective in extensive disease, follicular involvement, or in the immunocompromised host
- Infected household pets (especially cats and dogs) may transmit and should be treated

15

■ Pearl

Be wary of combination products containing antifungals and potent steroids; skin atrophy and reduced efficacy may result.

Reference

Gupta AK, Chaudhry M, Elewski B: Tinea corporis, tinea cruris, tinea nigra, and piedra. Dermatol Clin 2003;21:395, v. [PMID: 12956194]

Tinea Versicolor (Pityriasis Versicolor)

- **Essentials of Diagnosis**
  - Finely scaling patches on upper trunk and upper arms, usually asymptomatic
  - Lesions yellowish or brownish on pale skin, or hypopigmented on dark skin
  - Caused by yeast of the genus *Malassezia*
  - Short, thick hyphae and large numbers of spores on microscopic examination
  - Wood's light helpful in defining extent of lesions

- **Differential Diagnosis**
  - Seborrheic dermatitis
  - Pityriasis rosea
  - Pityriasis alba
  - Hansen's disease (leprosy)
  - Secondary syphilis (macular syphilid)
  - Vitiligo
  - Postinflammatory pigmentary alteration from another inflammatory dermatosis

- **Treatment**
  - Topical agents in limited disease (selenium sulfide shampoos or lotions, zinc pyrithione shampoos, imidazole shampoos, topical allylamines)
  - Oral agents in more diffuse involvement (single-dose ketoconazole repeated after 1 week, or 5–7 days of itraconazole)
  - Oral terbinafine not effective
  - Dyspigmentation may persist for months after effective treatment
  - Relapse likely if prophylactic measures not taken; a single monthly application of topical agent may be effective

- **Pearl**

Scrapings resemble "spaghetti and meatballs;" no other disorder does so.

Reference

Gupta AK, Batra R, Bluhm R, Faergemann J: Pityriasis versicolor. Dermatol Clin 2003;21:413, v. [PMID: 12956196]

Urticaria (Hives) & Angioedema

■ Essentials of Diagnosis

- Pale or red, evanescent, edematous papules or plaques surrounded by red halo with severe itching or stinging; appear suddenly and resolve in hours
- Acute (complete remission within 6 weeks) or chronic
- Subcutaneous swelling (angioedema) occurs alone or with urticaria; eyelids and lips often affected; respiratory tract involvement may produce airway obstruction, and gastrointestinal involvement may cause abdominal pain; anaphylaxis possible
- Can be induced by drugs (penicillins, aspirin, other NSAIDs, opioids, radiocontrast dyes, ACE inhibitors)
- Foods a frequent cause of acute urticaria (nuts, strawberries, shellfish, chocolate, tomatoes, melons, pork, garlic, onions, eggs, milk, azo dye additives)
- Infections also a cause (streptococcal upper respiratory infections, viral hepatitis, helminthic infections, or infections of the tonsils, a tooth, sinuses, gallbladder, prostate)

■ Differential Diagnosis

- Hereditary or acquired complement-mediated angioedema
- Physical urticarias (pressure, cold, heat, solar, vibratory, cholinergic, aquagenic)
- Urticarial hypersensitivity reactions to insect bites
- Urticarial vasculitis
- Bullous pemphigoid
- Erythema multiforme
- Granuloma annulare
- Lyme borreliosis (erythema migrans)

■ Treatment

- Treat acute urticaria with antihistamines and avoid identified triggers; short course of prednisone in some cases
- Chronic urticaria treated with antihistamines on a regular rather than as-needed basis; chronic prednisone discouraged
- Nonsedating antihistamines during waking hours
- Work-up to rule out usual triggers

■ Pearl

Angiotensin-converting enzyme (ACE) inhibitor-induced angioedema may occur at any time—even years—after beginning the medicine.

Reference

Dibbern DA Jr, Dreskin SC: Urticaria and angioedema: an overview. Immunol Allergy Clin North Am 2004;24:141, v. [PMID: 15120145]

15

Vitiligo

- **Essentials of Diagnosis**
    - Depigmented white patches surrounded by a normal, hyperpigmented, or occasionally inflamed border
    - Hairs in affected area usually turn white
    - Localized form may or may not be segmental
    - Often treatment resistant
    - Generalized form most common; involvement symmetric and tends to affect skin around orifices
    - Universal form depigments entire body surface
    - Acrofacial form affects the distal fingers and facial orifices
    - Ocular abnormalities (iritis, uveitis, and retinal pigmentary abnormalities) often present
    - Associated with insulin-dependent diabetes, pernicious anemia, autoimmune thyroiditis, alopecia areata, and Addison's disease

- **Differential Diagnosis**
    - Leukoderma associated with metastatic melanoma
    - Occupational vitiligo from phenols or other chemicals
    - Lichen sclerosis
    - Tinea versicolor
    - Pityriasis alba
    - Postinflammatory hypopigmentation
    - Hansen's disease (leprosy)
    - Cutaneous T-cell lymphoma
    - Lupus erythematosus
    - Piebaldism
    - Tuberous sclerosis

- **Treatment**
    - Spontaneous repigmentation infrequently occurs
    - Cosmetic camouflage
    - Potent topical steroids in focal lesions may help repigment; topical tacrolimus and pimecrolimus sometimes effective on the face
    - Psoralen plus UVA may help in generalized disease, but inadvertent burns are common
    - Total permanent depigmentation with monobenzone an option in extensive disease
    - Patient education, emotional support

- **Pearl**

An underappreciated part of the endocrine immunopathies; its presence should call for consideration of thyroid, adrenal, and gastric antibody studies.

Reference

Njoo MD, Westerhof W: Vitiligo. Pathogenesis and treatment. Am J Clin Dermatol 2001;2):167. [PMID: 11705094]

Zoster (Herpes Zoster, Shingles)

- ■ Essentials of Diagnosis
  - Occurs unilaterally within the distribution of a sensory nerve with some spillover into neighboring dermatomes
  - Prodrome of pain and paresthesias followed by papules and plaques of erythema which quickly develop vesicles
  - Vesicles become pustular, crust over, and heal
  - May disseminate (20 or more lesions outside the primary dermatome) in the elderly, debilitated, or immunosuppressed; visceral involvement (lungs, liver, or brain) may follow
  - Involvement of the nasal tip (Hutchinson's sign) a harbinger of ophthalmic zoster
  - Ramsay Hunt syndrome (ipsilateral facial paralysis, zoster of the ear, and auditory symptoms) from facial and auditory nerve involvement
  - Postherpetic neuralgia more common in older patients
  - Tzanck smears useful but cannot differentiate zoster from zosteriform herpes simplex
  - Direct fluorescent antibody test rapid and specific

- ■ Differential Diagnosis
  - Herpes simplex infection
  - Prodromal pain can mimic the pain of angina, duodenal ulcer, appendicitis, and biliary or renal colic
  - Zoster 30 times more common in the HIV-infected; ascertain HIV risk factors

- ■ Treatment
  - Heat or topical anesthetics locally
  - Therapy with acyclovir, famciclovir, or valacyclovir
  - Intravenous acyclovir for disseminated or ocular zoster
  - Bed rest to reduce risk of neuralgia in the elderly
  - Prednisone does not prevent neuralgia
  - Topical capsaicin, local anesthetics, nerve blocks, analgesics, tricyclic antidepressants, and gabapentin for postherpetic neuralgia
  - Patients with active lesions should avoid contact with neonates and immunosuppressed individuals

15

- ■ Pearl

"Shingles"—the word—is a linguistic corruption from Latin cingulum ("girdle"), reflecting the common thoracic presentation of this disorder.

Reference

Johnson RW, Dworkin RH: Treatment of herpes zoster and postherpetic neuralgia. BMJ 2003;326:748. [PMID: 12676845]

Gynecologic, Obstetric, & Breast Disorders

Abnormal Uterine Bleeding

- **Essentials of Diagnosis**
  - Excessive menses, intermenstrual bleeding, or both; post-menopausal bleeding
  - Common soon after menarche, 4–6 years premenopause

- **Differential Diagnosis**
  - Pregnancy (especially ectopic), spontaneous abortion
  - Anovulation (eg, polycystic ovaries, hypothyroidism)
  - Uterine myoma or carcinoma, polyp, trauma
  - Cervicitis, carcinoma of the cervix
  - Adenomyosis
  - Exogenous hormones (eg, unopposed estrogen, depo-medroxyprogesterone acetate, oral contraceptives)
  - Coagulation disorders (eg, von Willebrand's disease)

- **Treatment**
  - Papanicolaou smear (all ages) and endometrial biopsy (all post-menopausal women and those over age 35 with chronic anovulation or more than 6 months of bleeding)
  - Active bleeding with significant anemia: High-dose estrogen (25 mg intravenously or oral contraceptive taper; two pills twice daily for 3 days tapering over 2 weeks to one daily); high-dose progestin when high-dose estrogen contraindicated
  - Chronic bleeding: NSAIDs (any type, around the clock for 5 days) plus oral contraceptives, levonorgestrel intrauterine system, or cyclic progestin
  - Hysterectomy, uterine artery embolization or endometrial ablation for bleeding refractory to hormonal therapy
  - Hysterectomy if endometrial cancer, hyperplasia with atypia

- **Pearl**

If a reproductive-aged woman has abnormal bleeding, a pregnancy test is the obligatory first test.

Reference

Munro MG: Dysfunctional uterine bleeding: advances in diagnosis and treatment. Curr Opin Obstet Gynecol 2001;13:475.

Amenorrhea

- **Essentials of Diagnosis**
  - Absence of menses for over 3 cycles in women with past menses (secondary); absence of menarche by age 16 (primary)
  - May be anatomic, ovarian, or hypothalamic-pituitary-ovarian
  - Anatomic causes: congenital anomalies of the uterus, imperforate hymen, cervical stenosis
  - Ovarian failure: causes include autoimmune diseases, Turner's syndrome, ovarian dysgenesis, radiation or chemotherapy
  - Hypothalamic-pituitary-ovarian causes most common; include hyperandrogenic disorders, hypothalamic anovulation, hyperprolactinemia, hypothyroidism, and hypothalamic or pituitary lesions
  - Exclude pregnancy; measure TSH, prolactin
  - Check for withdrawal bleeding after progestin (10 mg medroxyprogesterone acetate for 10 days); bleeding indicates that the ovarian estrogen, normal uterus, and outflow tract are intact; no bleeding suggests hypothalamic-pituitary causes, premature ovarian failure
  - FSH and LH to evaluate for premature ovarian failure
  - Dehydroepiandrosterone sulfate and testosterone only in women with clitoromegaly, other signs of masculinization
  - Polycystic ovary syndrome is a diagnosis of exclusion; withdrawal bleeding, hirsutism, acne, insulin resistance

- **Differential Diagnosis**
  - Pregnancy
  - Physiologic (adolescence, perimenopause)
  - Causes as outlined above

- **Treatment**
  - Polycystic ovarian syndrome: oral contraceptives for cycle regularity decrease the risk of endometrial cancer; weight loss to induce spontaneous ovulation
  - Hypoestrogenic causes: treat underlying disorder (eg, anorexia); estrogen treatment to prevent osteoporosis
  - Hyperprolactinemia: surgery for macroadenoma, otherwise treat with bromocriptine or expectant management

16

- **Pearl**

Despite an extensive differential, three processes top the list: pregnancy, pregnancy, and pregnancy.

Reference

Gordon CM, Nelson LM: Amenorrhea and bone health in adolescents and young women. Curr Opin Obstet Gynecol 2003;15:377.

Cervical Dysplasia

- **Essentials of Diagnosis**
  - Risk factors: Early intercourse and multiple partners
  - Includes low- and high-grade squamous intraepithelial lesions or cervical intraepithelial neoplasia (CIN 1–3)
  - Seventy-five percent of low-grade (CIN 1) regress spontaneously; only 35% of high-grade (CIN 2–3) regress
  - Atypical squamous cells of undetermined significance (ASCUS) associated with underlying dysplasia in 10%; other causes are benign reparative changes, inflammation
  - Atypical glandular cells of undetermined significance (AGUS, AGCUS) associated with significant abnormality (eg, endometrial hyperplasia, adenocarcinoma, or high-grade dysplasia) in 40%
  - Over 90% of squamous dysplasia and cancer due to sexually transmitted infection with human papillomavirus (HPV)
  - Colposcopy confirms and excludes invasive cancer

- **Differential Diagnosis**
  - Inflammation due to vaginitis, cervicitis, or atrophy
  - Inaccurate interpretation of cytology or histology

- **Treatment**
  - Excision (loop electrosurgical excision procedure, cone biopsy) or ablation (cryotherapy, laser) for high-grade lesions and persistent low-grade lesions
  - Atypical cells: If atypical, favor dysplasia and perform colposcopy; if inflammatory, treat vaginitis or atrophy when suspected
  - Repeat Pap smear every 4–6 months until three consecutive normal results are reported; routine screening thereafter; or HPV typing can be used to triage ASCUS: Colposcopy if positive for high-risk HPV; routine screening if negative
  - Low-grade lesions: Colposcopy with biopsy confirms diagnosis; expectant management versus ablation or excision
  - High-grade lesions: Colposcopy with biopsy to confirm diagnosis; treat with ablation or excision
  - Atypical glandular cells: Colposcopy, endocervical curettage, and if abnormal bleeding is present, endometrial biopsy

- **Pearl**

Do not confuse atypical glandular cells with atypical squamous cells: the former may indicate malignancy.

Reference

Wright TC, Jr., Schiffman M, Solomon D et al: Interim guidance for the use of human papillomavirus DNA testing as an adjunct to cervical cytology for screening. Obstet Gynecol 2004;103:304.

16

Chronic Pelvic Pain

- ■ Essentials of Diagnosis
  - Subacute pelvic pain of more than 6 months' duration
  - Etiology often multifactorial
  - Up to 40% have been physically or sexually abused
  - Pain that resolves with ovulation suppression suggests gynecologic cause; some nongynecologic conditions also improve with ovulation suppression
  - Concomitant depression very common
  - Ultrasound and physical exam often not diagnostic
  - Half of women who undergo laparoscopy have no visible pathology

- ■ Differential Diagnosis
  - Gynecologic: Endometriosis, adenomyosis, pelvic adhesions, prior PID or chronic PID, leiomyomas
  - Gastrointestinal: Irritable bowel syndrome, inflammatory bowel disease, diverticular disease, constipation, neoplasia, hernia
  - Urologic: Detrusor overactivity, interstitial cystitis, urinary calculi, urethral syndrome, bladder carcinoma
  - Musculoskeletal: Myofascial pain, low back pain, disk problems, nerve entrapment, muscle strain or spasm
  - Psychiatric: Somatization, depression, physical or sexual abuse, anxiety

- ■ Treatment
  - Evaluate for and treat the above causes, including psychiatric
  - NSAIDs; avoid opioids
  - Ovulation suppression with oral contraceptives, depomedroxyprogesterone acetate, or a short course of leuprolide acetate can be both diagnostic and therapeutic
  - Diagnostic laparoscopy if gynecologic cause is suspected, medical management fails, or diagnosis remains in question
  - Hysterectomy with bilateral oophorectomy for refractory gynecologic pain in women who have completed childbearing

16

- ■ Pearl
  One of the most challenging conditions in all of gynecology; therapy is often not gratifying.

Reference
Scialli AR: Evaluating chronic pelvic pain. A consensus recommendation. Pelvic Pain Expert Working Group. J Reprod Med 1999;44:945. [PMID: 10589405]

Dysmenorrhea

- **Essentials of Diagnosis**
  - Occurs in 50% of menstruating women
  - Low, midline, cramping pelvic pain radiating to back or legs; pain starting before or with menses, peaking after 24 hours, and subsiding after 2 days; often associated with nausea, diarrhea, headache, and flushing
  - Primary dysmenorrhea: Pain without pelvic pathology and beginning within 1–2 years after menarche
  - Secondary dysmenorrhea: Pain with underlying pathology such as endometriosis or adenomyosis, developing years after menarche

- **Differential Diagnosis**
  - Endometriosis
  - Adenomyosis
  - Uterine myoma
  - Cervical stenosis, uterine anomalies
  - Chronic endometritis or pelvic inflammatory disease
  - Copper intrauterine device

- **Treatment**
  - NSAIDs or COX-2 inhibitors prior to the onset of bleeding, continued for 2–3 days
  - Suppression of ovulation with oral contraceptives, depomedroxyprogesterone acetate, or levonorgestrel intrauterine system
  - In secondary dysmenorrhea, laparoscopy may be needed diagnostically
  - Hysterectomy with or without bilateral salpingo-oophorectomy for severe refractory dysmenorrhea

16

- **Pearl**

Endometriosis is the most important cause in younger women; think adenomyosis if they're older.

Reference

Deligeoroglou E: Dysmenorrhea. Ann N Y Acad Sci 2000;900:237.

Ectopic Pregnancy

■ Essentials of Diagnosis

- Pregnancy implantation outside uterine cavity
- Occurs in 2% of pregnancies; most commonly presents 6–8 weeks after last menstrual period
- Symptoms of pregnancy, missed menstrual period, vaginal bleeding or spotting
- Pelvic pain may be absent, mild, or significant
- Tenderness on pelvic or abdominal examination; adnexal mass sometimes palpable
- Cardiovascular collapse, shock with rupture in some
- Serum β-hCG fails to rise appropriately during follow-up
- Transvaginal ultrasound to identify intrauterine gestation when β-hCG is above about 2000 mU/mL; an empty uterine cavity when β-hCG > 2000 is highly suspicious
- Transvaginal ultrasound often cannot demonstrate an extrauterine pregnancy
- Diagnosis confirmed by lack of placental villi after suction curettage or by laparoscopy

■ Differential Diagnosis

- Intrauterine pregnancy (threatened abortion)
- Ruptured corpus luteum cyst
- Appendicitis
- Pelvic inflammatory disease (rare during pregnancy)
- Gestational trophoblastic neoplasia
- Urinary calculi

■ Treatment

- Suction curettage
- Methotrexate for compliant patients with small, unruptured ectopic pregnancies
- Surgical removal of larger or complicated ectopic pregnancies
- Emergent laparotomy if hemodynamically unstable with acute abdomen
- Rh_o immune globulin to Rh-negative patients
- Periodically repeat β-hCG until it falls to nonpregnant level
- Early ultrasound confirmation of future pregnancies (repeat ectopic pregnancy occurs in about 10% of cases)

16

■ Pearl

Shock of unapparent cause in a reproductive-aged woman is ruptured ectopic until proven otherwise.

Reference

Della-Giustina D, Denny M: Ectopic pregnancy. Emerg Med Clin North Am 2003;21:565.

Endometriosis

■ Essentials of Diagnosis
- Seen in 10% of all menstruating women, 25% of infertile women
- Progressive, recurrent, characterized by aberrant growth of endometrium outside the uterus
- Classic triad: Cyclic pelvic pain, dysmenorrhea, and dyspareunia
- May be associated with infertility or pelvic mass (endometrioma)
- Pelvic examination may or may not be normal
- Hematochezia, painful defecation, or hematuria if bowel or bladder invaded
- Ultrasound often normal
- Laparoscopy confirms diagnosis

■ Differential Diagnosis
- Other causes of chronic pelvic pain
- Primary dysmenorrhea
- Adenomyosis

■ Treatment
- NSAIDs
- Ovulation suppression with continuous oral contraceptives until fertility is desired; second line: Progestin-only methods (depo-medroxyprogesterone acetate, levonorgestrel intrauterine system)
- If OCPs ineffective, GnRH analogs (eg, leuprolide) with add-back estrogen can be used for up to 6 months followed by continuous OCPs
- Laparoscopy with ablation of lesions for refractory pain helpful in up to two-thirds of patients; 50% recur
- Hysterectomy with bilateral salpingo-oophorectomy for those who have completed childbearing

■ Pearl

The only benign disease in medicine which behaves like metastatic carcinoma; endometriosis can occur anywhere in the body, including fingers, lungs, and other organs.

Reference

Mahutte NG, Arici A: Medical management of endometriosis-associated pain. Obstet Gynecol Clin North Am 2003;30:133.

Mammary Dysplasia (Fibrocystic Disease)

- ■ Essentials of Diagnosis
  - • Common age 30–50
  - • Painful, often multiple, usually bilateral masses in the breasts
  - • Rapid fluctuation in size of masses
  - • Pain, increase in size during premenstrual phase of cycle
  - • Rare in postmenopausal women not on hormonal therapy
  - • Eighty percent of women have histologic fibrocystic changes

- ■ Differential Diagnosis
  - • Breast carcinoma
  - • Fibroadenoma
  - • Fat necrosis
  - • Intraductal papilloma

- ■ Treatment
  - • A diagnostic work-up of any dominant mass is necessary
  - • Biopsy (fine-needle aspiration or core needle biopsy) to exclude carcinoma and determine if cystic or solid
  - • In women less than 35, ultrasound can be used instead of biopsy to differentiate cystic from solid masses
  - • Mammography in women older than 40
  - • Frequent follow-up of all women with breast masses even if work-up is negative
  - • For breast thickening or ill-defined masses, follow-up breast exam in different stage of menstrual cycle
  - • For mastalgia: Supportive brassiere (night and day), NSAIDs, oral contraceptives; for severe pain, danazol (100–200 mg bid), bromocriptine (2.5 mg bid) or tamoxifen (10 mg/day)

- ■ Pearl

All women fear breast cancer in this condition: medical management is only one part of the therapy.

16

Reference

Hindle WH: Breast mass evaluation. Clin Obstet Gynecol 2002;45:750.

Menopausal Syndrome

- ■ Essentials of Diagnosis
  - • Cessation of menses without other cause, usually due to aging or bilateral oophorectomy
  - • Average age is 51; earlier in women who smoke
  - • Perimenopause: Declining ovarian function over 4–6 years
  - • Menstrual irregularity, hot flushes, night sweats, vaginal dryness
  - • Elevated serum FSH and LH

- ■ Differential Diagnosis
  - • Other causes of amenorrhea, especially pregnancy
  - • Hyperthyroidism or hypothyroidism
  - • Pheochromocytoma
  - • Uterine neoplasm
  - • Sjögren's syndrome
  - • Depression
  - • Anorexia

- ■ Treatment
  - • Short-term hormonal therapy to treat hot flushes; second-line therapies include megestrol acetate, clonidine, SSRIs and gabapentin
  - • Hot flushes often resolve by 2–4 years after menopause
  - • For irregular bleeding in the perimenopause, oral contraceptives, levonorgestrel intrauterine system, cyclic or combined continuous estrogen plus progestin, or progestins alone
  - • Estrogen cream and nonhormonal lubricants for vaginal dryness
  - • Although long-term use of combined hormonal therapy decreases osteoporosis and colon cancer, it increases the risk of breast cancer and thromboembolism

- ■ Pearl

16

Sleep disturbances are an often overlooked symptom of menopause; short-term hormonal therapy may help.

Reference

Fitzpatrick LA: Alternatives to estrogen. Med Clin North Am 2003;87:1091.

Mucopurulent Cervicitis

■ Essentials of Diagnosis

- A sexually transmitted infection most commonly caused by *Neisseria gonorrhoeae* or *Chlamydia;* endocervical inflammation can result from herpesvirus, *Trichomonas,* or *Candida*
- Usually asymptomatic but may have abnormal vaginal discharge, or postcoital bleeding
- Red, friable cervix with purulent, often blood-streaked endocervical discharge
- Must be distinguished from physiologic ectopy of columnar epithelium common in young women

■ Differential Diagnosis

- Pelvic inflammatory disease
- Cervical carcinoma or dysplasia
- Cervical ulcer secondary to syphilis, chancroid, or granuloma inguinale
- Normal epithelial ectopy
- Cervical inflammation due to vaginal infection

■ Treatment

- In general, treat only if tests are positive for *N gonorrhoeae* or *Chlamydia;* empirically in a high-risk or noncompliant patient
- Gonorrhea: Ceftriaxone 125 mg IM or cefixime 400 mg po
- Chlamydia: Azithromycin 1 g single dose or doxycycline 100 mg bid for 14 days (once pregnancy excluded)
- Sexual abstinence until treatment completed; provide or refer partner for therapy

■ Pearl

All patients with cervicitis should be tested for HIV, syphilis, and hepatitis C, no matter the history.

16

Reference

Miller KE, Ruiz DE, Graves JC: Update on the prevention and treatment of sexually transmitted diseases. Am Fam Physician 2003;67:1915.

Myoma of the Uterus
(Fibroid Tumor, Leiomyoma, Fibromyoma)

- ■ Essentials of Diagnosis
  - Irregular enlargement of uterus caused by benign smooth muscle tumors
  - Occurs in 40–50% of women over age 40
  - May be asymptomatic or cause heavy or irregular vaginal bleeding, anemia, urinary frequency, pelvic pressure, dysmenorrhea
  - Acute pelvic pain rare
  - May be intramural, submucosal, subserosal, cervical, or parasitic (ie, deriving its blood supply from an adjacent organ)
  - Pelvic ultrasound confirms diagnosis

- ■ Differential Diagnosis
  - Pregnancy
  - Adenomyosis
  - Ovarian or adnexal mass
  - Abnormal uterine bleeding due to other causes
  - Leiomyosarcoma
  - Renal infarct
  - Tamoxifen therapy

- ■ Treatment
  - Exclude pregnancy
  - Papanicolaou smear and endometrial biopsy (if > 35 and irregular bleeding)
  - NSAIDs to reduce blood loss; hormonal therapy to reduce endometrial volume (oral contraceptives, depo-medroxyprogesterone acetate, levonorgestrel intrauterine system)
  - GnRH agonists for 3–6 months for women planning surgery or nearing menopause
  - Medical therapies often ineffective for large or submucosal myomas; resection or hysterectomy may be necessary

16

- ■ Pearl

Bleeding associated with fibroids is often due to infarction; serum CPK and LDH elevation may be diagnostic.

Reference

Manyonda I, Sinthamoney E, Belli AM: Controversies and challenges in the modern management of uterine fibroids. BJOG 2004;111:95.

Pelvic Inflammatory Disease
(PID, Salpingitis, Endometritis, Tubo-ovarian Abscess)

- **Essentials of Diagnosis**

  - Most common in young, sexually active women with multiple partners
  - Upper genital tract associated with *Neisseria gonorrhoeae* and *Chlamydia trachomatis,* anaerobes, *Haemophilus influenzae,* enteric gram-negative rods, and streptococci
  - A major cause of chronic pelvic pain, infertility and pelvic adhesions
  - Symptoms and severity vary from asymptomatic to toxic
  - Lower abdominal, adnexal, cervical motion tenderness; fever, abnormal cervical discharge, leukocytosis
  - Absence of competing diagnosis
  - Right upper quadrant pain (Fitz-Hugh and Curtis syndrome) from associated perihepatitis
  - Pelvic ultrasound may reveal a tubo-ovarian abscess
  - Laparoscopy for cases with uncertain diagnosis or no improvement despite antibiotic therapy

- **Differential Diagnosis**

  - Any cause of acute abdominal-pelvic pain or peritonitis
  - Appendicitis, diverticulitis
  - Ruptured ovarian cyst, ovarian torsion
  - Ectopic pregnancy
  - Acute cystitis, urinary calculi

- **Treatment**

  - Oral antibiotics for mild cases (14-day course) covering *N gonorrhoeae* and *Chlamydia* (ceftriaxone 250 mg IM plus doxycycline 100 mg bid for 14 days)
  - Hospitalization and intravenous antibiotics for toxic, adolescent, HIV-infected, or pregnant patients
  - Surgical drainage of tubo-ovarian abscess
  - Screen for HIV, hepatitis, syphilis
  - Sexual abstinence until treatment completed; partner should be treated

16

- **Pearl**

Do not rely on cervical cultures; often negative, they should not be used to guide management.

Reference

Beigi RH, Wiesenfeld HC: Pelvic inflammatory disease: new diagnostic criteria and treatment. Obstet Gynecol Clin North Am 2003;30:777.

Pelvic Organ Prolapse

- **Essentials of Diagnosis**
  - Common in older multiparous women as a delayed result of childbirth injury to pelvic floor
  - Includes prolapse of the uterus, bladder, rectum, small bowel, or vaginal cuff
  - Often asymptomatic; may have pelvic pressure or pulling, vaginal bulge, low back pain; difficulties with sexual function, defecation, or voiding
  - Pelvic examination confirms the diagnosis
  - Prolapse may be slight, moderate, or marked
  - Attenuation of pelvic structures with aging can accelerate development

- **Differential Diagnosis**
  - Vaginal or cervical neoplasm
  - Rectal prolapse
  - Rectal carcinoma

- **Treatment**
  - Supportive measures (eg, Kegel exercises), limit straining and lifting
  - Treat predisposing factors such as obesity, obstructive airway disease, constipation, and pelvic masses
  - Conjugated estrogen creams to decrease vaginal irritation
  - Pessaries may reduce prolapse and its symptoms; ineffective for very large prolapse
  - Corrective surgery for symptomatic prolapse that significantly affects quality of life

- **Pearl**

16

Ulcerations of the protruding cervix or vagina should be biopsied; prolapse does not exclude malignancy.

Reference

Thakar R, Stanton S: Management of genital prolapse. BMJ 2002;324:1258.

Preeclampsia-Eclampsia

- **Essentials of Diagnosis**
  - Progressive, multisystem condition affecting 5–10% of pregnant women
  - Preeclampsia is hypertension plus proteinuria; addition of seizures means eclampsia
  - Headache, blurred vision or scotomas, right upper quadrant pain, altered mental status
  - Intrauterine growth restriction, oligohydramnios
  - Funduscopic evidence of acute hypertension, hyperreflexia; encephalopathy
  - Thrombocytopenia, elevated AST or ALT, hemoconcentration or hemolysis
  - Pulmonary edema, oliguria, or DIC can occur
  - HELLP syndrome: Hemolysis, elevated liver enzymes, and low platelets
  - Increased in primiparas and patients with history of preeclampsia, hypertension, diabetes, chronic renal disease, autoimmune disorders

- **Differential Diagnosis**
  - Chronic hypertension due to other cause
  - Chronic renal disease due to other cause
  - Primary seizure disorder
  - Hemolytic-uremic syndrome
  - Thrombotic thrombocytopenic purpura

- **Treatment**
  - The only treatment is delivery of the fetus
  - Induce labor for severe disease regardless of gestational age
  - Remote from term, mild cases can be observed in the hospital with induction of labor for worsening disease; at term, mild cases should have labor induced
  - Antihypertensives if blood pressure > 180/110 mm Hg; goal is 150/90 mm Hg
  - For eclampsia, intravenous magnesium sulfate to prevent recurrent seizures

16

- **Pearl**

Deliver the baby, cure the disease.

Reference

Visser W et al: Prediction and prevention of pregnancy-induced hypertensive disorders. Baillieres Best Pract Res Clin Obstet Gynaecol 1999;13:131. [PMID: 10746098]

Puerperal Mastitis

- ■ **Essentials of Diagnosis**
  - • Occurs in nursing mothers within 3 months after delivery
  - • Unilateral inflammation of breast or one quadrant of breast
  - • Sore or fissured nipple with surrounding redness, tenderness, induration, warmth, fever, malaise
  - • Increased incidence in first-time mothers
  - • *Staphylococcus aureus* and streptococci are usual causative agents
  - • May progress to breast abscess
  - • Ultrasound can confirm abscess diagnosis

- ■ **Differential Diagnosis**
  - • Local irritation or trauma
  - • Nondraining duct
  - • Benign or malignant tumors (inflammatory carcinoma)
  - • Subareolar abscess (occurs in nonlactating women)
  - • Fat necrosis

- ■ **Treatment**
  - • For very mild cases, warm compresses and increased frequency of breastfeeding
  - • Oral dicloxacillin or first-generation cephalosporin
  - • Hospitalize for intravenous antibiotics if no improvement in 48 hours in toxic patients
  - • Increase frequency of breastfeeding
  - • Incision and drainage for abscess; stop breastfeeding from affected breast (may pump milk and discard)

- ■ **Pearl**

Women with this disorder may appear surprisingly toxic systemically, diverting attention from the diagnosis.

16

Reference

Marchant DJ: Inflammation of the breast. Obstet Gynecol Clin North Am 2002;29:89.

Spontaneous Abortion

- ■ Essentials of Diagnosis
  - Vaginal bleeding, pelvic pain and cramping before the 20th week of pregnancy
  - Occurs in up to 20% of pregnancies
  - Threatened abortion: Pregnancy may continue or abortion may ensue; cervix closed, bleeding and cramping mild, intrauterine pregnancy confirmed
  - Inevitable or incomplete abortion: Cervix dilated and products of conception may or may not be partially expelled; brisk uterine bleeding
  - Complete abortion: Products of conception completely expelled; cervix closed, cramping and bleeding decreased
  - Missed abortion (blighted ovum): Failed pregnancy detected by ultrasound; cervix closed, absent or minimal bleeding and cramping
  - Serum β-hCG fails to rise appropriately (except in threatened abortion)
  - Pelvic ultrasonography contraindicated when bleeding heavy or cervix open because it delays treatment

- ■ Differential Diagnosis
  - Ectopic pregnancy
  - Menorrhagia, menses, prolapsed uterine myoma
  - Gestational trophoblastic neoplasia
  - Cervical neoplasm or lesion

- ■ Treatment
  - Follow hematocrit closely
  - Confirm intrauterine pregnancy with ultrasound; if unable to confirm intrauterine location, follow closely until ectopic pregnancy is ruled out
  - Threatened abortion: β-hCG in 2–3 days; immediate follow-up if brisk bleeding develops
  - Limiting activity ineffective
  - Inevitable or incomplete abortion: Immediate suction curettage
  - Missed abortion: Suction curettage or wait for spontaneous abortion
  - Rh_o immune globulin to Rh-negative mothers
  - Follow-up to ensure patient is no longer pregnant

16

- ■ Pearl

Although this condition is common, this presentation is ectopic pregnancy until proved otherwise.

Reference

Creinin MD, Schwartz JL, Guido RS, Pymar HC: Early pregnancy failure–current management concepts. Obstet Gynecol Surv 2001;56:105.

Urinary Incontinence

- **Essentials of Diagnosis**
    - Uncontrolled loss of urine; classified as stress, urge, mixed, or overflow
    - Stress incontinence: urine loss during coughing or exercising; leakage observed on examination during cough or with Valsalva's maneuver
    - Urge incontinence due to spontaneous bladder contractions; accompanied by urgency, associated with frequency and nocturia, normal examination
    - Overflow incontinence is very unusual in women and is caused by overdistention of bladder due to neurologic lesion or outflow obstruction; postvoid residual markedly elevated
    - Urinary tract infections commonly cause transient incontinence or worsening of preexisting incontinence
    - Urodynamic evaluation indicated when diagnosis is uncertain or prior to surgical correction

- **Differential Diagnosis**
    - Urinary tract infection
    - Mobility disorders affecting ability to get to the toilet
    - Neurologic causes as outlined above
    - Urinary fistula, urethral diverticulum
    - Medications: diuretics, anticholinergics, antihistamines, α-adrenergic blockers

- **Treatment**
    - Exclude urinary tract infection
    - A diary of voiding aids in diagnosis and guides therapy
    - Kegel exercises, formal training of the pelvic muscles (biofeedback)
    - For urge incontinence: timed voids, limit fluid intake and caffeine, anticholinergic medications (oxybutynin chloride, tolterodine)
    - Surgical treatment is effective in up to 85% for stress incontinence refractory to conservative management

- **Pearl**

Urinary incontinence is socially isolating and depressing; treatment is simple, and quality of life is enhanced.

Reference

Sutherland SE, Goldman HB: Treatment options for female urinary incontinence. Med Clin North Am 2004;88:345.

16

Vaginitis

- **Essentials of Diagnosis**
  - Vaginal burning, pain, pruritus, discharge
  - Results from atrophy, infection, or allergic reaction
  - Common infectious causes include *Candida albicans, Trichomonas vaginalis,* bacterial vaginosis (*Gardnerella* and other anaerobes)
  - *Trichomonas* is sexually transmitted and causes profuse, malodorous discharge and vaginal irritation
  - Bacterial vaginosis may be asymptomatic or associated with a thin, gray, "fishy" discharge
  - *C albicans* associated with pruritus, burning, and a thick, white, nonmalodorous discharge
  - Wet mount with KOH, saline, and pH are usually diagnostic: Trichomonads are motile, pH > 4.5; bacterial vaginosis reveals clue cells, pH > 4.5; hyphae and spores with a normal pH (< 4.5) mean *Candida*

- **Differential Diagnosis**
  - Physiologic discharge, ovulation
  - Atrophic vaginitis, vulvar dystrophies (lichen sclerosis), and vulvar neoplasia in older women
  - Cervicitis, syphilis, herpesvirus outbreak
  - Cervical carcinoma
  - Foreign body (retained tampon)
  - Contact dermatitis (eg, condoms, perfumed products, soap)
  - Pubic lice, scabies

- **Treatment**
  - Limit vaginal irritants
  - Culture cervix for *Neisseria gonorrhoeae* and *Chlamydia* if no other cause for symptoms
  - For *T vaginalis:* Metronidazole (2 g as a single dose) for both patient and partner
  - For *C albicans:* Antifungal (eg, clotrimazole) vaginal cream or suppository or single-dose oral fluconazole (150 mg)
  - For bacterial vaginosis: Metronidazole (500 mg twice daily for 7 days or vaginal gel twice daily for 5 days)
  - For atrophic vaginitis, estrogen cream per vagina twice per week

16

- **Pearl**

Symptoms alone do not diagnose vaginitis; a wet mount must be done in all.

Reference

Egan ME et al: Diagnosis of vaginitis. Am Fam Physician 2000;62:1095. [PMID: 10997533]

Common Surgical Disorders

Abdominal Aortic Aneurysm

- **Essentials of Diagnosis**
  - More than 90% originate below the renal arteries
  - Most asymptomatic, discovered incidentally
  - Back or abdominal pain often precedes rupture
  - Diameter is the most important predictor of aneurysm rupture (up to a 40% risk of rupture over 5 years for aneurysms > 5 cm)
  - Most rupture leftward and posteriorly; left knee jerk disappears
  - Generalized arteriomegaly in many patients (many with associated iliac artery, femoral, or popliteal aneurysms)

- **Differential Diagnosis**
  - Pancreatic pseudocyst, pancreatitis
  - Multiple myeloma
  - Renal colic
  - Penetrating (posterior) duodenal ulcer

- **Treatment**
  - In asymptomatic healthy patients, surgery is recommended when the aneurysm is > 5 cm
  - Resection may be beneficial even for aneurysms as small as 4 cm (high-risk aneurysms are ulcerated or saccular)
  - In symptomatic patients, immediate repair regardless of size
  - Endovascular repair (transfemoral insertion of a prosthetic graft) considered if the anatomy of aneurysm is suitable; durability unknown

- **Pearl**

In brisk upper gastrointestinal hemorrhage in patients over age 60 with a normal upper endoscopy, consider aortoenteric fistula.

Reference

Brewster DC, Cronenwett JL, Hallett JW Jr, et al; Joint Council of the American Association for Vascular Surgery and Society for Vascular Surgery: Guidelines for the treatment of abdominal aortic aneurysms. J Vasc Surg 2003;37:1106. [PMID: 12756363]

Acute Appendicitis

- **Essentials of Diagnosis**
    - Consider in all patients with unexplained abdominal pain; 6% of the population will have appendicitis in their lifetime
    - Anorexia invariable
    - Abdominal pain, onset not abrupt, initially poorly localized or periumbilical, then focal in the right lower quadrant over 4–48 hours in two-thirds of patients
    - Low-grade fever, right lower quadrant tenderness at McBurney's point with or without peritoneal signs
    - Pelvic and rectal examinations may reveal tenderness
    - Mild leukocytosis (10,000–18,000/µL) with PMN predominance; if WBC > 18,000/mL, rupture with localized abscess or phlegmon should be considered
    - Microscopic hematuria or pyuria common
    - Consider pelvic ultrasound (in women) and CT scan to differentiate from nonsurgical conditions

- **Differential Diagnosis**
    - Gynecologic pathology (eg, ectopic pregnancy, pelvic inflammatory disease, endometriosis, mittelschmerz, ovarian torsion)
    - Urologic pathology (eg, testicular torsion)
    - Nephrolithiasis
    - Urinary tract infection or pyelonephritis
    - Perforated peptic ulcer
    - Crohn's disease
    - Meckel's diverticulitis
    - Mesenteric adenitis
    - Acute cholecystitis
    - Right lower lobe pneumonia

- **Treatment**
    - Open or laparoscopic appendectomy
    - CT guided drainage of localized abscess for an abscess or phlegmon with interval appendectomy
    - Certainty in diagnosis remains elusive (10–30% of patients are found to have a normal appendix at operation)
    - When diagnosis unclear, observe for several hours with serial examinations, or (if the patient is reliable) schedule return in 8–12 hours for reevaluation

17

- **Pearl**

The most common cause of the acute abdomen in every decade of life.

Reference

Shelton T, McKinlay R, Schwartz RW: Acute appendicitis: current diagnosis and treatment. Curr Surg 2003;60:502. [PMID: 14972214]

Acute Cholecystitis

■ Essentials of Diagnosis
- Abrupt onset of steady right upper quadrant or midabdominal pain; nausea, food intolerance common
- Classic finding is Murphy's sign, an inspiratory arrest with palpation in the right upper quadrant
- Fever, leukocytosis, slight elevation in liver function studies, and occasionally an elevation in amylase and lipase
- Biliary colic and acute cholecystitis often overlap; clinical distinction may be difficult
- Abdominal ultrasound is the diagnostic procedure of choice, showing stones, ductal anatomy, and inflammation (thickened gallbladder wall and pericholecystic fluid); however, may be acalculous
- Radionuclide (HIDA) scan shows a nonopacified gallbladder and diagnoses acute cholecystitis accurately in 97% of cases

■ Differential Diagnosis
- Acute appendicitis
- Acute pancreatitis
- Peptic ulcer disease
- Acute hepatitis
- Right lower lobe pneumonia
- Myocardial infarction
- Radicular pain in thoracic dermatome, eg, preeruptive zoster

■ Treatment
- Bowel rest, intravenous fluids, and analgesics; parenteral antibiotics to cover coliform organisms
- Early laparoscopic cholecystectomy leads to reduced morbidity and mortality
- Immediate cholecystectomy for gallbladder ischemia, perforation, emphysematous cholecystitis; percutaneously placed cholecystostomy catheters used initially in severely ill or patients with high surgical risk
- Endoscopic retrograde cholangiopancreatography (ERCP) with sphincterotomy performed when there are associated common bile duct stones, pancreatitis, or cholangitis

■ Pearl
In cholecystitis, the patient precisely identifies the time of onset of symptoms; not so in appendicitis.

Reference

Yusoff IF, Barkun JS, Barkun AN: Diagnosis and management of cholecystitis and cholangitis. Gastroenterol Clin North Am 2003;32:1145. [PMID: 14696301]

17

Acute Lower Extremity Arterial Occlusion

- **Essentials of Diagnosis**
  - Typical patient has valvular, hypertensive, or ischemic heart disease, often peripheral vascular disease as well
  - Some occur following posterior knee dislocation, iatrogenic catheter injury, placement of femoral arterial line
  - Abrupt onset of pain, dysesthesia
  - Classic symptoms and signs recalled easily using the 5 P's: Pulseless, pallor, paresthesias, paralysis, poikilothermia
  - Occasional atrial fibrillation on cardiac examination
  - Leukocytosis; elevated CK and LDH

- **Differential Diagnosis**
  - Neuropathic pain
  - Deep venous thrombosis
  - Reflex sympathetic dystrophy
  - Systemic vasculitis
  - Cholesterol atheroembolic syndrome

- **Treatment**
  - Surgical embolectomy
  - Thrombolytics for patients with preexisting peripheral vascular occlusive disease with delayed surgical bypass as needed
  - Fasciotomy if compartment syndrome develops
  - Heparin if limb judged not to be threatened; occasionally, vasospasm gives a false impression of total occlusion, and heparin may help

- **Pearl**

In a patient with an intra-arterial femoral line in the ICU on a ventilator, there will be no history; check distal pulses frequently.

Reference

Henke PK: Approach to the patient with acute limb ischemia: diagnosis and therapeutic modalities. Cardiol Clin 2002;20:513. [PMID: 12472039]

17

Cerebral Vascular Occlusive Disease

- ■ Essentials of Diagnosis
    - Most common in patients with standard risk factors for atherosclerosis (eg, hypertension, hypercholesterolemia, diabetes, smoking)
    - Many patients asymptomatic
    - Symptoms include amaurosis fugax, transient hemiparesis with or without aphasia or sensory changes; stroke diagnosed if focal findings persist for more than 24 hours
    - Bruit may be present but correlates poorly with degree of stenosis
    - Duplex ultrasound useful in assessing stenosis; gadolinium angiography is indicated only when the anatomy is not clearly delineated on ultrasound

- ■ Differential Diagnosis
    - Carotid artery dissection
    - Giant cell arteritis
    - Takayasu's arteritis
    - Lipohyalinosis
    - Radiation fibrosis
    - Cardiac source
    - Brain tumor or abscess (in patient with stroke)

- ■ Treatment
    - Aspirin
    - Thrombolytic agents in carefully selected patients with cerebral ischemia: Less than 3 hours of symptoms, no hemorrhage on CT
    - Carotid endarterectomy in stenosis > 80% without symptoms or in stenosis > 60% with symptoms (based on duplex ultrasound evaluation)

- ■ Pearl

Only one in four untreated patients with > 70% stenosis will have a stroke; of patients found to have 100% occlusion, only half have suffered a neurologic event.

17

Reference

Barnett HJ, Meldrum HE, Eliasziw M; North American Symptomatic Carotid Endarterectomy Trial (NASCET) collaborators: The appropriate use of carotid endarterectomy. CMAJ 2002;166:1169. [PMID: 12000252]

Diverticulitis

- **Essentials of Diagnosis**
  - Acute, intermittent cramping left lower abdominal pain; constipation in some cases alternating with diarrhea
  - Fever, tenderness in left lower quadrant, with palpable abdominal mass in some patients
  - Leukocytosis
  - Radiographic evidence of diverticula, thickened interhaustral folds, narrowed lumen
  - CT scan is the safest and most cost-effective diagnostic method

- **Differential Diagnosis**
  - Colorectal carcinoma
  - Appendicitis
  - Strangulating colonic obstruction
  - Colitis due to any cause
  - Pelvic inflammatory disease
  - Ruptured ectopic pregnancy or ovarian cyst
  - Inflammatory bowel disease

- **Treatment**
  - Liquid diet (10 days) and oral antibiotics (metronidazole plus fluoroquinolone or trimethoprim-sulfamethoxazole) for mild first attack
  - Nasogastric suction and broad-spectrum intravenous antibiotics for patients requiring hospitalization (eg, failed outpatient management, inadequate analgesia)
  - Percutaneous catheter drainage for intra-abdominal abscess
  - Emergent laparotomy with colonic resection and diversion for generalized peritonitis, uncontrolled sepsis, visceral perforation, and acute clinical deterioration
  - High-residue diet, stool softener, psyllium mucilloid for chronic therapy
  - Elective sigmoid colectomy for recurrent attacks or complicated diverticulitis treated with drainage and intravenous antibiotics

17

- **Pearl**

Left-sided diverticula are more common and more likely to become inflamed; right-sided diverticula are less common and more likely to bleed.

Reference

Stollman N, Raskin JB: Diverticular disease of the colon. Lancet 2004;363:631. [PMID: 14987890]

External Hernia

- **Essentials of Diagnosis**
    - Protrusion of a viscus through an opening in the wall of the cavity in which it is contained
    - Lump or swelling in the groin, sometimes associated with sudden pain and bulging during heavy lifting or straining
    - Discomfort is worse at the end of the day, relieved when patient reclines and hernia reduces
    - Clinically distinguishing an indirect from a direct hernia is unimportant, since repair is the same
    - Early symptoms of incarceration are those of partial bowel obstruction; the early discomfort will be periumbilical
    - A femoral hernia is an acquired protrusion of a peritoneal sac through the femoral ring; it is smaller, more difficult to palpate and to diagnose

- **Differential Diagnosis**
    - Hydrocele
    - Varicocele
    - Inguinal lymphadenopathy
    - Lipoma of the spermatic cord
    - Testicular torsion
    - Femoral artery aneurysm

- **Treatment**
    - In general, all hernias should be repaired unless local or systemic conditions preclude a safe outcome
    - Elective outpatient surgical repair for reducible hernias
    - Attempt reduction of incarcerated (irreducible) hernias (when peritoneal signs are absent) with conscious sedation, Trendelenburg position, and steady, gentle pressure
    - Emergent repair for nonreducible, incarcerated, or strangulated hernias

- **Pearl**

In inguinal hernia, the incidence of incarceration or strangulation is 1% per year.

Reference

Kingsnorth A, LeBlanc K: Hernias: inguinal and incisional. Lancet 2003; 362:1561. [PMID: 14615114]

Functional Intestinal Obstruction (Adynamic Ileus, Paralytic Ileus)

■ Essentials of Diagnosis

- History of precipitating factor (eg, recent surgery, peritonitis, other serious medical illness, anticholinergic drugs, hypokalemia, narcotic use)
- Continuous abdominal pain, distention, vomiting, and obstipation
- Minimal abdominal tenderness; decreased to absent bowel sounds
- Radiographic images show diffuse gastrointestinal distention, no obvious transition point, and air in the rectum

■ Differential Diagnosis

- Mechanical obstruction due to any cause
- Specific diseases associated with functional obstruction (ie, perforated viscus, pancreatitis, cholecystitis, appendicitis, nephrolithiasis)
- Colonic pseudo-obstruction (Ogilvie's syndrome)

■ Treatment

- Restriction of oral intake; nasogastric suction in severe cases
- Minimize narcotics and anticholinergic drugs
- Attention to electrolyte and fluid imbalance (ie, hypokalemia, dehydration)
- Prokinetic drugs (metoclopramide, erythromycin) may be tried
- For Ogilvie's syndrome, decompressive colonoscopy or intravenous neostigmine often attempted, the latter with marginal benefit and potential toxicity
- Serial abdominal radiographs to measure cecal distension (significantly increased risk of perforation when > 11 cm)
- Make every attempt to avoid surgery; adynamic ileus may persist for 7–10 days

■ Pearl

In any ileus, look at the chest film carefully; lower lobe pneumonias may cause it.

17

Reference

Kahi CJ, Rex DK: Bowel obstruction and pseudo-obstruction. Gastroenterol Clin North Am 2003;32:1229. [PMID: 14696305]

Malignant Tumors of the Esophagus

- **Essentials of Diagnosis**
  - Progressive dysphagia—initially during ingestion of solid foods, later with liquids; progressive weight loss ominous
  - Smoking, alcohol, asbestos, gastroesophageal reflux disease are risk factors
  - Adenocarcinoma (often associated with reflux-induced Barrett's esophagus) now has an incidence greater than that of squamous cell carcinoma
  - Classic radiographic appearance with irregular mucosal pattern and narrowing, with shelflike upper border or concentrically narrowed esophageal lumen
  - CT scan delineates extent of disease

- **Differential Diagnosis**
  - Benign tumors of the esophagus (< 1%)
  - Benign esophageal stricture
  - Esophageal diverticulum
  - Esophageal web
  - Achalasia (may be associated)
  - Globus hystericus

- **Treatment**
  - In 75–80% of patients, local tumor invasion or distant metastasis at the time of presentation precludes cure
  - For mid-esophageal lesions, bronchoscopy required to rule out direct extension into the trachea
  - For patients with localized primary, resection (when feasible) provides the best palliation
  - Adjuvant chemotherapy with radiation therapy or surgical resection results in cure for only 10–15%
  - Neoadjuvant chemotherapy and radiation can improve resectability for large tumors
  - Expandable metallic stent placement, laser fulguration, feeding tube placement with or without radiation therapy for additional palliation

17

- **Pearl**

True dysphagia—food sticking upon swallowing—has a nearly 100% association with anatomic lesions, a symptom always to be taken seriously.

Reference

Enzinger PC, Mayer RJ: Esophageal cancer. N Engl J Med 2003;349:2241. [PMID: 14657432]

Mesenteric Ischemia

■ Essentials of Diagnosis

Acute:

- Causes are emboli (eg, in atrial fibrillation); thrombosis (eg, in patients with atherosclerosis), or nonocclusive insufficiency (eg, congestive heart failure, hypovolemia)
- With occlusion, diffuse abdominal pain out of proportion to physical exam findings; evidence of vascular disease common historically or by exam
- Metabolic acidosis may suggest bowel infarction but is a late finding; studies may be normal early in the course

Chronic:

- Results from atherosclerotic plaques of superior mesenteric, celiac axis, and inferior mesenteric; more than one of the above major arteries must be involved because of collateral circulation
- Epigastric or periumbilical postprandial pain; patients limit intake to avoid pain, with weight loss and less pain

Ischemic colitis:

- Occurs primarily with inferior mesenteric artery ischemia; episodic bouts of crampy lower abdominal pain and mild, often bloody diarrhea; lactic acidosis or colonic infarction do not occur

■ Differential Diagnosis

- Diverticulitis and appendicitis
- Myocardial infarction
- Pancreatitis
- Inflammatory bowel disease and colitis due to other causes
- Visceral malignancy
- Polyarteritis nodosa
- Renal colic
- Cholecystitis

■ Treatment

- Decision to operate for suspected occlusive cause is challenging given comorbidities
- Laparotomy with removal of necrotic bowel and embolectomy or bypass of the superior mesenteric artery
- Intra-arterial infusion of papaverine if nonocclusive ischemia is present, along with maximizing hemodynamic status

17

■ Pearl

Abdominal pain in a patient with heart failure receiving digitalis and diuretics is nonocclusive mesenteric ischemia until proven otherwise.

Reference

Sreenarasimhaiah J: Diagnosis and management of intestinal ischaemic disorders. BMJ 2003;326:1372. [PMID: 12816826]

Pancreatic Pseudocyst

- **Essentials of Diagnosis**
  - Collection of pancreatic fluid in or around the pancreas; may occur as a complication of acute or chronic pancreatitis
  - Characterized by occasional fever, epigastric pain with back radiation, early satiety
  - Abdominal tenderness, and often a firm mass that may transmit aortic pulsations
  - Leukocytosis, persistent serum amylase elevation may be present; however, laboratory studies can be normal
  - Pancreatic cyst demonstrated by sonography or CT scan
  - Complications include hemorrhage, infection, rupture, fistula formation, pancreatic ascites, obstruction of surrounding intestine

- **Differential Diagnosis**
  - Pancreatic phlegmon or abscess (related processes)
  - Resolving pancreatitis
  - Pancreatic carcinoma
  - Abdominal aortic aneurysm

- **Treatment**
  - Up to two-thirds spontaneously resolve
  - Avoidance of alcohol; treatment of other causes of the initial pancreatitis (eg, hypercalcemia, hypertriglyceridemia, medications, gallstones)
  - Percutaneous catheter drainage with nutritional support while avoiding oral feedings effective in many cases but high recurrence rate
  - Endoscopic retrograde cholangiopancreatography (ERCP) with sphincterotomy and pancreatic duct stent for proximal decompression can aid in spontaneous resolution
  - Decompression into an adjacent hollow viscus (cystojejunostomy or cystogastrostomy) may be necessary
  - Octreotide to inhibit pancreatic secretion not of benefit

17

- **Pearl**

There are only two causes of pulsatile abdominal masses: pancreatic pseudocyst and aneurysm.

Reference

Tsuei BJ, Schwartz RW: Current management of pancreatic pseudocysts. Curr Surg 2003;60:587. [PMID: 14972194]

Pharyngoesophageal Diverticulum (Zenker's Diverticulum)

■ Essentials of Diagnosis

- Most prevalent in the fifth to eighth decades of life
- Results from herniation of the mucosa through a weak point in the muscle layer between the oblique fibers of the thyropharyngeus and the horizontal fibers of the cricopharyngeus (Killian's triangle)
- Dysphagia worsening as more is eaten; regurgitation of undigested food, halitosis
- Gurgling sounds in the neck on auscultation
- Barium swallow confirms diagnosis by demonstrating the sac

■ Differential Diagnosis

- Esophageal, mediastinal, or neck tumor
- Esophageal duplication cyst
- Cricopharyngeal achalasia (occasionally associated)
- Esophageal web
- Achalasia or lower esophageal stricture
- Epiphrenic diverticulum (lower esophagus)

■ Treatment

- There is no medical therapy; all patients should be considered candidates for cricopharyngeal myotomy extending onto the esophagus with either a diverticulopexy (< 2 cm) or a diverticular resection (> 2 cm)

■ Pearl

Unsuspected Zenker's diverticulum may be inadvertently perforated at upper endoscopy, a reason to perform contrast radiography prior to elective esophagoduodenoscopy.

Reference

Veenker E, Cohen JI: Current trends in management of Zenker diverticulum. Curr Opin Otolaryngol Head Neck Surg 2003;11:160. [PMID: 12923356]

17

Small Bowel Obstruction (SBO)

- **Essentials of Diagnosis**
  - Partial or complete obstruction of the intestinal lumen by an intrinsic or extrinsic lesion
  - Etiology: Adhesions (eg, from prior surgery or pelvic inflammatory disease) 60%, malignancy 20%, hernia 10%, inflammatory bowel disease 5%, volvulus 3%, other 2%.
  - Crampy abdominal pain, vomiting (often feculent in complete obstruction), abdominal distention, constipation or obstipation
  - Distended, tender abdomen with or without peritoneal signs; high-pitched tinkling or peristaltic rushes audible
  - Patients often intravascularly volume-depleted secondary to emesis, decreased oral intake, and sequestration of fluid into the bowel wall, bowel lumen, and the peritoneal cavity
  - Plain films of the abdomen show dilated small bowel with more than three air-fluid levels

- **Differential Diagnosis**
  - Adynamic ileus due to any cause (eg, hypokalemia, pancreatitis, nephrolithiasis, recent operation or trauma)
  - Colonic obstruction
  - Intestinal pseudo-obstruction

- **Treatment**
  - Nasogastric suction
  - Fluid and electrolyte (especially potassium) replacement with isotonic crystalloid
  - Most management decisions are based on the distinction between partial and complete obstruction
  - Surgical exploration for suspected strangulated hernia, obstruction not responsive to conservative therapy, or the development of peritoneal signs

17

- **Pearl**

Although Osler referred to adhesions as "the refuge of the diagnostically destitute," they remain the most common cause of small bowel obstruction.

Reference

Kahi CJ, Rex DK: Bowel obstruction and pseudo-obstruction. Gastroenterol Clin North Am 2003;32:1229. [PMID: 14696305]

18

Common Pediatric Disorders*

Acute Lymphoblastic Leukemia (ALL)

- Essentials of Diagnosis
  - Cause of childhood leukemias; peak at ages 2–6 years
  - Chromosomal abnormalities (eg, Down's syndrome)
  - Intermittent fever, bone pain, petechiae, purpura, pallor, mild splenomegaly without hepatomegaly, and lymphadenopathy
  - Anemia and thrombocytopenia are common; leukocyte counts often less than $10,000/\mu L$; lymphocytes described as atypical
  - Bone marrow shows homogeneous infiltration of more than 25% of leukemic blasts; most express common ALL antigen (CALLA)

- Differential Diagnosis
  - EBV or CMV infection
  - Immune thrombocytopenic purpura
  - Aplastic anemia

- Treatment
  - Induction with prednisone, vincristine, asparaginase, and occasionally daunorubicin; intrathecal methotrexate and/or cytarabine if at high risk for relapse
  - CNS therapy (intrathecal chemotherapy, sometimes cranial irradiation) to treat lymphoblasts present in meninges, and to prevent CNS relapse
  - Maintenance therapy with mercaptopurine, weekly methotrexate, and monthly vincristine or prednisone
  - Bone marrow transplant considered in selected patients
  - Younger children, WBC > 100,000 have worse prognosis; likewise (t9;22) and (t4;11) translocations

- Pearl

"Spontaneous cures" of ALL in older literature are likely cases of severe infectious mononucleosis.

Reference

Pui CH, Relling MV, Downing JR: Acute lymphoblastic leukemia. N Engl J Med 2004;350:1535. [PMID: 15071128]

---

* The following common childhood diseases are discussed in other chapters: aspiration of foreign body and cystic fibrosis, Chapter 2; pharyngitis, mumps, poliomyelitis, varicella and zoster, infectious mononucleosis, rabies, and rubella, Chapter 8; appendicitis, Chapter 17; otitis media and otitis externa, Chapter 21.

Bacterial Meningitis

■ **Essentials of Diagnosis**

- Signs of systemic illness (fever, malaise, poor feeding); headache, stiff neck, and altered mental status in older children
- In infants and young children, signs of meningeal irritation (Kernig's and Brudzinski's signs) may be absent
- Predisposing factors include ear infection, sinusitis, recent neurosurgical procedures, and skull fracture
- No symptom or sign reliably distinguishes bacterial cause from meningitis due to viruses, fungi, or other pathogens
- Organisms depend upon the age
- Age less than 2 months: Group B or D streptococci, gram-negative bacilli, *Listeria*
- Ages 2 months to 12 years: *Haemophilus influenzae, Streptococcus pneumoniae,* and *Neisseria meningitidis*
- Cerebrospinal fluid shows elevated protein, low glucose, elevated WBC (> 1000/μL) with a high proportion of PMNs (> 50%)
- Gram's stain and culture often lead to the definitive diagnosis

■ **Differential Diagnosis**

- Meningitis due to nonbacterial organisms
- Brain abscess
- Encephalitis
- Sepsis without meningitis
- Intracranial mass or hemorrhage

■ **Treatment**

- Prompt empiric antibiotics can be life-saving
- Exact antibiotic regimen depends upon age of patient; therapy narrowed once the susceptibilities of the organism are known
- Concomitant dexamethasone decreases morbidity and mortality in patients with meningitis secondary to *H influenzae;* unclear benefit if meningitis is due to other bacterial causes
- Patients monitored for acidosis, syndrome of inappropriate secretion of antidiuretic hormone, and hypoglycemia
- Coagulopathies may require platelets and fresh frozen plasma
- Mortality can be up to 10% in neonates; severe neurologic sequelae may occur in 10–25% of affected patients

18

■ **Pearl**

In an ill-appearing child with a history concerning for meningitis, administer antibiotics, perform lumbar puncture, and obtain a CT if the tap is nondiagnostic.

Reference

Saez-Llorens X, McCracken GH Jr: Bacterial meningitis in children. Lancet 2003;361:2139. [PMID: 12826449]

Colic

- ■ Essentials of Diagnosis
  - A syndrome characterized by severe and paroxysmal crying that usually worsens in the late afternoon and evening
  - Abdomen sometimes distended, the facies pained, fists often clenched; infant unresponsive to soothing
  - An abnormal sensitivity of the gastrointestinal tract to stimuli may contribute to its pathogenesis, but its exact etiology is unknown
  - Most cases present prior to age 2–3 months

- ■ Differential Diagnosis
  - Normal crying in an infant
  - Intussusception
  - Volvulus
  - Gastroenteritis
  - Constipation
  - Any illness in the infant causing distress (eg, otitis media, corneal abrasion)
  - Food allergy

- ■ Treatment
  - Reassurance to parents; education regarding the baby's cues
  - Elimination of cow's milk from formula (or from the mother's diet if she is nursing) in refractory cases to rule out milk protein allergy
  - Soothing with massage, creating a comfortable environment (eg, playing soothing music), avoidance of overfeeding may be useful adjuncts
  - Hypoallergenic diet or soy formula have not been demonstrated to have clear benefit, but may be helpful in difficult cases
  - Phenobarbital elixir and dicyclomine not recommended

- ■ Pearl

Rule of Threes: during the first 3 months, a healthy infant cries more than 3 hours a day, for more than 3 days a week, for more than 3 weeks.

Reference

Kilgour T, Wade S: Infantile colic. Clin Evid 2002;8:348. [PMID: 12603889]

18

Constipation

- **Essentials of Diagnosis**
  - Defined as infrequent bowel movements associated with difficulty passing; stools are hard in consistency
  - Can lead to painful defecation and eventually stool withholding and encopresis
  - Often caused by anatomic abnormalities, neurologic problems, or endocrine disorders; usually no cause is identified
  - A positive family history is often elicited
  - Rectal examination to evaluate fissures and assess rectal tone
  - Abdominal radiograph may confirm the diagnosis

- **Differential Diagnosis**
  - Hirschsprung's disease
  - Hypothyroidism
  - Hyperparathyroidism
  - Congenital gastrointestinal malformation
  - Infantile botulism
  - Lead intoxication

- **Treatment**
  - Impacted children will usually require a clean-out; although enemas are sometimes used, severe impaction may require oral polyethylene glycol electrolyte solution
  - Mainstay of therapy is behavioral; long course of toilet sitting and positive feedback necessary; biofeedback may be helpful
  - Close follow-up with families for support is critical
  - Dietary changes (increased fiber and lower milk and caffeine intake) usually beneficial
  - Mineral oil titrated to one or two soft stools per day is a recommended first-line agent
  - Lactulose or docusate sodium may be useful in difficult cases
  - Laxatives should not be used as a long-term solution
  - Families need to be reassured that functional constipation is difficult to cure and that months to years of treatment may be necessary

18

- **Pearl**

As always in constipation, accurate definition and structural causes come first.

Reference

Youssef NN, Di Lorenzo C: Childhood constipation: evaluation and treatment. J Clin Gastroenterol 2001;33:199. [PMID: 11500607]

Croup

- ■ Essentials of Diagnosis
  - Affects children predominantly between ages 3 months and 5 years; more common during fall and winter
  - Children often febrile, but not toxic appearing
  - Barking cough, stridor, and hoarseness following upper respiratory infection symptoms, typically worse at night
  - Lateral neck films can be useful; viral croup shows subglottic narrowing (steeple sign), normal epiglottis
  - Direct laryngoscopy may cause airway obstruction if bacterial epiglottitis present
  - Croup may recur, but usually lessens in severity with age as airway diameter increases

- ■ Differential Diagnosis
  - Foreign body in the esophagus or larynx
  - Retropharyngeal abscess
  - Epiglottitis

- ■ Treatment
  - Mist therapy utility is anecdotal
  - Corticosteroids reduce the number of return visits to the emergency department, but may not shorten course of disease
  - Oxygen and racemic epinephrine are accepted therapy

- ■ Pearl

Every mother knows that a walk with a child in the cool night air is the treatment of choice.

Reference

Knutson D, Aring A: Viral croup. Am Fam Physician 2004;69:535. [PMID: 14971835]

18

Down's Syndrome

- **Essentials of Diagnosis**
  - Occurs in 1:600–800 newborns, with increasing incidence in children of mothers over 35 years of age
  - Ninety-five percent of patients have 47 chromosomes with trisomy 21
  - Characteristic findings include small, broad head; upward slanting palpebral fissures; inner epicanthal folds; speckled irides (Brushfield's spots); flat nasal bridge; transverse palmar crease (simian crease); and short hands
  - One-third to one-half have congenital heart disease (AV canal defects most common)
  - Atlantoaxial subluxation and sensorineural hearing loss more frequent than in the general population
  - Leukemia is 20 times more common, and there is an increased susceptibility to infections

- **Differential Diagnosis**
  - There is none; the combination of phenotypic abnormalities and chromosomal analysis confirms the diagnosis

- **Treatment**
  - Goal of therapy is to help affected patients develop full potential
  - Therapy directed toward correction of specific problems (eg, cardiac surgery, antibiotics)
  - No evidence exists to support use of megadoses of vitamins or intensive exercise programs
  - Electrocardiography and echocardiography in the neonatal period to evaluate for congenital heart disease
  - Cervical spine radiography recommended once during the preschool years to evaluate for atlantoaxial instability
  - Patients with Down's syndrome should have annual vision and hearing examinations, and thyroid screening

- **Pearl**

18

Chromosome 21 codes the beta-amyloid seen ubiquitously in brains of patients with Down's syndrome and adults with Alzheimer's disease.

Reference

Roizen NJ, Patterson D: Down's syndrome. Lancet 2003;361:1281. [PMID: 12699967]

Enuresis

■ Essentials of Diagnosis

- Involuntary urination at an age at which control is expected (cognitive age of approximately 5 years), mostly occurring at night
- Primary enuresis occurs in children who have never had control and accounts for nearly 90% of cases; secondary in children with at least 6 months of prior control
- Symptoms must be present at least twice per week for at least 6 months for the diagnosis
- Approximately 75% of children with enuresis have at least one parent who had similar difficulties as a child
- Affects 7% of boys and 3% of girls at age 5; decreasing to 3% of boys and 2% of girls by age 10
- Secondary enuresis often caused by psychosocial stressors
- Medical problems, including UTI and diabetes mellitus, must be excluded

■ Differential Diagnosis

- Urinary tract infection
- Diabetes mellitus
- Congenital genitourinary anomalies
- Constipation
- Child abuse
- Behavioral difficulties

■ Treatment

- Therapy for causative medical problems
- Support and positive reinforcement for children and families
- Fluid restriction and bladder emptying prior to bedtime
- Alarm systems effective, but may take weeks to work
- Desmopressin works quickly but does not provide long-term control
- Imipramine not recommended due to side effects and overdose potential

■ Pearl

Careful clinical, developmental, and family history, as well as a thorough understanding of a family's psychosocial environment, are essential in helping patients and families successfully treat this disorder.

Reference

Thiedke CC: Nocturnal enuresis. Am Fam Physician 2003;67:1499. [PMID: 12722850]

Febrile Seizures

■ **Essentials of Diagnosis**

- Occur in 2–5% of children
- Peak between 14 and 18 months of age; most common between age 9 months and 5 years
- Last less than 15 minutes, are generalized, and occur in developmentally normal children
- Seizures lasting more than 15 minutes, persistent neurological deficits, or recurrent seizures are considered complex
- Risk factors include positive family history or previous personal history of febrile seizures
- One in three will have a recurrent seizure, 75% within a year
- Risk of developing epilepsy is approximately 1% in children without risk factors; up to 9% of children with risk factors (eg, positive family history, atypical seizure type or duration, underlying neurological disease) will develop epilepsy

■ **Differential Diagnosis**

- Meningitis
- Encephalitis
- Intracranial hemorrhage
- Intracranial tumor
- Trauma

■ **Treatment**

- No treatment for simple febrile seizures
- Electroencephalography not recommended in the initial evaluation
- Lumbar puncture indicated in children under 12 months of age if no source of infection can be found
- Prophylactic anticonvulsants may lower the risk of recurrence, but are not recommended routinely

■ **Pearl**

An excellent case can be made for brain CT or MRI following any first-time seizure regardless of age.

18

Reference

Baulac S, Gourfinkel-An I, Nabbout R, et al: Fever, genes, and epilepsy. Lancet Neurol 2004;3:421. [PMID: 15207799]

Henoch-Schönlein Purpura (Anaphylactoid Purpura)

- **Essentials of Diagnosis**
    - A small-vessel vasculitis affecting skin, gastrointestinal tract, and kidney
    - Typically occurs between ages 2 and 8 years; boys affected more often than girls (2:1); occasionally observed in adults
    - Two-thirds of patients have a preceding upper respiratory tract infection
    - Skin lesions often begin as urticaria and progress to a maculopapular eruption, finally becoming a symmetric purpuric rash
    - Eighty percent develop migratory polyarthralgias or polyarthritis; edema of the hands, feet, scalp, and periorbital areas occurs commonly
    - Colicky abdominal pain occurs in two-thirds, and it may be complicated by intussusception
    - Renal involvement in 25–50%
    - Platelet count, prothrombin time, and partial thromboplastin time normal; urinalysis may reveal hematuria and proteinuria; serum IgA often elevated

- **Differential Diagnosis**
    - Immune thrombocytopenic purpura
    - Meningococcemia
    - Rocky Mountain spotted fever
    - Other hypersensitivity vasculitides
    - Juvenile rheumatoid arthritis
    - Kawasaki's disease
    - Child abuse

- **Treatment**
    - Pain medications and NSAIDs to treat joint pain and inflammation
    - Corticosteroid therapy decreases duration of abdominal pain, but does not appear to alter skin or renal manifestations
    - No satisfactory specific treatment
    - Prognosis is generally good; less than 1% of patients have residual renal disease

18

- **Pearl**

Remember this diagnosis in adults with abdominal pain and palpable purpura.

Reference

Ballinger S: Henoch-Schönlein purpura. Curr Opin Rheumatol 2003;15:591. [PMID: 12960486]

Intussusception

- **Essentials of Diagnosis**
  - Telescoping of one part of the bowel into another, leading to edema, hemorrhage, ischemia, and eventually infarction
  - The most common cause of intestinal obstruction in the first 6 years of life; boys are affected more commonly than girls (4:1)
  - Majority (80%) of cases occur prior to 2 years of age
  - Lead points include hypertrophied Peyer's patches, intestinal polyps, lymphoma, or other tumors; in children over 6, lymphoma most common lesion
  - Most (90%) are ileocolic; ileoileal or colocolic may occur
  - Symptoms include intermittent colicky abdominal pain, vomiting, and bloody stool (currant jelly stools); children are often asymptomatic between bouts of pain
  - Plain films may show signs of obstruction, but a barium or air-barium enema is the standard for diagnosis

- **Differential Diagnosis**
  - Volvulus
  - Incarcerated hernia
  - Acute appendicitis
  - Acute gastroenteritis
  - Urinary tract infection
  - Small bowel obstruction due to other cause
  - Henoch-Schönlein Purpura

- **Treatment**
  - Patients stabilized with fluid; decompressed with a nasogastric tube
  - Surgical consultation to exclude perforation
  - Air-barium enema has a reduction rate of up to 90%, but it is never performed if perforation is suspected; reduction by enema may result in perforation in 1%
  - If perforation occurs or if enema fails, surgical decompression may be necessary
  - Recurs in up to 10% of cases if reduced via enema, usually in the first day after reduction; recurrence rate following surgical reduction is between 2% and 5%

18

- **Pearl**

Think of this diagnosis in a toddler with paroxysmal colicky abdominal pain who acts normally in between episodes and later develops increasing lethargy and bloody stools.

Reference

Daneman A, Navarro O: Intussusception. Part 2: An update on the evolution of management. Pediatr Radiol 2004;34:97; quiz 187. Epub 2003 Nov 21. [PMID: 14634696]

Juvenile Rheumatoid Arthritis (Still's Disease)

- ■ Essentials of Diagnosis
  - Useful diagnostic criteria: Age of onset less than 16 years; duration greater than 6 weeks; true arthritis must be present; other etiologies that cause arthritis must be excluded
  - Three types: Oligoarticular, polyarticular, and systemic
  - Oligoarticular: Fewer than 5 joints involved, predominantly large joints in the lower extremities
  - Polyarticular: More than 5 joints involved; affects both large and small joints; rheumatoid nodules are often present
  - Systemic: Arthritis characterized by quotidian fever; fevers may be accompanied by evanescent salmon-colored rash; pervasive visceral involvement including hepatosplenomegaly, lymphadenopathy, and serositis
  - ESR, CRP often elevated but nonspecific; ANA elevated in 40–85% of cases, more commonly in oligo- and polyarthritis

- ■ Differential Diagnosis
  - Rheumatic fever
  - Infective arthritis
  - Reactive arthritis due to various causes
  - Lyme disease
  - SLE
  - Dermatomyositis
  - Leukemia
  - Inflammatory bowel disease
  - Bone tumors
  - Osteomyelitis

- ■ Treatment
  - Stepwise approach to therapy is essential; goals of treatment are to restore function, relieve pain, and maintain joint function
  - NSAIDs and physical therapy are the mainstays
  - Methotrexate, hydroxychloroquine, sulfasalazine, and local corticosteroid injections for those symptomatic after NSAIDs
  - Azathioprine, cyclophosphamide, and systemic steroids may be necessary for treatment of refractory cases

18

- ■ Pearl

Systemic Still's disease is one of the few causes of biquotidian fever spikes.

Reference

Ilowite NT: Current treatment of juvenile rheumatoid arthritis. Pediatrics 2002;109:109. [PMID: 11773549]

Kawasaki's Disease
(Mucocutaneous Lymph Node Syndrome)

- **Essentials of Diagnosis**
    - Illness of unknown etiology characterized by sometimes severe vasculitis primarily of medium-sized arteries; 80% of cases occur before the age of 5 years
    - Criteria for diagnosis include fever for 5 days and at least four of the following: Bilateral nonexudative conjunctivitis; involvement of mucous membranes (eg, fissuring of lips, strawberry tongue); cervical lymphadenopathy of at least 1.5 cm; rash; and changes in extremities (edema, desquamation)
    - Arthritis common
    - Cardiovascular complications include myocarditis, pericarditis, and arteritis predisposing to coronary artery aneurysm formation
    - Acute myocardial infarction may occur; 1–2% of patients die from this complication during the initial phase of the disease
    - Thrombocytosis, elevated sedimentation rate typical
    - Patients require echocardiogram to evaluate for coronary aneurysms
    - No specific test is yet available; the diagnosis of Kawasaki's disease is based on clinical criteria and exclusion of other possibilities

- **Differential Diagnosis**
    - Acute rheumatic fever
    - Juvenile rheumatoid arthritis
    - Viral exanthems
    - Infectious mononucleosis
    - Streptococcal pharyngitis
    - Measles
    - Toxic shock syndrome

- **Treatment**
    - Intravenous immune globulin and high-dose aspirin are the mainstays of therapy
    - Corticosteroids contraindicated

18

- **Pearl**

Kawasaki's disease and anomalous origin of the left coronary artery from the pulmonary artery are the most likely causes of Q-wave infarction in childhood.

Reference

Burns JC, Glode MP: Kawasaki syndrome. Lancet 2004;364:533. [PMID: 15302199]

Otitis Media

■ **Essentials of Diagnosis**

- Peak incidence between the ages of 6 months and 3 years
- History may include fever, ear pain, and other nonspecific systemic symptoms (eg, vomiting, poor feeding)
- Tympanometry shows an opaque, bulging, hyperemic tympanic membrane with a loss of landmarks; pneumatic otoscopy shows loss of mobility
- Breastfeeding probably protective
- Exposure to tobacco smoke and pacifier use thought to increase incidence; other risk factors include craniofacial or congenital anomalies (eg, cleft palate)
- Although caused by viruses, most cases assumed to be bacterial
- Bacterial causes are (1) *Streptococcus pneumoniae,* 40–50%; (2) *Haemophilus influenzae,* 20–30%; (3) *Moraxella catarrhalis,* 10–15%

■ **Differential Diagnosis**

- Otitis externa
- Cholesteatoma
- Foreign body

■ **Treatment**

- Treatment controversial; most children with otitis media not treated in Europe
- CDC recommendations: (1) Children > 2 not in day care and not exposed to antibiotics in the last 3 months, amoxicillin 40–45 mg/kg per day for 5 days; (2) children < 2 in day care or with recent antibiotic exposure, high-dose amoxicillin 80–100 mg/kg per day for 10 days; (3) second-line therapy includes amoxicillin-clavulanate, cefuroxime, or intramuscular ceftriaxone
- Three or more episodes in 6 months or four episodes in a year warrant prophylactic antibiotics; tympanostomy tubes considered with persistent infection

■ **Pearl**

Nasotracheal intubation is an overlooked cause of otitis media.

18

Reference

American Academy of Pediatrics Subcommittee on Management of Acute Otitis Media: Diagnosis and management of acute otitis media. Pediatrics 2004;113:1451. [PMID: 15121972]

Pyloric Stenosis

- **Essentials of Diagnosis**
  - Increase in size of the muscular layer of the pylorus of unknown etiology
  - Occurs in approximately 3 per 1000 births; boys:girls 4:1; Caucasians more commonly affected than African-Americans or Asians
  - Vomiting usually begins between 2 and 8 weeks of age but may occur as early as 1 week of age or as late as 5 months
  - Emesis often described by parents as projectile; rarely bilious
  - Infant is hungry and nurses avidly, but weight gain is poor and growth retardation occurs
  - Dehydration and hypokalemic hypochloremic alkalosis are characteristic
  - Palpable olive-sized mass in the subhepatic region best felt after the child has vomited
  - Ultrasound is 90% sensitive
  - Barium studies, not commonly performed, demonstrate increased pyloric channel and bulge of pyloric muscle into antrum (shoulder sign)

- **Differential Diagnosis**
  - Gastroesophageal reflux disease
  - Esophageal stenosis or achalasia
  - Duodenal stenosis
  - Small bowel obstruction due to other causes
  - Antral web
  - Adrenal insufficiency
  - Pylorospasm
  - Inborn errors of metabolism

- **Treatment**
  - Ramstedt's pyloromyotomy is curative and the treatment of choice
  - Dehydration and electrolyte abnormalities should be corrected prior to surgery
  - Excellent prognosis after surgery

18

- **Pearl**

Pyloric stenosis: an epigastric mass in a vomiting infant with metabolic alkalosis? Game, set, match for this diagnosis.

Reference

Hernanz-Schulman M: Infantile hypertrophic pyloric stenosis. Radiology 2003;227:319. Epub 2003 Mar 13. [PMID: 12637675]

Respiratory Syncytial Virus (RSV) Bronchiolitis

- **Essentials of Diagnosis**
  - The major cause of bronchiolitis and pneumonia in children less than 1 year of age
  - Epidemics with seasonal variability most common from late fall to early spring
  - Clinical presentation of bronchiolitis is characterized by variable fever, cough, tachypnea, diffuse wheezing, inspiratory retractions, and difficulty feeding
  - Apnea may be the presenting symptom, especially in newborns and infants
  - Chest x-ray shows hyperinflation and peribronchiolar thickening with occasional atelectasis
  - RSV antigen detected in nasal or pulmonary secretions is diagnostic
  - Diagnosis often made clinically

- **Differential Diagnosis**
  - Bronchiolitis due to other viruses or bacteria
  - Asthma
  - Community-acquired pneumonia
  - Pertussis
  - Foreign body aspiration
  - Chlamydial pneumonitis
  - Laryngomalacia

- **Treatment**
  - Severely ill children should be hospitalized, given humidified oxygen, and kept in respiratory isolation to prevent spread to other patients
  - Bronchodilator therapy, while usually instituted, has not been demonstrated to reduce the severity of symptoms or shorten the course of disease
  - Corticosteroid use considered in hospitalized patients, though they may not reduce symptom severity or shorten disease course
  - Ribavirin may be given to selected patients at very high risk for complications (eg, those with complex congenital heart disease)

18

- **Pearl**

When croup lasts for more than a week, turn to this diagnosis.

Reference

Steiner RW: Treating acute bronchiolitis associated with RSV. Am Fam Physician 2004;69:325. [PMID: 14765771]

Roseola Infantum (Exanthema Subitum)

- ■ Essentials of Diagnosis
  - A benign illness typically caused by human herpes virus 6, occurring with a peak incidence between 6 and 15 months of age; 95% of cases occur before the third year
  - Abrupt onset of fever (as high as 40°C) lasting from 3 to 5 days in an otherwise mildly ill child; dissociation between systemic symptoms and febrile course
  - No conjunctivitis or pharyngeal exudate; mild cough or coryza occasionally present
  - Fever ceases abruptly; a characteristic rash develops with 12–24 hours after becoming afebrile in 20%, consisting of rose-pink maculopapules beginning on the trunk and spreading outward with disappearance in 1–2 days
  - Rash may occur without fever

- ■ Differential Diagnosis
  - Erythema infectiosum
  - EBV
  - Measles
  - Rubella
  - Enterovirus infection
  - Scarlet fever
  - Drug allergy
  - Kawasaki's disease

- ■ Treatment
  - Supportive care only; antipyretics for fever control
  - Reassurance for parents
  - Febrile seizures occur, but no more commonly than with other self-limited infections
  - Children are no longer infectious once afebrile

- ■ Pearl
  Appearance of rash following defervescence in an otherwise well child clinches the diagnosis.

18

Reference

Dockrell DH: Human herpesvirus 6: molecular biology and clinical features. J Med Microbiol 2003;52(Pt 1):5. [PMID: 12488560]

Tetralogy of Fallot

- **Essentials of Diagnosis**
  - Most common cause of cyanotic heart disease after 1 week of age
  - Components include: Obstruction to right ventricular outflow tract, overriding aorta, ventricular septal defect, and right ventricular hypertrophy
  - Varying cyanosis after the neonatal period, dyspnea on exertion, easy fatigability, growth retardation
  - Exam may be notable for right ventricular lift, harsh systolic ejection murmur maximal at the left sternal border, single loud S_2
  - Studies may demonstrate an elevated hematocrit, boot-shaped heart with diminished pulmonary vascularity on chest x-ray
  - Echocardiography, cardiac catheterization, and angiocardiography all useful in confirming the diagnosis

- **Differential Diagnosis**

  Other cyanotic heart diseases:
  - Pulmonary atresia with intact ventricular septum
  - Tricuspid atresia
  - Hypoplastic left heart syndrome
  - Complete transposition of the great arteries
  - Total anomalous pulmonary venous return
  - Persistent truncus arteriosus

- **Treatment**
  - Acute treatment of cyanotic episodes ("tet" spells) includes supplemental oxygen, placing the patient in the knee-chest position; consideration of intravenous propanolol, morphine
  - Palliation with oral beta-blockers or surgical anastomosis between the subclavian and pulmonary artery (Blalock-Taussig shunt) recommended for very small infants with severe symptoms and in those who are not candidates for complete correction
  - Surgical correction (closure of ventricular septal defect and right ventricular outflow tract reconstruction) is the treatment of choice in selected patients; patients are still at risk for sudden death because of arrhythmias
  - Complete repair in childhood has a 10-year survival rate of more than 90% and a 30-year survival rate of 85%

- **Pearl**

  The combination of right ventricular hypertrophy, small pulmonary arteries, and pulmonary oligemia is seen in no other condition.

18

Reference

Waldman JD, Wernly JA: Cyanotic congenital heart disease with decreased pulmonary blood flow in children. Pediatr Clin North Am 1999;46:385. [PMID: 10218082]

Urinary Tract Infection

- ■ Essentials of Diagnosis
  - Girls at higher risk than boys
  - Circumcision decreases rates of urinary tract infection only during the first year of life
  - Bacterial infection of the urinary tract, defined as $> 10^3$ colony-forming units/mL by suprapubic aspiration, $> 10^4$ CFU/mL by catheter, or $> 10^5$ CFU/mL clean catch
  - Most common pathogens are *E coli, Klebsiella,* enterococci, and *Proteus mirabilis*
  - Urinalysis usually positive for leukocytes and bacteria
  - Symptoms may be nonspecific in younger children and infants (eg, intermittent fever, poor feeding, emesis, diarrhea)
  - Difficult to differentiate lower tract infections from pyelonephritis
  - Risk factors include uncircumcised boys (during first year of life), female gender, presence of vesicoureteral reflux or obstructive uropathy, constipation, genitourinary anatomic abnormality

- ■ Differential Diagnosis
  - Appendicitis
  - Gastroenteritis
  - Pelvic inflammatory disease (adolescents)
  - Diabetes mellitus
  - Urethral irritation

- ■ Treatment
  - Empiric antibiotics such as penicillins or cephalosporins are first-line therapies; trimethoprim-sulfamethoxazole may be used in older children
  - Voiding cystourethrogram for infants and children once free of infection to exclude vesicoureteral reflux
  - Prophylactic antibiotics continued until voiding cystourethrogram performed

- ■ Pearl

Urinary tract infections in boys are invariably due to anatomic abnormalities; a thorough investigation is obligatory.

18

Reference

Riccabona M: Urinary tract infections in children. Curr Opin Urol 2003;13:59. [PMID: 12490817]

Wilms' Tumor (Nephroblastoma)

■ Essentials of Diagnosis

- Second most common abdominal tumor in children
- Presents between ages 2 and 5 years; occasionally may be seen in neonates or adolescents
- Occurs sporadically or as part of a malformation syndrome or cytogenic abnormality (eg, Beckwith-Wiedemann)
- Often discovered incidentally as an asymptomatic abdominal mass; occasionally presents with intermittent fever, abdominal pain, hematuria
- Abdominal ultrasound or CT reveals a solid intrarenal mass; 5–10% are bilateral
- Metastatic lesions in lung often present on chest x-ray

■ Differential Diagnosis

- Neuroblastoma
- Rhabdomyosarcoma
- Germ cell tumor/teratoma
- Lymphoma
- Polycystic kidneys
- Renal abscess
- Hydronephrosis

■ Treatment

- Once the diagnosis is made, almost all patients undergo surgical exploration of the abdomen with attempted excision of the tumor and possible nephrectomy
- Vincristine, dactinomycin, and doxorubicin are mainstays of chemotherapy
- Irradiation to sites of known disease prevent recurrence

■ Pearl

This is the diagnosis in a toddler with a nontender abdominal mass discovered incidentally.

Reference

Kalapurakal JA, Dome JS, Perlman EJ, et al: Management of Wilms' tumour: current practice and future goals. Lancet Oncol 2004;5:37. [PMID: 14700607]

18

Selected Genetic Disorders*

Acute Intermittent Porphyria

- **Essentials of Diagnosis**
  - Autosomal dominant with variable expressivity
  - Symptoms begin in the teens or twenties, usually in young women; rare after menopause; most asymptomatic
  - Caused by deficiency of porphobilinogen deaminase activity, with increased urinary aminolevulinic acid and porphobilinogen
  - Abdominal pain, peripheral or central nervous system dysfunction, psychiatric illness; no skin photosensitivity
  - Attacks precipitated by drugs (eg, barbiturates, sulfonamides, estrogens), intercurrent infections, and alcohol
  - Profound hyponatremia occasionally occurs; diagnosis confirmed by demonstrating increasing porphobilinogen in urine during acute attack
  - Absence of fever and leukocytosis

- **Differential Diagnosis**
  - Other causes of acute abdominal pain (appendicitis, peptic ulcer disease, cholecystitis, diverticulitis, ruptured ectopic pregnancy, familial Mediterranean fever)
  - Polyneuropathy due to other causes
  - Guillain-Barré syndrome
  - Heavy metal poisoning (eg, lead)
  - Psychosis due to other causes
  - Other causes of hyponatremia

- **Treatment**
  - High-carbohydrate diet may prevent attacks
  - Flares require analgesics, intravenous glucose, and hematin

- **Pearl**

In a young woman with abdominal pain and multiple surgical scars, think acute intermittent porphyria before adding another one.

Reference

Badminton MN, Elder GH: Management of acute and cutaneous porphyrias. Int J Clin Pract 2002;56:272. [PMID: 12074210]

* The following genetic disorders are discussed in other chapters. Chapter 2: Cystic fibrosis; Chapter 5: sickle cell anemia, thalassemia, von Willebrand's disease; Chapter 12: Huntington's chorea; Chapter 18: Down's syndrome

Alkaptonuria

■ Essentials of Diagnosis

- Recessively inherited deficiency of the enzyme homogentisic acid oxidase; leads to accumulation of an oxidation product in cartilage and degenerative joint disease of the spine with purplish joints
- A slight, darkish blue color below the skin in areas overlying cartilage such as ears ("ochronosis"); some have more hyperpigmentation in sclerae and conjunctivae
- Aortic or mitral stenosis due to accumulation of metabolites in heart valves; predisposition to coronary artery disease occasionally
- Back pain in spondylitis
- Diagnosed by demonstrating homogentisic acid in the urine, which turns black spontaneously on air exposure

■ Differential Diagnosis

- Ankylosing spondylitis or other spondyloarthropathies
- Osteoarthritis
- Amiodarone toxicity
- Argyria
- Rheumatic heart disease

■ Treatment

- Similar to that for other arthropathies
- Rigid dietary restriction may be used but of unproven benefit

■ Pearl

The only disease in medicine causing black cartilage.

Reference

Phornphutkul C, Introne WJ, Perry BM, et al: Natural history of alkaptonuria. N Engl J Med 2002;347:2111. [PMID: 12501223]

19

Gaucher's Disease

■ Essentials of Diagnosis

- Autosomal recessive; over 200 mutations have been found to cause this disease
- Deficiency of beta-glucocerebrosidase causes accumulation of sphingolipid within phagocytic cells throughout the body
- Infiltration primarily involves the liver, spleen, bone marrow, and lymph nodes
- Uncommon forms of Gaucher's disease, type II and type III, involve sphingolipid accumulation in neurological tissue and thus lead to various neurological problems
- Anemia, thrombocytopenia, and splenomegaly are common; erosion of bones due to local infarction with bone pain (painful episodes termed "crises")
- Bone marrow aspirates reveal typical Gaucher cells, with eccentric nucleus, PAS-positive inclusions; elevated serum acid phosphatase
- Definitive diagnosis requires demonstration of deficient glucose cerebrosidase activity in leukocytes

■ Differential Diagnosis

- Hepatomegaly, splenomegaly, lymphadenopathy due to other causes
- Idiopathic avascular necrosis of bone, especially the hip
- Metastatic malignancy to bone

■ Treatment

- Recombinant form of the enzyme glucocerebrosidase (imiglucerase) given intravenously on a regular basis improves orthopedic and hematologic problems; major drawback is exceptional cost; neurological abnormalities seen in type II and type III disease do not improve with enzyme replacement
- Largely supportive in nonresponders
- Splenectomy for those with bleeding problems due to platelet sequestration

■ Pearl

A Jewish patient with a hip fracture and splenomegaly has Gaucher's disease until proven otherwise.

Reference

Niederau C, Haussinger D: Gaucher's disease: a review for the internist and hepatologist. Hepatogastroenterology 2000;47:984. [PMID: 11020862]

Hemochromatosis

- ■ Essentials of Diagnosis
  - The most common genetic disease among white North Americans
  - Autosomal recessive disease caused by *C282Y* mutation in most, with symptoms and signs of hepatic, pancreatic, cardiac, articular, and gonadal dysfunction
  - Hyperabsorption of iron and its parenchymal storage results in tissue injury
  - Symptoms typically occur after age 50 in men and after age 60 in women and depend on which organs are prominently involved
  - Clinical manifestations variably include cirrhosis and often hepatocellular carcinoma, congestive heart failure, diabetes mellitus, erectile dysfunction, arthropathy, and hypopituitarism
  - Elevated serum iron, normal transferrin, percentage saturation of iron > 50%, and increased ferritin
  - Genetic testing indicated in those with coinfected hemochromatosis and siblings of diagnosed patients
  - Liver biopsy characteristic, with iron stain identifying accumulation in parenchymal cells

- ■ Differential Diagnosis
  - Other causes of cirrhosis or heart failure
  - Diabetes mellitus
  - Other causes of hypopituitarism
  - Other causes of iron overload, especially multiple transfusions (more than 100 units) as in homozygous beta-thalassemia

- ■ Treatment
  - Genetic screening recommend for all first-order relatives
  - Early recognition and diagnosis (precirrhotic state) is crucial
  - Low-iron diet
  - Weekly phlebotomy to deplete iron stores, followed by maintenance phlebotomy or intramuscular deferoxamine
  - Treat manifestations of liver disease, congestive heart failure, diabetes, and arthropathy
  - Liver transplantation for decompensated cirrhosis

- ■ Pearl

Widespread iron fortification of foods is arguably carcinogenic, given that hepatocellular carcinoma is the most common cause of death in this disease.

19

Reference

Pietrangelo A: Hereditary hemochromatosis—a new look at an old disease. N Engl J Med 2004;350:2383. [PMID: 15175440]

Homocystinuria

- ■ Essentials of Diagnosis
  - • Autosomal recessive disease resulting in extreme elevations of plasma and urinary homocystine levels, a basis for diagnosis for this disorder
  - • Patients often present in second and third decades of life with evidence of arterial or venous thromboses without underlying risk factors for hypercoagulability
  - • Ectopia lentis almost always present; mental retardation common
  - • Repeated venous and arterial thromboses common; reduced life expectancy from myocardial infarction, stroke, and pulmonary embolism

- ■ Differential Diagnosis
  - • Marfan's syndrome
  - • Other causes of mental retardation
  - • Other causes of hypercoagulability

- ■ Treatment
  - • Treatment in infancy with pyridoxine and folate helps some
  - • Pyridoxine nonresponders treated with dietary reduction in methionine and supplementation of cysteine, also from infancy
  - • Betaine may also be useful
  - • Anticoagulation as appropriate for thrombosis

- ■ Pearl

Ninety-five percent of ectopia lentis occurs in Marfan's syndrome, with upward lens displacement; the remaining 5% have this disorder, with downward lens dislocation.

Reference

Yap S: Classical homocystinuria: vascular risk and its prevention. J Inherit Metab Dis 2003;26:259. [PMID: 12889665]

Marfan's Syndrome

- **Essentials of Diagnosis**
  - Autosomal dominant; a systemic connective tissue disease due to mutations in the fibrillin gene on chromosome 15
  - Characterized by abnormalities of the skeletal system, eye, and cardiovascular system
  - Spontaneous pneumothorax, ectopia lentis, and myopia are characteristic; patients have disproportionately tall stature with long extremities and arachnodactyly, thoracic deformity, and joint laxity or contractures
  - Aortic dilation and dissection most worrisome complication; mitral valve prolapse seen in 85%; mitral regurgitation seen occasionally

- **Differential Diagnosis**
  - Homocystinuria
  - Aortic dissection due to other causes
  - Mitral or aortic regurgitation due to other causes
  - Ehlers-Danlos syndrome
  - Klinefelter's syndrome

- **Treatment**
  - Children should have periodic vision surveillance and annual orthopedic consultation
  - Patients of all ages require echocardiography—often annually—to monitor aortic diameter and mitral valve function
  - Endocarditis prophylaxis required
  - Beta-blockade may retard the rate of aortic dilation; vigorous exercise avoidance protects some from aortic dissection
  - Prophylactic replacement of aortic root recommended when diameter becomes 50–55 mm (normal is less than 40 mm)
  - Most untreated patients die in their fourth or fifth decade from dissection or congestive heart failure (due to aortic regurgitation)

- **Pearl**

One of the few disorders in medicine immediately diagnosable by inspection.

Reference

Dean JC: Management of Marfan syndrome. Heart 2002;88:97. [PMID: 12067963]

19

Neurofibromatosis

■ Essentials of Diagnosis

- Sporadic or autosomal dominant
- Two distinct forms: Type 1 (von Recklinghausen's disease), characterized by multiple hyperpigmented macules and neurofibromas; type 2, characterized by eighth cranial nerve tumors and occasionally other intracranial or intraspinal tumors
- Often presents with symptoms and signs of tumor of the spinal or cranial nerves; superficial cutaneous nerve examination reveals palpable mobile nodules
- Associated cutaneous lesions include axillary freckling and patches of cutaneous pigmentation (café au lait spots)
- Malignant degeneration of neurofibromas possible, leading to peripheral sarcoma
- Also associated with meningioma, bone cysts, pheochromocytomas, or scoliosis

■ Differential Diagnosis

- Intracranial or intraspinal tumor due to other causes
- Albright's syndrome

■ Treatment

- Genetic counseling important
- Disfigurement may be corrected by plastic surgery
- Intraspinal or intracranial tumor and tumors of peripheral nerves treated surgically if symptomatic

■ Pearl

Up to six café au lait spots are allowed before von Recklinghausen's disease is considered.

Reference

Kandt RS: Tuberous sclerosis complex and neurofibromatosis type 1: the two most common neurocutaneous diseases. Neurol Clin 2003;21:983. [PMID: 14743661]

19

Wilson's Disease (Hepatolenticular Degeneration)

- ### Essentials of Diagnosis
  - Rare autosomal recessive disorder with onset between first and third decades and symptoms of acute or chronic liver or neuropsychiatric dysfunction
  - Excessive deposition of copper in the liver and brain due to a genetic defect on chromosome 13; genetic testing impractical since over 200 different mutations in the Wilson's disease gene have been identified
  - Physiologic aberration is excessive copper absorption from small intestine and decreased hepatic excretion of copper
  - Symptoms of cirrhosis and basal ganglia dysfunction
  - Kayser-Fleischer rings in the cornea (in all cases of neurologic Wilson's disease), hepatomegaly, parkinsonian tremor and rigidity, psychiatric abnormalities
  - Elevated urinary copper excretion (> 100 micrograms/24 h), elevated hepatic copper concentration (> 250 micrograms/g of dry liver), decreased serum ceruloplasmin (< 20 micrograms/dL) before cirrhosis develops

- ### Differential Diagnosis
  - Other causes of fulminant hepatic failure
  - Other causes of cirrhosis
  - Other causes of psychiatric and neurologic disturbances, especially Parkinson's disease

- ### Treatment
  - Early treatment intended to remove excess copper crucial
  - Restrict dietary copper (shellfish, organ foods, legumes)
  - Oral penicillamine facilitates urinary excretion of chelated copper; pyridoxine supplementation necessary
  - Trientine if penicillamine cannot be tolerated
  - Oral zinc acetate promotes fecal copper excretion
  - Ammonium tetrathiomolybdate promising as initial therapy for neurological Wilson's disease
  - Liver transplantation for fulminant hepatitis, decompensated cirrhosis, and perhaps intractable neurologic disease
  - Family members (especially siblings) require screening tests (serum ceruloplasmin, liver tests, slitlamp eye examination)

19

- ### Pearl
One percent of Wilson's disease patients present with hemolytic anemia; copper is toxic to red cell membranes.

Reference
Gitlin JD: Wilson disease. Gastroenterology 2003;125:1868. [PMID: 14724838]

Common Disorders of the Eye

Acute Conjunctivitis

- **Essentials of Diagnosis**
  - Acute onset of red, itchy, burning eyes with tearing, eyelid crusting, foreign body sensation, and discharge
  - Conjunctival injection and edema, mucoid or purulent discharge, lid edema and possible preauricular lymph node enlargement
  - Vision may be normal or slightly decreased
  - Causes include bacterial and viral (including herpetic) infections and allergy

- **Differential Diagnosis**
  - Acute anterior uveitis
  - Acute angle-closure glaucoma
  - Corneal abrasion or infection
  - Dacryocystitis
  - Nasolacrimal duct obstruction
  - Chronic conjunctivitis
  - Scleritis in autoimmune disease

- **Treatment**
  - Topical broad-spectrum ophthalmic antibiotic (eg, fluoroquinolone, cool compresses, artificial tears
  - Ophthalmology follow-up for persistent symptoms or decreased visual acuity

- **Pearl**

There are many causes of the red eye; be careful with potentially damaging empiric therapy.

Reference

Rietveld RP, van Weert HC, ter Riet G, Bindels PJ: Diagnostic impact of signs and symptoms in acute infectious conjunctivitis: systematic literature search. BMJ 2003;327:789. [PMID: 14525879]

Acute (Angle-Closure) Glaucoma

■ Essentials of Diagnosis

- Less than 5% of all glaucoma
- Acute onset of eye pain and redness, photophobia, blurred vision with colored halos around lights, headaches, nausea, or abdominal pain
- Decreased vision, conjunctival injection, steamy cornea, mid-dilated and nonreactive pupil, and elevated intraocular pressure by tonometry
- Preexisting narrow anterior chamber angle predisposes; older patients, hyperopes, Asians, and Inuits more susceptible
- Precipitated by pupillary dilation caused by stress, pharmacologic mydriasis, dark environment (eg, movie theater)

■ Differential Diagnosis

- Acute conjunctivitis
- Acute anterior uveitis
- Corneal abrasion or infection
- Other types of glaucoma

■ Treatment

- Prompt ophthalmologic referral
- Pharmacotherapy includes: Topical beta-blocker (timolol), alpha-agonist (brimonidine), carbonic anhydrase inhibitor (dorzolamide); if elevated intraocular pressure does not respond to topical therapy, systemic carbonic anhydrase inhibitor (acetazolamide) or hyperosmotic agent (eg, glycerol or mannitol)
- Laser peripheral iridotomy usually curative

■ Pearl

Don't avoid a dilated funduscopic examination for fear of precipitating acute glaucoma; you will do the patient a favor by identifying this treatable disease early.

Reference

Congdon NG, Friedman DS: Angle-closure glaucoma: impact, etiology, diagnosis, and treatment. Curr Opin Ophthalmol 2003;14:70. [PMID: 12698044]

20

Age-Related Macular Degeneration

- ■ Essentials of Diagnosis
  - Non-neovascular ("dry") form: Central or paracentral blind spot and gradual loss of central vision; may be asymptomatic
  - Small and hard or large and soft drusen, geographic atrophy of the retinal pigment epithelium, and pigment clumping
  - Neovascular ("wet") form: Distortion of straight lines or edges, central or paracentral blind spot, and rapid loss of central vision
  - Gray-green choroidal neovascular membrane, lipid exudates, subretinal hemorrhage or fluid, pigment epithelial detachment, and fibrovascular disciform scars
  - Risk factors include age, positive family history, cigarette smoking, hyperopia, light iris color, hypertension, and cardiovascular disease

- ■ Differential Diagnosis
  - Dominant drusen
  - Choroidal neovascularization from other causes (eg, ocular histoplasmosis, angioid streaks, myopic degeneration, traumatic choroidal rupture, optic disk drusen, choroidal tumors, laser scars, and inflammatory chorioretinal lesions)

- ■ Treatment
  - Prompt ophthalmologic referral
  - Micronutrient supplementation with Age Related Eye Disease Study formulation (eg, Ocuvite Preservision) slows progression in patients with moderate to severe disease
  - Laser photocoagulation, photodynamic therapy, submacular surgery, and macular translocation for choroidal neovascularization

- ■ Pearl

Age-related macular degeneration is the leading cause of blindness in America for patients over 65 years of age.

Reference

Chopdar A, Chakravarthy U, Verma D: Age related macular degeneration. BMJ 2003;326:485. [PMID: 12609947]

20

Blepharitis & Meibomitis

- **Essentials of Diagnosis**
  - Chronic itching, burning, mild pain, foreign body sensation, tearing, and crusting around the eyes on awakening
  - Crusty, red, thickened eyelids with prominent blood vessels or inspissated oil glands in the eyelid margins, conjunctival injection, mild mucoid discharge, and acne rosacea

- **Differential Diagnosis**
  - Sebaceous gland carcinoma

- **Treatment**
  - Warm compresses for 10 minutes, followed by scrubbing the eyelid margins with dilute baby shampoo at least twice daily
  - Artificial tears for ocular surface irritation
  - Topical antibiotic ointment at bedtime
  - Recurrent or persistent meibomitis may be treated with doxycycline for 6–8 weeks, followed by slow taper; in women, negative pregnancy test before and contraception during treatment are essential

- **Pearl**

No precaution is too prudent when contemplating treatment of young women with tetracycline.

Reference

McCulley JP, Shine WE: Changing concepts in the diagnosis and management of blepharitis. Cornea 2000;19:650. [PMID: 11009317]

20

Cataract

- **Essentials of Diagnosis**
  - Slowly progressive, painless visual loss or blurring, with glare from oncoming headlights, reduced color perception, and decreased contrast sensitivity
  - Lens opacification grossly visible or seen by ophthalmoscopy
  - Causes include aging, trauma, drugs (steroids, anticholinesterases, antipsychotics), uveitis, radiation, tumor, retinitis pigmentosa, systemic diseases (diabetes mellitus, hypoparathyroidism, Wilson's disease, myotonic dystrophy, galactosemia, Down's syndrome, atopic dermatitis), congenital

- **Differential Diagnosis**
  - Generally unmistakable
  - Ectopia lentis may cause some diagnostic confusion

- **Treatment**
  - Surgical removal with intraocular lens implant for visual impairment or occupational requirement

- **Pearl**

When bilateral cataracts are removed in succession, the patient is always most grateful for the first procedure because color vision returns.

Reference

Snellingen T, Evans JR, Ravilla T, Foster A: Surgical interventions for age-related cataract. Cochrane Database Syst Rev 2002;2:CD001323. [PMID: 12076405]

Corneal Ulceration

- **Essentials of Diagnosis**
  - Acute eye pain, photophobia, redness, tearing, discharge, and blurred vision
  - Upper eyelid edema, conjunctival injection, mucopurulent discharge, white corneal infiltrate with overlying epithelial defect that stains with fluorescein dye, hypopyon (if severe)
  - Causes include trauma, contact lens wear, infection (bacterial, herpetic, fungal, *Acanthamoeba*)

- **Differential Diagnosis**
  - Acute anterior uveitis
  - Acute angle-closure glaucoma
  - Acute conjunctivitis
  - Sterile or immunologic ulcer
  - Corneal abrasion or foreign body

- **Treatment**
  - Frequent topical broad-spectrum antibiotics and daily ophthalmologic follow-up
  - Prompt ophthalmologic referral for any central ulcer or a peripheral ulcer > 2 mm in diameter

- **Pearl**

Never patch a corneal ulcer!

Reference

Cohen EJ: Cornea and external disease in the new millennium. Arch Ophthalmol 2000;118:979. [PMID: 10900114]

Diabetic Retinopathy

- **Essentials of Diagnosis**
  - May have decreased or fluctuating vision or floaters; often asymptomatic early in the course of the disease.
  - Nonproliferative: Dot and blot hemorrhages, microaneurysms, hard exudates, cotton-wool spots, venous beading, and intraretinal microvascular abnormalities
  - Proliferative: Neovascularization of optic disk, retina, or iris; preretinal or vitreous hemorrhages; tractional retinal detachment

- **Differential Diagnosis**
  - Hypertensive retinopathy
  - HIV retinopathy
  - Radiation retinopathy
  - Central or branch retinal vein occlusion
  - Ocular ischemic syndrome
  - Sickle cell retinopathy
  - Retinopathy of severe anemia
  - Embolization from intravenous drug abuse (talc retinopathy)
  - Collagen-vascular disease
  - Sarcoidosis
  - Eales' disease

- **Treatment**
  - Ophthalmologic referral and regular follow-up in all diabetics
  - Laser photocoagulation for macular edema and proliferative disease
  - Pars plana vitrectomy for nonclearing vitreous hemorrhage and tractional retinal detachment involving or threatening the macula

- **Pearl**

Aggressive glycemic control is critical in preventing disease progression; be sure your patients know their HbA_{1c}!

Reference

Frank RN: Diabetic retinopathy. N Engl J Med 2004;350:48. [PMID: 14702427]

Giant Cell (Temporal) Arteritis

- **Essentials of Diagnosis**
  - Sudden painless unilateral loss of vision in a patient over 50 years of age in association with ipsilateral temporal headache; may also have diplopia, visual field deficits
  - Review of systems positive for any or all of the following: Jaw claudication, ear pain, scalp tenderness, proximal muscle and joint aches (polymyalgia rheumatica), fever, anorexia, weight loss
  - Palpable, tender, nonpulsatile temporal artery may be present
  - Afferent pupillary defect (Marcus-Gunn pupil), pale swollen optic nerve and possibly a macular cherry-red spot
  - Erythrocyte sedimentation rate (ESR) and C-reactive protein (CRP) often significantly elevated

- **Differential Diagnosis**
  - Nonarteritic ischemic optic neuropathy
  - Optic neuritis
  - Compressive optic nerve tumor
  - Central retinal artery occlusion

- **Treatment**
  - High-dose IV or oral steroids should be started immediately to prevent vision loss in the contralateral eye
  - Prompt ophthalmologic referral for temporal artery biopsy (but start the steroids while making these arrangements)

- **Pearl**

An elderly woman with a headache and ophthalmologic symptoms has giant cell (temporal) arteritis until proven otherwise.

Reference

Su GW, Foroozan R: Update on giant cell arteritis. Curr Opin Ophthalmol 2003;14:332. [PMID: 14615636]

20

HIV Retinopathy

- ■ Essentials of Diagnosis
  - • Cotton-wool spots, intraretinal hemorrhages, microaneurysms seen on funduscopic examination in a patient with known or suspected HIV infection
  - • Typically asymptomatic unless accompanied by other HIV-related retinal pathology (eg, CMV retinitis)

- ■ Differential Diagnosis
  - • Diabetic retinopathy
  - • Hypertensive retinopathy
  - • Radiation retinopathy
  - • Retinopathy of severe anemia
  - • Central or branch retinal vein occlusion
  - • Sickle cell retinopathy
  - • Embolization from intravenous drug abuse (talc retinopathy)
  - • Sarcoidosis
  - • Eales' disease

- ■ Treatment
  - • Treat the underlying HIV disease
  - • Ophthalmologic referral is appropriate for any patient with HIV, especially with a low CD4 count and/or visual symptoms

- ■ Pearl

HIV retinopathy is the most common ophthalmologic manifestation of HIV infection; it usually indicates a low CD4 count.

Reference

Kramer M, Lynn W, Lightman S: HIV/AIDS and the eye. Hosp Med 2003;64:421. [PMID: 12886853]

Hordeolum & Chalazion

- ■ Essentials of Diagnosis
  - Eyelid lump, swelling, pain, and redness
  - Visible or palpable, well-defined subcutaneous nodule within the eyelid; eyelid edema, erythema, and point tenderness with or without preauricular node
  - Hordeolum: Acute obstruction and infection of eyelid gland (meibomian gland—internal hordeolum; gland of Zeis or Moll—external hordeolum), associated with *Staphylococcus aureus*
  - Chalazion: Chronic obstruction and inflammation of meibomian gland with leakage of sebum into surrounding tissue and resultant lipogranuloma; rosacea may be associated

- ■ Differential Diagnosis
  - Preseptal cellulitis
  - Sebaceous cell carcinoma
  - Pyogenic granuloma

- ■ Treatment
  - Warm compresses for 15–20 minutes at least four times daily
  - Topical antibiotic ointment twice daily
  - Incision and curettage for persistent chalazion (> 6–8 weeks)
  - Intralesional steroid injection for chalazion near the nasolacrimal drainage system

- ■ Pearl

Avoid early surgical treatment with its risk of scarring; most will resolve with conservative treatment.

Reference

Lederman C, Miller M: Hordeola and chalazia. Pediatr Rev 1999;20:283. [PMID: 10429150]

20

Hypertensive Retinopathy

- **Essentials of Diagnosis**
  - Usually asymptomatic; may have decreased vision
  - Generalized or localized retinal arteriolar narrowing, almost always bilateral
  - Arteriovenous crossing changes (AV nicking), retinal arteriolar sclerosis (copper or silver wiring), cotton-wool spots, hard exudates, flame-shaped hemorrhages, retinal edema, arterial macroaneurysms, chorioretinal atrophy
  - Optic disk edema in malignant hypertension

- **Differential Diagnosis**
  - Diabetic retinopathy
  - Radiation retinopathy
  - HIV retinopathy
  - Central or branch retinal vein occlusion
  - Sickle cell retinopathy
  - Retinopathy of severe anemia
  - Embolization from intravenous drug abuse (talc retinopathy)
  - Autoimmune disease
  - Sarcoidosis
  - Eales' disease

- **Treatment**
  - Treat the hypertension
  - Ophthalmologic referral

- **Pearl**

The only pathognomonic funduscopic change of hypertension is focal arteriolar narrowing, and it is typically seen in hypertensive crisis.

Reference

Luo BP, Brown GC: Update on the ocular manifestations of systemic arterial hypertension. Curr Opin Ophthalmol 2004;15:203. [PMID: 15118507]

20

Open-Angle (Chronic) Glaucoma

- **Essentials of Diagnosis**
  - Ninety-five percent or more of glaucoma
  - Insidious onset resulting in eventual complete loss of vision; asymptomatic early; common in blacks, elderly, and myopic patients
  - Tonometry reveals elevated intraocular pressure (> 21 mm Hg) but highly variable
  - Pathologic cupping of optic disk seen funduscopically, can be asymmetric
  - Loss of peripheral visual field

- **Differential Diagnosis**
  - Normal diurnal variation of intraocular pressure
  - Other types of glaucoma; congenital optic nerve abnormalities; ischemic, compressive, or toxic optic neuropathy
  - Bilateral retinal disorders (chorioretinitis, retinoschisis, retinitis pigmentosa)

- **Treatment**
  - Prostaglandin analog (latanoprost)
  - Beta-blocking agents (timolol)
  - α-Adrenergic agents (brimonidine, apraclonidine)
  - Carbonic anhydrase inhibitors (acetazolamide, dorzolamide)
  - Miotics (pilocarpine)
  - Laser trabeculoplasty, trabeculectomy, and aqueous shunt procedure

- **Pearl**

A patient referred by an ophthalmologist for evaluation of dyspnea has beta-blocker–induced asthma or congestive heart failure until proven otherwise.

Reference

Weinreb RN, Khaw PT: Primary open-angle glaucoma. Lancet 2004;363:1711. [PMID: 15158634]

20

Pingueculum & Pterygium

- ■ Essentials of Diagnosis
  - • Pingueculum: Yellow-white flat or slightly raised conjunctival lesion in the interpalpebral fissure adjacent to the limbus but not involving the cornea
  - • Pterygium: Wing-shaped fold of fibrovascular tissue arising from the interpalpebral conjunctiva and extending onto the cornea
  - • Irritation, redness, decreased vision; may be asymptomatic
  - • Both lesions can be highly vascularized and injected; their growth is associated with sunlight and chronic irritation

- ■ Differential Diagnosis
  - • Conjunctival intraepithelial neoplasia
  - • Dermoid
  - • Pannus

- ■ Treatment
  - • Protect the eyes from sun, dust, and wind with sunglasses or goggles
  - • Reduce ocular irritation with artificial tears or mild topical steroid
  - • Surgical removal for extreme irritation not relieved with above treatment, extension of pterygium to the pupillary margin, or irregular astigmatism

- ■ Pearl

Xanthomas always, xanthelasma sometimes, and pterygium and pingueculum are never associated with hyperlipidemia except coincidentally.

Reference

Hirst LW: The treatment of pterygium. Surv Ophthalmol 2003;48:145. [PMID: 12686302]

20

Retinal Artery Occlusion (Branch or Central)

■ Essentials of Diagnosis

- Sudden unilateral and painless loss of vision or visual field defect
- Focal wedge-shaped area of retinal whitening or edema within the distribution of a branch arteriole or diffuse retinal whitening with a cherry-red spot at the fovea; arteriolar constriction with segmentation of blood column; visible emboli
- Central vision may be spared by a cilioretinal artery (present in up to 30% of individuals)
- Associated underlying diseases include carotid plaque or cardiac-source emboli; giant cell (temporal) arteritis
- Less common than vein occlusion in hypercoagulable states

■ Differential Diagnosis

- Ophthalmic artery occlusion
- Inherited metabolic or lysosomal storage disease
- Ocular migraine

■ Treatment

- Medical emergency calling for immediate ophthalmologic referral
- Digital ocular massage, systemic acetazolamide or topical beta-blocker to lower intraocular pressure, anterior chamber paracentesis, and carbogen by facemask
- Check erythrocyte sedimentation rate (ESR) and C-reactive protein (CRP) to rule out giant cell (temporal) arteritis as an underlying etiology
- Consider ophthalmic artery thrombolysis if within 6–12 hours of onset of symptoms and no contraindications

■ Pearl

The retina is part of the central nervous system, and this disorder is thus treated as one does a stroke.

Reference

Rumelt S, Brown GC: Update on treatment of retinal arterial occlusions. Curr Opin Ophthalmol 2003;14:139. [PMID: 12777932]

20

Retinal Vein Occlusion
(Branch, Hemiretinal, or Central)

- ■ **Essentials of Diagnosis**
  - Sudden, unilateral, and painless visual loss or field defect
  - Local or diffuse venous dilation and tortuosity, retinal hemorrhages, cotton-wool spots, and edema; optic disk edema and hemorrhages; neovascularization of disk, retina, or iris by funduscopy and slitlamp examination
  - Associated underlying diseases include atherosclerosis and hypertension, glaucoma, hypercoagulable state including factor V Leiden or natural anticoagulant deficiency (AT-III, protein S, protein C), lupus anticoagulant; hyperviscosity (polycythemia or Waldenström), Behçet's disease, lupus
  - Retrobulbar external venous compression (thyroid disease, orbital tumor) and migraine also may be responsible

- ■ **Differential Diagnosis**
  - Venous stasis
  - Ocular ischemic syndrome
  - Diabetic retinopathy
  - Papilledema
  - Radiation retinopathy
  - Hypertensive retinopathy
  - Retinopathy of anemia
  - Leukemic retinopathy

- ■ **Treatment**
  - Prompt ophthalmologic referral
  - Laser photocoagulation for iris or retinal neovascularization or persistent macular edema
  - Surveillance and treatment of underlying diseases

- ■ **Pearl**

Think of hemoglobin SC disease in a pregnant woman with this disorder.

Reference

Sharma A, D'Amico DJ: Medical and surgical management of central retinal vein occlusion. Int Ophthalmol Clin 2004;44:1. [PMID: 14704516]

20

Retinal Detachment

■ Essentials of Diagnosis

- Risk factors include lattice vitreoretinal degeneration, posterior vitreous separation (especially with vitreous hemorrhage), high myopia, trauma, and previous ocular surgery (especially with vitreous loss)
- Acute onset of photopsias (flashes of light), floaters ("cobwebs"), or shadow ("curtain") across the visual field, with peripheral or central visual loss
- Elevation of the retina with a flap tear or break in the retina, vitreous pigmented cells or hemorrhage seen by ophthalmoscopy

■ Differential Diagnosis

- Retinoschisis
- Choroidal detachment
- Posterior vitreous separation

■ Treatment

- Immediate ophthalmologic referral
- Repair of small tears by laser photocoagulation or cryopexy
- Repair of retinal detachment by pneumatic retinopexy, scleral buckling, pars plana vitrectomy with drainage of subretinal fluid, endolaser, cryopexy, gas or silicone oil injection

■ Pearl

A patient complaining of new-onset flashes, floaters, and visual field defects has a retinal detachment until proven otherwise.

Reference

Gariano RF, Kim CH: Evaluation and management of suspected retinal detachment. Am Fam Physician 2004;69:1691. [PMID: 15086041]

20

Subconjunctival Hemorrhage

- ■ Essentials of Diagnosis
    - • Acute painless onset of bright red blood in the white part of the eye. Striking appearance, but painless with minimal to no effect on vision
    - • Most often occur in patients on aspirin or anticoagulation who have a recent history of severe coughing, sneezing, heavy lifting or constipation (Valsalva)
    - • Often seen in eye trauma, even a minor finger poke or aggressive eye rubbing
    - • Can have associated conjunctival edema (chemosis)

- ■ Differential Diagnosis
    - • Kaposi's sarcoma
    - • Conjunctival neoplasms such as lymphoma

- ■ Treatment
    - • None: Just like a bruise, the blood will change color and eventually be absorbed within a month; artificial tears if irritation present
    - • Hold aspirin, other NSAIDs, anticoagulation if possible
    - • Cough suppressant
    - • Stool softener
    - • Hematologic work-up and ophthalmologic referral if recurrent

- ■ Pearl

In the setting of trauma, 360 degrees of subconjunctival hemorrhage with associated chemosis is a sign of occult open globe; prompt ophthalmologic referral is indicated.

Reference

Shields SR: Managing eye disease in primary care. Part 2. How to recognize and treat common eye problems. Postgrad Med 2000;108:83, 91. [PMID: 11043082]

Uveitis

■ Essentials of Diagnosis

- Inflammation of the uveal tract, including the iris (iritis), ciliary body (cyclitis), and choroid (choroiditis); categorized as anterior (iridocyclitis), posterior (chorioretinitis), or diffuse (panuveitis)
- Acute onset of eye pain and redness, photophobia, tearing, and blurred vision (anterior uveitis); gradual visual loss with floaters, but otherwise asymptomatic (posterior uveitis); may be unilateral or bilateral
- Injected conjunctiva or sclera with flare and inflammatory cells on slitlamp examination, white cells on corneal endothelium, and iris nodules (anterior uveitis); white cells and opacities in the vitreous, retinal, or choroidal infiltrates, edema, and vascular sheathing (posterior uveitis)
- Multiple causes: post-trauma or surgery, lens-induced, HLA-B27–associated autoimmune diseases (ankylosing spondylitis, Reiter's syndrome, psoriatic arthritis, inflammatory bowel disease), infectious (herpes simplex or zoster, syphilis, tuberculosis, toxoplasmosis, toxocariasis, histoplasmosis, leprosy, Lyme disease, CMV, candidal), sarcoidosis, Behçet's disease, Vogt-Koyanagi-Harada syndrome

■ Differential Diagnosis

- Acute conjunctivitis
- Corneal abrasion or infection
- Retinal detachment
- Retinitis pigmentosa
- Intraocular tumor (eg, retinoblastoma, leukemia, malignant melanoma, lymphoma)
- Retained intraocular foreign body
- Scleritis

■ Treatment

- Prompt ophthalmologic referral in all cases
- Anterior disease: frequent topical steroids, periocular steroid injection, dilation of the pupil with cycloplegic agent (eg, cyclopentolate, scopolamine, homatropine)
- Posterior disease: more commonly requires systemic steroids and immunosuppressive agents

■ Pearl

The most common ocular manifestation of systemic disease.

Reference

Durrani OM, Meads CA, Murray PI: Uveitis: a potentially blinding disease. Ophthalmologica 2004;218:223. [PMID: 15258410]

20

Common Disorders of the Ear, Nose, & Throat

Acute Otitis Media

- **Essentials of Diagnosis**
  - Ear pain, with sensation of fullness in ear and hearing loss; fever and chills; onset often follows upper respiratory syndrome or barotrauma
  - Dullness and hyperemia of eardrum with loss of landmarks and light reflex
  - Most common organisms in both children and adults include *Streptococcus pneumoniae, Haemophilus influenzae, Moraxella catarrhalis,* and group A streptococcus
  - Complications include mastoiditis, petrous ridge osteomyelitis, sigmoid sinus thromboses, meningitis, brain abscess

- **Differential Diagnosis**
  - Bullous myringitis (associated with mycoplasmal infection)
  - Acute external otitis
  - Otalgia referred from other sources (especially pharynx)
  - Serous otitis

- **Treatment**
  - Antibiotics versus supportive care controversial; oral decongestants and anti-inflammatories (NSAIDs)
  - Tympanostomy tubes for refractory cases, with audiology and otolaryngology referral

- **Pearl**

With unexplained fever in an intubated patient, look in the ears; otitis media can result from eustachian tube obstruction by the nasotracheal tube.

Reference

Rovers MM, Schilder AG, Zielhuis GA, Rosenfeld RM: Otitis media. Lancet 2004;363:465. Erratum in: Lancet 2004;363:1080. [PMID: 14962529]

Acute Sialadenitis
(Parotitis, Submandibular Gland Adenitis)

■ Essentials of Diagnosis

- Inflammation of parotid or submandibular gland due to salivary stasis, sialolithiasis, and infection
- Facial swelling and pain overlying the parotid or submandibular gland
- Often seen in dehydration
- Examination shows erythema and edema over affected gland and pus from affected duct
- May be confused with rapidly enlarging lymph node
- Complications: Parotid or submandibular space abscess

■ Differential Diagnosis

- Salivary gland tumor
- Facial cellulitis or dental abscess
- Sjögren's syndrome
- Mumps
- Lymphoepithelial cysts or Burkitt's lymphoma in immunocompromised patients

■ Treatment

- Antibiotics with gram-positive coverage
- Warm compresses
- Hydration
- Oral rinses

■ Pearl

Look for this in marathon runners after the race on hot days; hyper-amylasemia clinches the diagnosis.

Reference

Bradley PJ: Benign salivary gland disease. Hosp Med 2001;62:392. [PMID: 11480124]

21

Acute Sinusitis

- **Essentials of Diagnosis**
    - Nasal congestion, purulent discharge, facial pain, and headache; teeth may hurt or feel abnormal in maxillary sinusitis; history of allergic rhinitis, acute upper respiratory infection, or dental infection often present
    - Fever, toxicity; tenderness, erythema, and swelling over affected sinus; discolored nasal discharge and poor response to decongestants alone
    - Clouding of sinuses on imaging or by transillumination
    - Coronal CT scans have become the diagnostic study of choice
    - Pain not prominent in chronic sinusitis, a poorly defined entity
    - Typical pathogens include *Streptococcus pneumoniae,* other streptococci, *Haemophilus influenzae, Staphylococcus aureus, Moraxella catarrhalis; Aspergillus* in HIV patients and anaerobes in chronic sinusitis
    - Complications: Orbital cellulitis or abscess, meningitis, brain abscess

- **Differential Diagnosis**
    - Viral or allergic rhinitis
    - Dental abscess
    - Dacryocystitis
    - Carcinoma of sinus or inverting papilloma
    - Cephalalgia due to other causes, especially cluster headache

- **Treatment**
    - Oral and nasal decongestants, broad-spectrum antibiotics, nasal saline
    - Functional endoscopic sinus surgery or external sinus procedures for medically resistant sinusitis, nasal polyposis, sinusitis complications

- **Pearl**

Sphenoid sinusitis is the only cause in medicine of a nasal ridge headache radiating to the top of the skull.

Reference

Piccirillo JF: Clinical practice. Acute bacterial sinusitis. N Engl J Med 2004;351:902. [PMID: 15329428]

Allergic Rhinitis (Hay Fever)

- **Essentials of Diagnosis**
  - Seasonal or perennial occurrence of watery nasal discharge, sneezing, itching of eyes and nose
  - Pale, boggy mucous membranes with conjunctival injection
  - Peripheral eosinophilia on occasion also in nasal secretions

- **Differential Diagnosis**
  - Upper respiratory viral infections
  - Chronic sinusitis

- **Treatment**
  - Desensitization occasionally beneficial
  - Oral or nasal antihistamines; oral decongestants
  - Short-course systemic steroids and oral leukotriene inhibitors for severe cases
  - Nasal corticosteroids and nasal cromolyn sodium

- **Pearl**

A Wright's flambé of secretions is the best way to demonstrate eosinophils: Stain the smear, ignite it, decolorize it, and the cells will be seen readily at low power.

Reference

Gendo K, Larson EB: Evidence-based diagnostic strategies for evaluating suspected allergic rhinitis. Ann Intern Med 2004;140:278. [PMID: 14970151]

Benign Positional Vertigo

- **Essentials of Diagnosis**
  - Acute onset of vertigo with or without nausea, lasting for seconds to a minute
  - Provoked by changes in head positioning rather than by maintenance of a particular posture
  - Nystagmus with positive Dix-Hallpike test (delayed onset of symptoms by movement of head with habituation and fatigue of symptoms)

- **Differential Diagnosis**
  - Endolymphatic hydrops
  - Vestibular neuronitis
  - Posterior fossa tumor
  - Vertebrobasilar insufficiency
  - Migraines

- **Treatment**
  - Self-limiting with spontaneous recovery in weeks to months
  - Reassurance with otolaryngologic referral for persistent symptoms or other neurologic abnormalities
  - Single-session physical therapy protocols will be useful in most patients

- **Pearl**

Learn this well—it's the most common cause of vertigo encountered in primary care settings.

Reference

Korres SG, Balatsouras DG: Diagnostic, pathophysiologic, and therapeutic aspects of benign paroxysmal positional vertigo. Otolaryngol Head Neck Surg 2004;131:438. [PMID: 15467614]

Chronic Serous Otitis Media

- ■ Essentials of Diagnosis
  - • Allergic and immune factors probably contribute
  - • Due to obstruction of the eustachian tube, resulting in transudation of fluid
  - • More common in children, but can occur in adults following an upper respiratory tract infection, scuba diving, air travel, or eustachian tube obstruction by tumor
  - • Painless hearing loss with feeling of fullness or voice reverberation in affected ear
  - • Dull, immobile tympanic membrane with loss of landmarks and bubbles seen behind tympanic membrane; intact light reflex
  - • Fifteen- to twenty-decibel conductive hearing loss by audiometry and Weber tuning fork examination lateralizing to affected ear

- ■ Differential Diagnosis
  - • Acute otitis media
  - • Nasopharyngeal tumor (as causative agent)

- ■ Treatment
  - • Oral decongestants, antihistamines, oral or intranasal steroids, and antibiotics
  - • Tympanotomy tubes for refractory cases with audiology and otolaryngology referral

- ■ Pearl

Unilateral otitis media, especially in a patient of Asian ethnicity, is nasopharyngeal carcinoma until proved otherwise; mirror examination of the nasopharynx is obligatory.

Reference

American Academy of Family Physicians; American Academy of Otolaryngology-Head and Neck Surgery; American Academy of Pediatrics Subcommittee on Otitis Media With Effusion: Otitis media with effusion. Pediatrics 2004;113:1412. [PMID: 15121966]

21

Endolymphatic Hydrops (Ménière's Syndrome)

- **Essentials of Diagnosis**
  - Etiology is unknown
  - Due to distention of the endolymphatic compartment of the inner ear
  - The four tenets: Episodic vertigo and nausea (lasting 1–8 hours), aural pressure, continuous tinnitus, and fluctuating hearing loss
  - Sensorineural hearing loss by audiometry starting in the low frequencies

- **Differential Diagnosis**
  - Benign positional vertigo
  - Posterior fossa tumor
  - Vestibular neuronitis
  - Vertebrobasilar insufficiency
  - Psychiatric disorder
  - Multiple sclerosis
  - Syphilis

- **Treatment**
  - Low-salt diet and diuretic
  - Antihistamines, diazepam, and antiemetics may need to be given parenterally for acute attacks
  - Aminoglycoside ablation of unilateral vestibular function via middle ear infusion
  - Surgical treatment in refractory cases: Decompression of endolymphatic sac, vestibular nerve section, or labyrinthectomy if profound hearing loss present

- **Pearl**

One of the few unilateral diseases of paired organs.

Reference

Minor LB, Schessel DA, Carey JP: Meniere's disease. Curr Opin Neurol 2004; 17:9. [PMID: 15090872]

21

Epiglottitis

■ **Essentials of Diagnosis**

- More common in children but increasingly recognized in adults
- Sudden onset of stridor, odynophagia, dysphagia, and drooling
- Muffled voice, toxic-appearing and febrile patient
- Cherry-red, swollen epiglottis on indirect laryngoscopy, which should be done with airway back-up in children; pharynx typically normal or slightly injected
- Should be suspected when odynophagia is out of proportion to oropharyngeal findings
- *Haemophilus* most common specific cause in children; less often isolated in adults but should be considered

■ **Differential Diagnosis**

- Viral croup
- Foreign body in larynx
- Retropharyngeal abscess
- Lemierre's syndrome (septic thrombophlebitis of internal jugular vein)

■ **Treatment**

- Humidified oxygen with no manipulation of oropharynx or epiglottis
- Airway observation in a monitored setting, intubation with tracheotomy stand-by
- Children usually need intubation; adults need close airway observation
- Parenteral antibiotics active against *Haemophilus influenzae* and short course of systemic corticosteroids

■ **Pearl**

The patient with a severe sore throat and unimpressive pharyngeal examination by tongue blade has epiglottitis until proved otherwise.

Reference

Sack JL, Brock CD: Identifying acute epiglottitis in adults. High degree of awareness, close monitoring are key. Postgrad Med 2002;112:81,85. [PMID: 12146095]

21

External Otitis

■ Essentials of Diagnosis

- Often a history of water exposure or trauma to the ear canal
- Presents with otalgia, often accompanied by pruritus and purulent discharge
- Usually caused by *Pseudomonas aeruginosa, Staphylococcus aureus* or fungi (*Candida, Aspergillus*)
- Movement of the auricle elicits pain; erythema and edema of the ear canal with a purulent exudate on examination
- Tympanic membrane (TM) is red but moves normally with pneumatic otoscopy, but often not seen due to ear canal edema

■ Differential Diagnosis

- Malignant otitis externa (external otitis in an immunocompromised or diabetic patient, or one with osteomyelitis of the temporal bone); *Pseudomonas* causative in diabetes

■ Treatment

- Prevent additional moisture and mechanical injury to the ear canal
- Otic drops containing a mixture of an aminoglycoside or quinolones as well as a corticosteroid
- Purulent debris filling the canal should be removed; occasionally, a wick is needed to facilitate entry of the otic drops
- Analgesics

■ Pearl

A painful red ear in a toxic-appearing diabetic is assumed to be malignant otitis externa until proved otherwise.

Reference

Sander R: Otitis externa: a practical guide to treatment and prevention. Am Fam Physician 2001;63:927, 941. [PMID: 11261868]

Viral Rhinitis (Common Cold)

- ■ Essentials of Diagnosis
  - Headache, nasal congestion, watery rhinorrhea, sneezing, scratchy throat, and malaise
  - Due to a variety of viruses, including rhinovirus and adenovirus
  - Examination of the nares reveals erythematous mucosa and watery discharge

- ■ Differential Diagnosis
  - Acute sinusitis
  - Allergic rhinitis
  - Bacterial pharyngitis

- ■ Treatment
  - Supportive treatment only: anti-inflammatories, antihistamines, decongestants
  - Phenylephrine nasal sprays (should not be used for more than 5 days)
  - Zinc lozenges
  - Secondary bacterial infection suggested by a change of rhinorrhea from clear to yellow or green; cultures are useful to guide antimicrobial therapy

- ■ Pearl

To date, no cure has been discovered for the common cold; physicians should not anticipate one, and resist the temptation to give antibiotics.

Reference

Gentile DA, Skoner DP: Viral rhinitis. Curr Allergy Asthma Rep 2001;1:227. [PMID: 11892040]

22

Poisoning

Acetaminophen (Tylenol; Many Others)

- **Essentials of Diagnosis**
  - First 24 hours: may be asymptomatic
  - 24–48 hours: increased transaminases
  - 72–96 hours: enzymes peak, hepatic failure possible
  - Toxic dose: 150 mg/kg (children) or 7.5 g (adults)
  - Peak levels occur 30–60 minutes after ingestion
  - Measure serum acetaminophen level 4 hours postingestion
  - Plot on nomogram and treat if level above lower limit (> 150 µg/mL); if lab units in milligrams per deciliter, multiply by 10
  - Detectable serum acetaminophen level or elevated transaminases require treatment if presentation after 24 hours
  - Patients may not realize that combination analgesics (eg, Tylenol No. 3, Vicodin, Darvocet) contain acetaminophen

- **Differential Diagnosis**
  - Other hepatotoxin ingestion (eg, *Amanita* mushrooms, carbon tetrachloride)
  - Viral hepatitis

- **Treatment**
  - Activated charcoal with N-acetylcysteine (NAC; see below)
  - Gastric lavage if less than 1 hour since ingestion or large ingestion
  - NAC; repeat dose of NAC if vomited within 1 hour of administration
  - NAC should not be delayed due to charcoal; give both
  - Intravenous NAC may be given when the oral route is not possible; however, anaphylactoid reactions have occurred

- **Pearl**

A serum acetaminophen level should be obtained in all overdoses, regardless of the history of the ingestion.

Reference

Dargan PI, Jones AL: Acetaminophen poisoning: an update for the intensivist. Crit Care 2002;6:108. Epub 2002 Mar 14. [PMID: 11983032]

Amphetamines, Ecstasy, Cocaine

■ Essentials of Diagnosis
  • Sympathomimetic clinical scenario: anxiety, tremulousness, agitation, tachycardia, hypertension, diaphoresis, dilated pupils, muscular hyperactivity, hyperthermia
  • Psychosis, seizures
  • Metabolic acidosis may occur
  • With cocaine in particular, stroke and myocardial infarction
  • Ecstasy (MDMA) associated with serotonin syndrome (see antidepressants) and malignant hyperthermia
  • Obtain rectal temperature
  • Studies include glucose, chemistry panel, renal panel, urinalysis, ECG, cardiac monitoring, PT/PTT

■ Differential Diagnosis
  • Anticholinergic poisoning
  • Functional psychosis
  • Heat stroke
  • Other stimulant overdose (eg, ephedrine, phenylpropanolamine)

■ Treatment
  • Activated charcoal for oral ingestions
  • Gastric lavage if less than 1 hour since ingestion
  • For agitation or psychosis: Sedation with benzodiazepines may need large doses; titrate rapidly in first 30 minutes; neuroleptics lower seizure threshold and may worsen the clinical outcome
  • For hyperthermia: Remove clothing, cool mist spray, cooling blanket, benzodiazepines for muscle rigidity
  • For hypertension: Benzodiazepines; if refractory start nitroprusside infusion; avoid beta-blockers, as they may worsen hypertension due to unopposed alpha stimulation
  • For chest pain: Benzodiazepines, aspirin, nitroglycerin; give morphine if not responsive

■ Pearl
Amphetamine abuse is common; always consider in a hyperadrenergic patient.

Reference
Freese TE, Miotto K, Reback CJ: The effects and consequences of selected club drugs. J Subst Abuse Treat 2002;23:151. [PMID: 12220613]

22

Anticholinergics
(Atropine, Scopolamine, Antihistamines)

- **Essentials of Diagnosis**
  - Many drugs have anticholinergic effects, including antihistamines, antipsychotics, belladonna alkaloids, cyclic antidepressants, mushrooms, and some plants
  - Anticholinergic toxidrome: Dilated pupils, loss of accommodation, flushed skin, tachycardia, hyperthermia, altered mental status, myoclonus, decreased bowel sounds, distended bladder, seizures
  - The classic presentation: "Hot as hades, blind as a bat, dry as a bone, red as a beet, mad as a hatter"
  - Also complaints of dry mouth, thirst, difficulty in swallowing, blurring of vision
  - Prolonged QT interval and torsade de pointes with nonsedating antihistamines
  - Useful studies include electrolyte panel, creatinine, calcium, glucose, urinalysis, creatinine kinase, and ECG

- **Differential Diagnosis**
  - Amphetamines or other stimulant overdose
  - LSD or other hallucinogen ingestion
  - Delirium tremens
  - Acute psychosis
  - Jimsonweed or other ingestion of an anticholinergic-containing plant

- **Treatment**
  - Activated charcoal: repeated doses may cause abdominal distention
  - Consider gastric lavage if less than 1 hour since ingestion
  - In those with hyperthermia, benzodiazepines, cooling fan, ice water bath, intravenous hydration
  - The use of physostigmine is controversial and limited to severe symptomatology; contraindicated if conduction abnormalities seen on ECG or tricyclic coingestion suspected

- **Pearl**

To distinguish anticholinergic toxicity from sympathomimetic toxicity, check for skin moisture, eg, sweating in the axilla; anticholinergic toxicity yields a hot but dry axilla.

Reference

Estelle F, Simons R: H1-receptor antagonists: safety issues. Ann Allergy Asthma Immunol 1999;83:481. [PMID: 10582735]

Antidepressants: Atypical Agents (Serotonin Syndrome)

- ## Essentials of Diagnosis
  - Trazodone, bupropion, venlafaxine, and the SSRIs (fluoxetine, sertraline, paroxetine, fluvoxamine, and citalopram); well-tolerated in pure overdoses, high toxic:therapeutic ratios
  - Nausea, vomiting, dizziness, blurred vision, sinus tachycardia; citalopram may cause ECG changes
  - Serotonin syndrome: Mental status changes, agitation, myoclonus, hyperreflexia, diaphoresis, tremor, diarrhea, incoordination, fever
  - Useful studies include ECG, chemistry panel, urinalysis

- ## Differential Diagnosis
  - Alcohol withdrawal
  - Heatstroke
  - Hypoglycemia
  - Neuroleptic malignant syndrome

- ## Treatment
  - Activated charcoal
  - Gastric lavage if less than 1 hour since large ingestion or if a mixed drug ingestion
  - In those with hyperthermia, aggressive cooling, intravenous fluids, and benzodiazepines useful
  - Cardiac monitoring and ECG based on specific agent (eg, citalopram)
  - Benzodiazepines initially; bupropion, venlafaxine, and SSRIs associated with seizures
  - Serotonin syndrome typically self-limited; stop all offending agents
  - Cyproheptadine (an antiserotonergic agent) in serotonin syndrome has unproven benefit; consider only after cooling and sedation initiated

- ## Pearl

Remember that rave participants increase the risk by taking an SSRI ("preloading") followed by ecstasy.

Reference

Sarko J: Antidepressants, old and new. A review of their adverse effects and toxicity in overdose. Emerg Med Clin North Am 2000;18:637. [PMID: 11130931]

22

Antidepressants: Tricyclics

- **Essentials of Diagnosis**
  - Hypotension, tachydysrhythmias, and seizures are the most life-threatening presentation and develop within minutes of ingestion; other symptoms due to anticholinergic effects
  - Peripheral antimuscarinic: Dry mouth, dry skin, muscle twitching, decreased bowel activity, dilated pupils
  - Central antimuscarinic: Agitation, delirium, confusion, hallucinations, slurred speech, ataxia, sedation, coma
  - Cardiac: QRS-interval widening, terminal right axis deviation, prolonged QTc interval, sinus tachycardia
  - Generalized seizures from $GABA_A$-receptor antagonism
  - Toxicity can occur at therapeutic doses in combination with other drugs (antihistamines, antipsychotics)
  - Useful studies include ECG and telemetric monitoring, chemistry panel, renal panel, glucose, urinalysis, qualitative tricyclic determination, complete blood count

- **Differential Diagnosis**
  - Other drug ingestions: Carbamazepine, antihistamines, class Ia and Ic antiarrhythmics, propranolol, lithium; cocaine
  - Hyperkalemia

- **Treatment**
  - Activated charcoal
  - Gastric lavage if less than 1 hour since ingestion
  - Sodium bicarbonate for QRS > 100 ms, refractory hypotension, or ventricular dysrhythmia (1- to 2-mEq/kg boluses to goal serum pH 7.50–7.55, then infuse D_5W with three ampules sodium bicarbonate at 2–3 mL/kg per hour)
  - Hyperventilation may improve conduction delay, especially in patients with underlying CHF who cannot tolerate large amounts of sodium bicarbonate
  - Seizures usually respond to benzodiazepines; phenytoin not recommended for refractory seizures due to possible prodysrhythmic effects
  - Hypotension must be rapidly corrected with intravenous fluids, and vasopressors if necessary (eg, norepinephrine)

- **Pearl**

TCAs are responsible for more drug-related deaths than any other prescribed medications, and are the most difficult poisonings to treat.

Reference

Kerr GW, McGuffie AC, Wilkie S: Tricyclic antidepressant overdose: a review. Emerg Med J 2001;18:236. [PMID: 11435353]

22

Arsenic

■ Essentials of Diagnosis

- Symptoms appear within 1 hour after ingestion but may be delayed as long as 12 hours
- Symptoms depend on amount, time, and form ingested
- Acute ingestion: nausea, vomiting, abdominal pain, diarrhea, dysrhythmias, hypotension, fever, seizures neuropathy
- Chronic ingestion: headache, encephalopathy, neuropathy, malaise, peripheral edema, leukopenia
- Useful studies include abdominal x-ray (may demonstrate metallic ingestion), spot urine for arsenic, complete blood count (basophilic stippling of red cells), renal panel, liver panel, urinalysis, 24-hour urine, ECG

■ Differential Diagnosis

- Septic shock
- Other heavy metal toxicities, including thallium and mercury
- Other peripheral neuropathies, including Guillain-Barré syndrome
- Addison's disease
- Hypo- and hyperthyroidism

■ Treatment

- Intravenous fluids and vasopressors, if necessary, for hypotension
- Dysrhythmias: Lidocaine or defibrillation for ventricular tachycardia; intravenous magnesium or isoproterenol, overdrive pacing for torsade de pointes
- Benzodiazepines for seizures
- Chelation therapy should begin as soon as acute arsenic toxicity is suspected
- If radiopaque material visible on abdominal films, bowel decontamination recommended (gastric lavage followed by activated charcoal followed by whole-bowel irrigation until abdominal films are clear)

■ Pearl

At least suspect this poisoning in a repeatedly widowed woman with psychiatric problems.

Reference

Ratnaike RN: Acute and chronic arsenic toxicity. Postgrad Med J 2003;79:391. [PMID: 12897217]

22

Benzodiazepines

■ Essentials of Diagnosis
- Primarily CNS effects, including drowsiness, slurred speech, confusion, ataxia, respiratory depression, hypotension, coma
- Isolated benzodiazepine ingestion rarely results in death; mixed ingestions increase morbidity and mortality

■ Differential Diagnosis
- Other sedative-hypnotic agents, eg chloral hydrate, barbiturates
- Toxic alcohols
- Opioid ingestion
- Metabolic encephalopathy
- Encephalitis, meningitis, other medical diseases of the CNS

■ Treatment
- Patients who are unresponsive or confused should receive dextrose, thiamine, and naloxone
- Respiratory depression should be monitored closely; intubate if necessary
- Activated charcoal
- Flumazenil has an extremely limited role in patients with acute overdose due to the possibility of severe side effects (eg, seizures)

■ Pearl

Obtain the toxicology screening before giving benzodiazepines to treat any suspected withdrawal syndrome.

Reference

Chouinard G: Issues in the clinical use of benzodiazepines: potency, withdrawal, and rebound. J Clin Psychiatry 2004;65(Suppl 5):7. [PMID: 15078112]

Beta-Blockers

- ■ Essentials of Diagnosis
  - • Hypotension, bradycardia, atrioventricular block, cardiogenic shock, torsade de pointes (due to sotalol)
  - • Altered mental status, psychosis, seizures, and coma, most often in the setting of hypotension, but may also occur with propranolol and other lipophilic agents
  - • Onset of symptoms typically within hours of overdose
  - • Useful studies include ECG (prolonged PR interval, AV block, widened QRS interval) serum digoxin level, chemistry panel

- ■ Differential Diagnosis
  - • Calcium antagonist overdose
  - • Digitalis or other cardiac glycoside ingestion
  - • Tricyclic antidepressant toxicity
  - • Cholinergic toxicity

- ■ Treatment
  - • If endotracheal intubation or gastric lavage required, pretreat with atropine to limit vagal stimulation
  - • Gastric lavage is recommended for large overdoses, provided the patient presents within 1 hour of ingestion (even if asymptomatic)
  - • Whole bowel irrigation for ingestion of sustained-release formulation
  - • For bradycardia and hypotension, if refractory to normal saline bolus and atropine, then glucagon bolus
  - • If the above fails, then epinephrine, isoproterenol or dobutamine infusion, aortic balloon pump

- ■ Pearl

Beta-blocker toxicity commonly has mental status changes; calcium channel blocker toxicity doesn't; and digoxin toxicity maintains blood pressure and mental status.

Reference

Bailey B: Glucagon in beta-blocker and calcium channel blocker overdoses: a systematic review. J Toxicol Clin Toxicol 2003;41:595. [PMID: 14514004]

Calcium Antagonists (Calcium Channel Blockers)

- **Essentials of Diagnosis**
  - Bradycardia, hypotension, atrioventricular block, hyperglycemia, pulmonary edema; patients may be asymptomatic
  - Cardiac arrest or cardiogenic shock
  - Decreased cerebral perfusion leads to confusion or agitation, dizziness, lethargy, seizures
  - Useful studies include ECG, serum digoxin level, chemistry panel, and ionized calcium

- **Differential Diagnosis**
  - Beta-blocker toxicity
  - Tricyclic antidepressant toxicity
  - Digitalis toxicity
  - Hypotensive, bradycardiac shock typically distinct from hyper-dynamic shock of hypovolemia or sepsis

- **Treatment**
  - Gastric lavage often used
  - Multidose activated charcoal
  - Whole bowel irrigation for sustained-release preparations
  - Supportive therapy for coma, hypotension, and seizures
  - To reverse cardiotoxic effects: Fluid boluses and atropine, then calcium chloride boluses
  - Glucagon bolus: 2–5 mg over 60 seconds, repeat up to total of 10 mg; then begin intravenous infusion

- **Pearl**

Verapamil is the most potent negative inotrope of the calcium blockers; beware of its use in cardiomyopathic patients with arrhythmias.

Reference

Zimmerman JL: Poisonings and overdoses in the intensive care unit: general and specific management issues. Crit Care Med 2003;31:2794. [PMID: 14668617]

Carbon Monoxide

■ Essentials of Diagnosis

- May result from exposure to any incomplete combustion of any carbonaceous fossil fuel (eg, automobile exhaust, smoke inhalation, improperly vented gas heater)
- Symptoms nonspecific and flulike: Fatigue, headache, dizziness, abdominal pain, nausea, confusion
- With more severe intoxication, lethargy, syncope, seizures, coma
- Secondary injury from ischemia: myocardial infarction, rhabdomyolysis, noncardiogenic pulmonary edema, retinal hemorrhages, neurological deficits
- Survivors of severe poisoning may have permanent neurologic deficits
- Useful studies include carboxyhemoglobin level (can be venous), ECG, chemistry panel, renal panel, arterial blood gas; pulse oximetry can be falsely normal

■ Differential Diagnosis

- Cyanide poisoning
- Depressant drug ingestion
- Myocardial ischemia
- In chronic intoxication, headache of other cause

■ Treatment

- Remove from exposure
- Maintain airway and assist ventilation; intubation may be necessary
- 100% oxygen by nonrebreathing facemask
- Hyperbaric oxygen considered in patients with syncope, coma, seizures, Glasgow Coma Scale score < 15, myocardial ischemia, ventricular dysrhythmias, any focal neurological deficits or persistent headache, ataxia after 2–4 hours of oxygen treatment

■ Pearl

Think of carbon monoxide poisoning if several family members present with nonspecific symptoms during the winter months, and inquire about methods of heating.

Reference

Gorman D, Drewry A, Huang YL, Sames C: The clinical toxicology of carbon monoxide. Toxicology 2003;187:25. [PMID: 12679050]

22

Cardiac Glycosides (Digitalis)

■ Essentials of Diagnosis
  - Accidental ingestion, common in children
  - May be due to plant ingestions: oleander, foxglove, lily of the valley, red squill, dogbane
  - Age, coexisting disease, electrolyte disturbance (hypokalemia, hypomagnesemia, hypercalcemia), hypoxemia, and other cardiac medications (including diuretics) increase potential for digitalis toxicity
  - Acute overdose: nausea, vomiting, severe hyperkalemia, visual disturbances, syncope, confusion, delirium, bradycardia, supraventricular or ventricular dysrhythmias, atrioventricular block
  - Chronic toxicity: nausea, vomiting, ventricular arrhythmias
  - Elevated serum digoxin level in acute overdose; level may be normal with chronic toxicity
  - Useful studies include: ECG, serum digoxin level, chemistry panel, magnesium, calcium, renal panel

■ Differential Diagnosis
  - Beta-blocker toxicity
  - Calcium blocker toxicity
  - Tricyclic antidepressant ingestion
  - Clonidine overdose
  - Organophosphate insecticide poisoning

■ Treatment
  - Activated charcoal; multiple doses may be required due to enterohepatic circulation of digoxin
  - Gastric lavage if less than 1 hour since ingestion
  - Maintain adequate airway and assist ventilation as necessary
  - Correct hypomagnesemia, hypoxia, hypoglycemia, hyperkalemia or hypokalemia; calcium is contraindicated, as it may generate ventricular arrhythmias
  - Lidocaine, phenytoin, magnesium for ventricular arrhythmias
  - Atropine, pacemaker for bradycardia or atrioventricular block
  - Digoxin-specific antibody indicated if: Severe ventricular dysrhythmias, bradycardia unresponsive to atropine, digoxin level > 15 ng/mL, ingestion of > 10 mg in previously healthy adult, and serum potassium > 5 mEq/L

■ Pearl
The cause of the highest serum potassium in clinical medicine, and the most rapidly correctable.

22

Reference

Hauptman PJ, Kelly RA: Digitalis. Circulation 1999;99:1265. [PMID: 10069797]

Cyanide

- ■ Essentials of Diagnosis
  - Laboratory or industrial exposure (plastics, solvents, glues, fabrics), smoke inhalation in fires
  - By-product of the breakdown of nitroprusside, ingestion of cyanogenic glycosides in some plant products (apricot pits, bitter almonds)
  - Absorbed rapidly by inhalation, through skin, or gastrointestinally
  - Symptoms shortly after inhalation or ingestion; some compounds (acetonitrile, a cosmetic nail remover) metabolize to hydrogen cyanide, and symptoms may be delayed
  - Dose-dependent toxicity; headache, breathlessness, anxiousness, nausea to confusion, bradycardia, hypotension, shock, seizures, death
  - Disrupts the ability of tissues to use oxygen; picture mimics hypoxia, including profound lactic acidosis
  - High oxygen saturation of venous blood; retinal vessels bright red
  - Odor of bitter almonds on patient's breath or vomitus only present in 40% of population
  - Useful studies include: Chemistry panel, renal panel, serum glucose, arterial blood gas, serum lactate level

- ■ Differential Diagnosis
  - Carbon monoxide poisoning
  - Hydrogen sulfide poisoning
  - Other sources of acidosis in suspected ingestion: Methanol, ethylene glycol, salicylates, iron, metformin

- ■ Treatment
  - Remove patient from the source of exposure, decontaminate skin, 100% oxygen by face mask, intravenous fluid, cardiac monitoring
  - For ingestion, activated charcoal
  - Inhaled amyl nitrite or intravenous sodium nitrite plus sodium thiosulfate antidote; nitrites may exacerbate hypotension or cause massive methemoglobinemia
  - In case of fire exposure, consider thiosulfate alone, as methemoglobinemia and carbon monoxide may cause reduced oxygen-carrying capacity

- ■ Pearl

In a patient brought in from a theater fire with lactic acidosis, this is the diagnosis.

Reference

Cummings TF: The treatment of cyanide poisoning. Occup Med (Lond) 2004;54:82. [PMID: 15020725]

22

Ethanol (Alcohol)

- **Essentials of Diagnosis**
  - Odor of alcohol on breath or clothing
  - Slurred speech, nystagmus, decreased motor coordination, respiratory depression
  - With the development of tolerance, blood alcohol levels correlate poorly with degree of intoxication
  - Most common cause of an osmolar gap (significant acidosis, however, should not be assumed due to ethanol alone)

- **Differential Diagnosis**
  - Other alcohol ingestion (methanol, isopropanol)
  - Benzodiazepine ingestion

- **Treatment**
  - Supportive care including intubation for airway protection if indicated
  - Gastric lavage indicated only for massive ingestion within 30 minutes; activated charcoal does not adsorb ethanol
  - Bedside glucose check or empiric dextrose, thiamine, folate
  - Examination to evaluate for injuries or illness; check for hypothermia
  - Serial observation until clinically sober; consider other causes if further deterioration in mental status
  - Assessment and referral to treatment programs is appropriate when the patient is sober; referral to primary health care and services for housing, food, and jobs may also be appropriate

- **Pearl**

Healed rib fractures on chest films in patients without a history of trauma suggest cryptic alcoholism.

Reference

Etherington JM: Emergency management of acute alcohol problems. Part 2: Alcohol-related seizures, delirium tremens, and toxic alcohol ingestion. Can Fam Physician 1996;42:2423. [PMID: 8969860]

Gamma-Hydroxybutyrate

■ Essentials of Diagnosis

- An endogenous metabolite of GABA that is easily made at home, GHB is used recreationally and in involuntary intoxication (eg, date rape); it has no clinical use in the US
- Has been used as an anesthetic, in the treatment of alcohol withdrawal, and as an adjunctive agent for body builders
- An odorless, colorless, nearly tasteless liquid, powder, or capsule
- Dose-related response; euphoria, nystagmus, clonic jerking, mild hypothermia, bradycardia, nausea, vomiting, respiratory depression, coma, and seizures may occur
- Clinical clues include abrupt onset of uncharacteristic aggressive behavior with rapidly following drowsiness and marked agitation on stimulation despite prolonged apnea and hypoxia
- May be detectable in urine by mass spectrometry for up to 12 hours; may generate U waves on ECG

■ Differential Diagnosis

- Ethanol or other alcohol intoxication
- Opioid ingestion
- Other sedative-hypnotic ingestion (benzodiazepines, chloral hydrate, methaqualone)

■ Treatment

- Consider gastric lavage and activated charcoal; may be of limited value in small ingestions and due to rapid absorption
- Supportive care including intubation if needed for airway stabilization or respiratory assistance
- Check for mixed ingestion of alcohol or other agents
- Consider ABG and head CT in comatose patient with unreliable history
- Patient counseling and evidence collection in the setting of rape or assault; drug testing is also appropriate in this setting

■ Pearl

Imaginative street names for this dangerous drug include "liquid ecstasy," "grievous bodily harm," "Georgia home boy."

Reference

Gahlinger PM: Club drugs: MDMA, gamma-hydroxybutyrate (GHB), Rohypnol, and ketamine. Am Fam Physician 2004;69:2619. [PMID: 15202696]

22

Iron

- ■ Essentials of Diagnosis
  - Five clinical stages of acute iron toxicity occur: (1) local GI toxicity (within 6 hours), (2) latent, (3) systemic toxicity (begins 24–48 hours after ingestion), (4) hepatic failure (2–3 days), (5) gastric outlet obstruction (2–8 weeks)
  - Initially, GI irritation results in vomiting, diarrhea, abdominal pain, mucosal ulceration, and bleeding
  - Systemic effects begin with disruption of cellular metabolism resulting in acidosis, lethargy, hyperventilation, seizures, coma, coagulopathy, and hypovolemic shock
  - Elevated serum iron levels correlate somewhat with toxicity but falsely low levels may occur due to variable absorption rates and the presence of deferoxamine
  - Radiopaque tablets may be visible on plain abdominal radiographs; negative radiographs do not exclude iron ingestion (common children's chewables are not radiopaque)
  - Useful studies include complete blood count, abdominal x-ray, chemistry panel, renal panel, PT/PTT, serum glucose, arterial blood gas, blood type and screen

- ■ Differential Diagnosis
  - Arsenic, copper salt, mercurial salt poisoning
  - Salicylate or acetaminophen overdose
  - Theophylline overdose
  - Hepatotoxic mushroom ingestion
  - Infectious gastroenteritis, appendicitis, sepsis

- ■ Treatment
  - Consider GI lavage early after ingestion or if pill fragments still in stomach on abdominal x-ray
  - Whole bowel irrigation; endoscopic or surgical removal may be appropriate for large iron loads
  - Intravenous fluid and pressor support; correct coagulopathy with vitamin K and fresh frozen plasma
  - Chelation therapy with deferoxamine for anyone with toxic appearance and/or a very high serum iron level

- ■ Pearl

The potential for a toxic reaction is based on ingestion of elemental iron; moderate toxicity at a dose of 20–60 mg/kg, severe toxicity above 60 mg/kg.

Reference

22

Fine JS: Iron poisoning. Curr Probl Pediatr 2000;30:71. [PMID: 10742921]

Isoniazid (INH)

- ■ Essentials of Diagnosis
  - • Common triad: profound metabolic acidosis, persistent coma, refractory seizures
  - • Hyperglycemia commonly occurs and may mimic DKA
  - • Chronic therapeutic use results in peripheral neuritis, tinnitus, memory impairment, and hypersensitivity reactions
  - • Hepatic failure the most dangerous adverse reaction to chronic use
  - • Substantial genetic variability in the rate at which people metabolize INH; about half of US population is slow metabolizers

- ■ Differential Diagnosis
  - • Salicylate, cyanide, carbon monoxide, or anticholinergic overdose
  - • In the patient with seizures, acidosis, and coma, consider sepsis, diabetic ketoacidosis, head trauma
  - • Hepatitis due to other cause

- ■ Treatment
  - • Gastric lavage for large ingestion
  - • Activated charcoal
  - • Pyridoxine (vitamin B_6, 1 g for each gram of INH ingested; 5 g slow intravenous empiric dose)
  - • Benzodiazepines as adjunct in seizure control
  - • Supportive therapy for coma, hypotension

- ■ Pearl

Ten to twenty percent of patients using INH for chemoprophylaxis will have elevated serum aminotransferases; 1% overall will progress to overt hepatitis; the former have no symptoms, the latter have those of typical hepatitis.

Reference

Romero JA, Kuczler FJ Jr: Isoniazid overdose: recognition and management. Am Fam Physician 1998;57:749. [PMID: 9490997]

Lead

- **Essentials of Diagnosis**
  - Results from chronic exposure; sources include solder, batteries, paint (in homes built before 1970)
  - Symptoms and signs include colicky abdominal pain, gum lead line, constipation, headache, irritability, neuropathy, learning disorders in children, episodes of gout
  - Ataxia, confusion, obtundation, seizures
  - Useful studies include complete blood count, chemistry panel, renal panel, lead level, abdominal x-ray, long bone radiographs (looking for lead lines)
  - Blood lead > 10 µg/dL toxic, > 70 mg/dL severe

- **Differential Diagnosis**
  - Other heavy metal toxicity (arsenic, mercury)
  - Tricyclic antidepressant, anticholinergic, ethylene glycol, or carbon monoxide exposure
  - Other sources of encephalopathy: Alcohol withdrawal, sedative-hypnotic medications, meningitis, encephalitis, hypoglycemia
  - Medical causes of acute abdomen (eg, porphyria, sickle cell crisis)
  - For chronic toxicity: depression, iron deficiency anemia, learning disability
  - Idiopathic gout

- **Treatment**
  - Airway protection and ventilatory assistance as indicated; supportive therapy for coma and seizures
  - Lavage for acute ingestion; whole bowel irrigation, endoscopy, or surgical removal if a large lead-containing object is visible on abdominal radiograph
  - Chelation therapy based on clinical presentation and blood lead levels
  - Investigate the source and test other workers or family members who might have been exposed

- **Pearl**

A cause of nonsurgical acute abdomen in the places where illegal whiskey is made in car radiators.

Reference

Needleman H: Lead poisoning. Annu Rev Med 2004;55:209. [PMID: 14746518]

22

Lithium

- ■ Essentials of Diagnosis
  - Acute ingestion: cogwheel rigidity, tremor, hyperreflexia, nausea, vomiting, abdominal cramping
  - Chronic ingestion: confusion, which may progress to coma if unrecognized and patient continues lithium ingestion
  - Ventricular dysrhythmia, sinus arrest, asystole, nephrogenic diabetes insipidus
  - Elevated serum lithium levels (> 1.5 mEq/L); acute ingestions lead to higher serum levels than chronic overdose
  - U waves, flattened or inverted T waves, ST depression, and bradycardia may be seen on ECG
  - Multiple medications increase the risk of lithium toxicity (ACE inhibitors, loop diuretics, NSAIDs, phenothiazines), as do renal failure, volume depletion, gastroenteritis, and decreased sodium intake
  - Useful studies: Chemistry panel (a decreased anion gap may be seen), renal panel, urinalysis, ECG

- ■ Differential Diagnosis
  - Neurologic disease (cerebrovascular accident, postictal state, meningitis, parkinsonism, tardive dyskinesia)
  - Other psychotropic drug intoxication
  - Neuroleptic malignant syndrome
  - Delirium

- ■ Treatment
  - Airway protection, ventilatory and hemodynamic support as indicated
  - Gastric lavage if within first hour of ingestion
  - Activated charcoal not useful for lithium overdose, but may be useful for other ingested medications; whole bowel irrigation for sustained-release preparations
  - Sodium polystyrene sulfonate (Kayexalate) may be useful to bind lithium (monitor potassium if used)
  - Aggressive normal saline hydration with close management of volume and electrolytes
  - Indications for hemodialysis in acute ingestions: Decreased level of consciousness, seizures, or lithium level > 4 mEq/L; chronic ingestions: Symptomatic patient with lithium level > 2.5 mEq/L

- ■ Pearl

Consider lithium like sodium; it is handled identically by the kidney, and higher levels thus occur in volume depletion.

Reference

Timmer RT, Sands JM: Lithium intoxication. J Am Soc Nephrol 1999;10:666.
  [PMID: 10073618]

22

Methanol, Ethylene Glycol, & Isopropanol

- **Essentials of Diagnosis**
  - Methanol: windshield washer fluid, carburetor fluid, glass cleaners, lacquers, adhesives, inks
  - Ethylene glycol: antifreeze, deicing solutions, solvents
  - Isopropanol: rubbing alcohol, nail polish removers
  - Methanol: altered mental status, visual complaints (dense central scotoma) and metabolic acidosis
  - Ethylene glycol: CNS depression
  - Isopropranol: intoxication but with acetone on breath
  - Anion gap: renal dysfunction, urinalysis, increased serum osmolality, abnormal ECG, serum alcohol level
  - Urine fluoresces under Wood's lamp with ethylene glycol

- **Differential Diagnosis**
  - Ethanol ingestion
  - Other causes of an anion gap acidosis
  - Hypoglycemia

- **Treatment**
  - Gastric lavage only if patient presented within 30 minutes; activated charcoal will not bind alcohols
  - Maintain adequate airway and assist ventilation
  - Supportive therapy for coma and seizures
  - Consider contacting a regional poison control center, (800) 222–1222
  - Fomepizole (Antizol) in any symptomatic adult or child, and in an asymptomatic adult with methanol or ethylene glycol levels > 20 mg/dL; ethanol an alternative, blocks other alcohol metabolism
  - Methanol: 50 mg of leucovorin (folinic acid)
  - Ethylene glycol: thiamine and pyridoxine
  - Hemodialysis for metabolic acidosis, renal, visual symptoms (methanol); deterioration despite intensive supportive care, electrolyte imbalances unresponsive to conventional therapy, levels > 25 mg/dL for ethylene glycol and isopropanol
  - Isopropanol: Supportive

- **Pearl**

Ethylene glycol is colorless; antifreeze is dyed green or brown to discourage ingestion.

Reference

Abramson S, Singh AK: Treatment of the alcohol intoxications: ethylene glycol, methanol and isopropanol. Curr Opin Nephrol Hypertens 2000;9:695. [PMID: 11128434]

Methemoglobinemia

- ■ Essentials of Diagnosis
  - Cyanosis unresponsive to oxygen is hallmark of methemoglobinemia
  - Seen in infants, especially after diarrheal illness
  - Drugs that can oxidize normal ferrous (Fe^{2+}) hemoglobin to abnormal ferric (Fe^{3+}) hemoglobin (methemoglobin) include local anesthetics (lidocaine, benzocaine), aniline dyes, nitrates and nitrites, nitrogen oxides, chloroquine, trimethoprim, dapsone, and phenazopyridine
  - Methemoglobin cannot bind oxygen and decreases delivery of oxygen bound to normal heme (shifting the oxyhemoglobin dissociation curve to the left)
  - Dizziness, nausea, headache, dyspnea, anxiety, tachycardia, and weakness at low levels, to myocardial ischemia, arrhythmias, decreased mentation, seizures, coma
  - Saturation fixed at 85% even in severe hypoxemia
  - Definitive diagnosis is by co-oximetry (may be from a venous sample); routine blood gas analysis may be falsely normal
  - Blood may appear chocolate brown

- ■ Differential Diagnosis
  - Hypoxemia
  - Sulfhemoglobinemia
  - Carbon monoxide or hydrogen sulfide poisoning

- ■ Treatment
  - Activated charcoal for recent ingestion
  - Discontinue offending agent; high-flow oxygen
  - Intravenous methylene blue for symptomatic patients with high methemoglobin levels or methemoglobin levels > 30%; contraindicated in patients with G6PD deficiency
  - If methylene blue therapy fails or is contraindicated, then exchange transfusion or hyperbaric oxygen

- ■ Pearl

Whenever the oxygen saturation is 85%, especially after local anesthesia, think of this; it is an in vitro phenomenon, unrelated to tissue oxygenation.

Reference

Rehman HU: Methemoglobinemia. West J Med 2001;175:193. [PMID: 11527852]

22

Opioids

- **Essentials of Diagnosis**
  - Respiratory depression, miosis, altered mental status
  - Signs of intravenous drug abuse (needle marks, a tourniquet)
  - Some (propoxyphene, tramadol, dextromethorphan, meperidine) may cause seizures
  - Noncardiogenic pulmonary edema
  - Meperidine or dextromethorphan plus a monoamine oxidase inhibitor may produce serotonin syndrome

- **Differential Diagnosis**
  - Alcohol or sedative-hypnotic overdose
  - Clonidine overdose
  - Phenothiazine overdose
  - Organophosphate or carbamate insecticide exposure
  - Gamma-hydroxybutyrate overdose
  - Congestive heart failure
  - Infectious or metabolic encephalopathy
  - Hypoglycemia, hypoxia, postictal state

- **Treatment**
  - Naloxone for suspected overdose (0.4 mg IV for mildly sedated patients suspected of opioid overdose; 2 mg IV for severely sedated or comatose patient, repeat dose up to 10 mg IV)
  - Gastric lavage for very large ingestions presenting within 1 hour
  - Activated charcoal for oral ingestion
  - Maintain adequate airway and assist ventilation, including intubation
  - Supportive therapy for coma, hypothermia, and hypotension
  - Benzodiazepines for seizures
  - Acetaminophen level
  - Update tetanus for IV drug users

- **Pearl**

Be wary of unsuspected opioid toxicity in hospitalized patients who have progressive renal insufficiency while taking fixed doses of acetaminophen and codeine.

Reference

Zimmerman JL: Poisonings and overdoses in the intensive care unit: general and specific management issues. Crit Care Med 2003;31:2794. [PMID: 14668617]

Organophosphates and Carbamates

- **Essentials of Diagnosis**
  - Insecticides (eg, orthene, malathion, parathion) and agents of chemical warfare (sarin); inhibit red blood cell acetylcholinesterase (AchE) and plasma cholinesterase and may be inhaled, ingested, or absorbed through the skin
  - Organophosphates permanently inactivate AchE; carbamates will dissociate from AchE within 24 hours
  - Clinical manifestations include: Mydriasis, tachycardia, hypertension, muscle fasciculations, weakness, paralysis, confusion, seizures, coma

- **Differential Diagnosis**
  - Curare or neuromuscular blocker poisoning
  - Sympathomimetic toxicity
  - Asthma or COPD exacerbation

- **Treatment**
  - Decontaminate skin if exposed and avoid secondary exposure to health providers
  - Nasogastic tube suction if within 1 hour, charcoal if possible; however, administration may be difficult if patient is persistently vomiting
  - 100% oxygen; maintain adequate airway and assist ventilation as necessary, avoid succinylcholine if intubation required (use a non-depolarizing agent)
  - Atropine (2–4 mg IV doses in adults, 0.05 mg/kg doses in children) doubling dose every 5–10 minutes until response achieved, may require very large repeated doses or infusion
  - Pralidoxime 1–2 g over 30 minutes, may repeat in 1 hour and every 4–8 hours

- **Pearl**

Carbamates are reversible inhibitors of cholinesterases; cholinergic crises are shorter than with organophosphates, and atropine is the antidote of choice.

Reference

Rusyniak DE, Nanagas KA: Organophosphate poisoning. Semin Neurol 2004;24:197. [PMID: 15257517]

Salicylates

■ Essentials of Diagnosis
- Many over-the-counter products contain salicylates, including Pepto-Bismol, various liniments, oil of wintergreen
- Mild acute ingestion: hyperpnea, lethargy
- Moderate intoxication: severe hyperpnea, neurologic disturbances, severe lethargy
- Severe intoxication: agitation, confusion, severe hyperpnea, seizures
- Chronic pediatric ingestion: hyperventilation, volume depletion, acidosis, hypokalemia, metabolic acidosis, respiratory alkalosis; in adults: hyperventilation, confusion, tremor, paranoia, memory deficits

■ Differential Diagnosis
- Carbon monoxide poisoning
- Any cause of anion gap metabolic acidosis (eg, methanol or ethylene glycol ingestion)

■ Treatment
- Elevated serum salicylate level; treatment should always consider both serum level and clinical condition
- Gastrointestinal lavage or whole bowel irrigation for early, large, or sustained-release ingestions
- Activated charcoal
- Maintain adequate airway and assist ventilation
- Supportive therapy for coma, hyperthermia, hypotension, and seizures; correct hypoglycemia and hypokalemia
- Intravenous fluid resuscitation with normal saline to maintain urine output at 2–3 mL/kg per hour; urinary alkalinization with sodium bicarbonate to enhance salicylate excretion (urine pH 7.5–8)
- Indications for hemodialysis for: (1) serum salicylate levels > 100 mg/dL, coma, renal or hepatic failure, and pulmonary edema; (2) severe acid-base imbalance; (3) rising serum salicylate levels; or (4) failure to respond to the conservative treatment

■ Pearl

The classic triad of salicylate poisoning: wide anion-gap acidosis, contraction metabolic alkalosis, respiratory alkalosis.

Reference

Zimmerman JL: Poisonings and overdoses in the intensive care unit: general and specific management issues. Crit Care Med 2003;31:2794. [PMID: 14668617]

Theophylline

- ## Essentials of Diagnosis
  - Mild: nausea, vomiting, tachycardia, tremor
  - Severe: any tachyarrhythmia, hypokalemia, hyperglycemia, metabolic acidosis, hallucinations, hypotension, seizures
  - Chronic: vomiting, tachycardia, and seizures (may be the first and only sign of chronic toxicity), but no hypokalemia or hyperglycemia
  - Wide pulse pressure early
  - Theophylline level is essential to care

- ## Differential Diagnosis
  - Salicylate overdose
  - Caffeine overdose
  - Iron toxicity
  - Sympathomimetic poisoning
  - Anticholinergic toxicity
  - Thyroid storm
  - Alcohol or other drug withdrawal

- ## Treatment
  - Gastric lavage if presentation within 1 hour
  - Activated charcoal mainstay of therapy
  - Whole bowel irrigation if no charcoal response
  - Oxygen; maintain adequate airway and assist ventilation
  - Monitor for arrhythmias; correct hypokalemia
  - Treat seizures with benzodiazepines
  - Hypotension and tachycardia may respond to beta-blockade
  - Indications for hemodialysis or hemoperfusion: Acute theophylline level > 90 mg/L or rapidly approaching it; level of > 40 mg/L chronically in a patient with a poor response to oral activated charcoal and any patient with ongoing seizures, ventricular dysrhythmias, poorly responsive hypotension

- ## Pearl
  Inappropriate sinus tachycardia in a patient with COPD may be the only clue to the diagnosis; once seizures occur, the prognosis worsens appreciably.

Reference
Vassallo R, Lipsky JJ: Theophylline: recent advances in the understanding of its mode of action and uses in clinical practice. Mayo Clin Proc 1998;73:346. [PMID: 9559039]

22

Index